Library of Congress Cataloging-in-Publication Data

Medical management of radiation accidents / editors, Fred A. Mettler, Jr.,
    Charles A. Kelsey, Robert C. Ricks.
       p.   cm.
    Includes bibliographies and index.
    ISBN 0-8493-4865-X
    1. Radiation injuries. I. Mettler, Fred A., 1945-
II. Kelsey, Charles A. III. Ricks, Robert C.
    [DNLM: 1. Accidents. 2. Radiation Injuries—therapy. WN 610
M48653]
RA1231.R2M42   1990
617.1′24—dc19
DNLM/DLC   89-7737
for Library of Congress   CIP

International Standard Book Number 0-8493-4865-X

Library of Congress Card Number 89-7737
Printed in the United States   4 5 6 7 8 9 0

Printed on acid-free paper

Medical Management of Radiation Accidents

Editors

Fred A. Mettler, Jr., M.D., M.P.H.
Professor and Chairman
Department of Radiology
University of New Mexico School of Medicine
Albuquerque, New Mexico

Charles A. Kelsey, Ph.D.
Department of Radiology
University of New Mexico School of Medicine
Albuquerque, New Mexico

Robert C. Ricks, M.S., Ph.D.
Radiation Emergency Assistance Center/Training Site
Oak Ridge Associated Universities
Oak Ridge, Tennessee

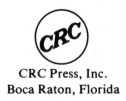

CRC Press, Inc.
Boca Raton, Florida

PREFACE

Radiation accidents are rare. They are often complex in nature and usually distressing to both the patient and involved medical staff. There are few if any comprehensive publications on the medical management of radiation accidents.

The purpose of this text is to provide the reader with information regarding the nature, number, and current medical management of radiation accidents. This is intended for persons with some previous background knowledge such as physicians, health physicists, or radiation safety officers. Basic concepts and historical aspects (including the accidents at Chernobyl and Goiania) are covered in the first several chapters. Special aspects related to reactor, transportation, and military accidents are covered next. Specific management of acute problems such as whole-body irradiation, internal and external contamination, skin decontamination, and wound management are discussed in separate chapters. Logistical aspects of emergency room management, instrumentation, and dose estimation are also covered. The last several chapters deal with long-term followup, carcinogenic risk estimation, studies of the Three Mile Island and Chernobyl reactor accidents, and legal issues. There is a glossary and a number of useful appendices with sample hospital procedures, suggested supply lists, emergency phone numbers, and tables with physical data related to dose estimation.

Fred A. Mettler, Jr.
Albuquerque, New Mexico

EDITORS

Fred A. Mettler, Jr., M.D., M.P.H., is professor and chairman of the Department of Radiology at the University of New Mexico School of Medicine in Albuquerque.

Dr. Mettler received an A.B. in mathematics from Columbia University in 1966. He received an M.D. degree from Thomas Jefferson University in 1970 and an M.P.H. degree in environmental health from Harvard University in 1975.

Dr. Mettler is a member of the National Council on Radiation Protection and Measurements (NCRP) and is the U.S. Representative to the United Nations Scientific Committee on the Effects of Atomic Radiation (UNSCEAR). He has published over 150 scientific papers and book chapters as well as seven books.

Charles A. Kelsey, Ph.D., is Chief of Biomedical Physics and Professor of Radiology at the University of New Mexico School of Medicine, and Radiation Safety Officer at the Veterans Administration Hospital in Albuquerque, New Mexico.

Dr. Kelsey graduated in 1957 from St. Edward's University in Austin, Texas with a B.S. degree in Physics (magna cum laude). He received his Ph.D. degree in Nuclear Physics from the University of Notre Dame in 1962.

Dr. Kelsey is a fellow of the American College of Radiology and is a Certified Radiological Physicist. He is a member of the American Association of Physicists in Medicine, the American College of Radiology, the Association of University Radiologists, the Radiological Society of North America, and the Health Physics Society.

He has served on the Radiation Study Section of the National Institutes of Health and as an advisor to the Food and Drug Administration, the National Science Foundation, and the U.S. Army. Dr. Kelsey has presented over 200 papers at scientific meetings and published over 100 scientific papers. His current major research interests include radiation protection and medical image perception.

Robert C. Ricks, M.S., Ph.D., is Director of the Radiation Emergency Assistance Center/Training Site (REAC/TS), Medical Sciences Division, Oak Ridge Associated Universities, Oak Ridge, Tennessee.

Dr. Ricks graduated from Lamar University in Beaumont, Texas, with a B.S. in biology and obtained his M.S. and Ph.D. from Texas A & M University, College Station, Texas. His major areas of interest include radiation biology and physiology.

Dr. Ricks is also Director of the World Health Organization (WHO) International Collaborating Center for Radiation Emergency Assistance. In this regard, he leads a team of physicians, nurses, and health physicists providing advice and consultation for worldwide radiation assistance and collaboration with other WHO centers.

Dr. Ricks is a member of the Health Physics Society. He has presented over 100 invited lectures at the national and international levels and conducted over 200 training courses in medical management of radiation accidents. He has presented numerous papers on radiation biology and emergency response and training. In 1989 Dr. Ricks received the Distinguished Lecturer Award presented by the Southwestern Chapter of the Society of Nuclear Medicine.

CONTRIBUTORS

Steve Nicholas Allen, B.A.
Associate Product Specialist
W. L. Core and Associates
Elkton, Maryland

David E. Drum, M.D., Ph.D.
Associate Professor
Department of Radiology
Harvard Medical School
Brigham and Women's Hospital
Boston, Massachusetts

Karl F. Hubner, M.D.
Director, Nuclear Medicine and
  Radiologic Research
Department of Radiology
University of Tennessee Medical Center
Knoxville, Tennessee

Carol B. Jankowski, B.S., M.Ed.
Educator
Radiation Safety Program
Brigham and Women's Hospital
Boston, Massachusetts

Robert M. Jefferson
Consultant
Albuquerque, New Mexico

Eugene E. Joiner, B.S., M.S.
Research Associate
Medical and Health Sciences Division
Oak Ridge Associated Universities
Oak Ridge, Tennessee

Phillip M. Kannan, B.S., M.S., J.D.
Assistant General Counsel
Martin Marietta Energy Systems, Inc.
Oak Ridge, Tennessee

Charles A. Kelsey, Ph.D.
Professor and Chief
Biomedical Physics
Department of Radiology
University of New Mexico School of
  Medicine
Albuquerque, New Mexico

L. Gayle Littlefield, Ph.D.
Director
Cytogenetics Laboratory
Medical Sciences Division
Oak Ridge Associated Universities
Oak Ridge, Tennessee

Jonathan C. Marshall, B.Sc., MB.BS.
University College Hospital and
  The Middlesex Hospital
London, England

Fred A. Mettler, Jr., M.D., M.P.H.
Professor and Chairman
Department of Radiology
University of New Mexico School of
  Medicine
Albuquerque, New Mexico

George A. Poda, M.D.
Clinical Associate
Department of Occupational Medicine
Oak Ridge Associated Universities
Oak Ridge, Tennessee

Joel M. Rappeport, M.D.
Professor
Department of Internal Medicine
Yale University School of Medicine
New Haven, Connecticut

Robert C. Ricks
REAC/Training Site
Oak Ridge Associated Universities
Oak Ridge, Tennessee

Robert Rosenberg, M.D.
Assistant Professor
Department of Radiology
University of New Mexico Hospital
Albuquerque, New Mexico

Henry D. Royal, M.D.
Associate Professor of Radiology
Washington University
  School of Medicine
Associate Director
Division of Nuclear Medicine
Mallinckrodt Institute of Radiology
St. Louis, Missouri

Eugene L. Saenger, M.D.
Professor Emeritus
Department of Radiology
University of Cincinnati College of
  Medicine
Cincinnati, Ohio

George L. Voelz, M.D.
Staff Member
Occupational Health Specialist
Occupational Medicine Group
Los Alamos National Laboratory
Los Alamos, New Mexico

This book is dedicated to those individuals, such as Drs. A. Guskova and L. A. Ilyin, who, at risk to their own safety, brought their professional expertise, courage, and compassion to the victims of Chernobyl.

TABLE OF CONTENTS

Chapter 1

FUNDAMENTALS OF RADIATION ACCIDENTS

Fred A. Mettler, Jr. and Charles A. Kelsey

TABLE OF CONTENTS

I. INTRODUCTION

Radiation accidents are matters of great concern not only to the individual involved but the media and public as well. This concern is a function of ignorance about radiation effects and mechanisms, as well as a general perception of the mysterious nature of radioactivity. It is often difficult to get people to separate in their own minds the differences between the relatively miniscule risks of a chest X-ray from those of full-scale nuclear war. The result of all of these factors makes it extremely important that a potential or real radiation accident be carefully, methodically, and scientifically assessed.

One of the most important aspects to determine is whether the potential accident is, in fact, a radiation accident alone or whether the patient has a combined injury, for example, physical trauma, myocardial infarction, or some other major medical problem in addition to radiation exposure. Under most, if not all circumstances, the immediate medical problems and treatment will supersede treatment for radiation injuries. Even acute life-threatening doses of radiation do not require medical attention within the first hour or so. Once immediate life-saving and medical stabilization needs have been attended to, evaluation and possible countermeasures to a potential radiation accident may proceed.[1]

II. RADIATION

Radiation generally refers to the transfer of energy. Radiation as a general term includes radio waves, radar, microwave, ultraviolet radiation, and even electric power (Figure 1). All these are part of the electromagnetic radiation spectrum. As the wavelength of most of these forms of radiation gets shorter, the energy increases. If the energy of the radiation is high enough then, as the energy is transferred to an atom in an absorbing material (such as tissue), the binding energy of an electron being held by that atom may be overcome and the electron may be ejected from the atom. This process is called *ionization*. *Ionizing radiation* includes X-rays, gamma rays, cosmic rays, and various particulate radiations such as alpha particles, beta particles, and neutrons.

The method by which incident radiation interacts with a tissue may be direct or indirect. Electromagnetic radiations such as X-rays or gamma photons are *indirectly ionizing* i.e., their energy is utilized to eject an electron. It is this electron that secondarily reacts with a target molecule. Charged particles (such as alpha and beta particles) strike the tissue and directly react with target molecules. Charged particulate radiations, therefore, are termed *directly ionizing* radiation. Uncharged particles such as neutrons are classed as indirectly ionizing.

The amount of energy deposited in a tissue can be measured as a function of distance along the track of the radiation (Figure 2). Ionizing radiation may be categorized into high-LET and low-LET radiation. *LET* refers to *Linear Energy Transfer* or the amount of energy deposited per unit of track length. LET is normally expressed in keV/μm of absorbing tissue. Low-LET radiations (gamma and X-rays) have a relatively uniform energy deposition along the track of the photon. High-LET radiations, such as alpha particles, deposit a large amount of energy in a very small volume of tissue. Thus with alpha particles there may be a lot of damage caused in a small volume of tissue, but this rapid deposition of energy causes the particle to slow down quickly and therefore not to penetrate deeply.

III. QUANTITIES AND UNITS

The amount or quantity of radiation may be expressed in several ways (see Table 1). The first of these is the measurement of *exposure*. Initially, the unit utilized was the *roentgen*. It is defined as the amount of low energy X- or gamma rays that produce a given amount

THE ELECTROMAGNETIC SPECTRUM

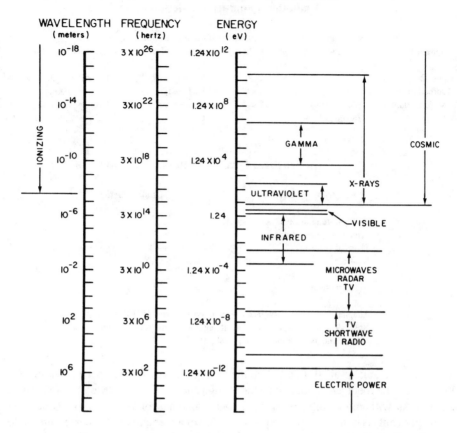

FIGURE 1. Comparison of the wavelength frequency and energy of the electromagnetic spectrum. Ionizing radiation represents that portion of the spectrum in which the energy exceeds approximately 10 eV. (From *Medical Effects of Ionizing Radiation,* Mettler, F. A. and Moseley, R. D., Eds., Grune & Stratton, New York, 1985. With permission.)

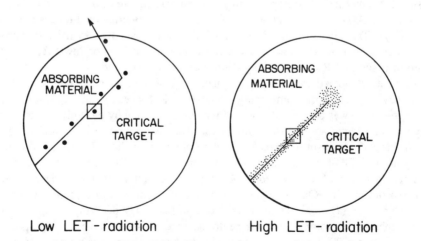

FIGURE 2. Comparison of high- and low-LET radiation. Low-LET radiation causes relatively sparse ionization along the track of the radiation, whereas high-LET radiation causes very dense ionization along the radiation path with a cluster or radiation at the end of the path (the Bragg peak). (From *Medical Effects of Ionizing Radiation,* Mettler, F. A. and Moseley, R. D., Eds., Grune & Stratton, New York, 1985. With permission.)

TABLE 1
Radiation Quantities and Units

Quantity	New named unit and symbol	In other SI Units	Old special unit and symbol	Conversion factor
Exposure	—	$C\ kg^{-1}$	Roentgen (R)	$1\ C\ kg^{-1} \sim 3876\ R$
Absorbed dose	Gray (Gy)	$J\ kg^{-1}$	Rad (rad)	$1\ Gy = 100\ rad$
Dose equivalent	Sievert (Sv)	$J\ kg^{-1}$	Rem (rem)	$1\ Sv = 100\ rem$
Activity	Becquerel (Bq)	s^{-1}	Curie (Ci)	$1\ Bq \sim 2.7 \times 10^{-11}\ Ci$

TABLE 2
Practical Quality Factors

Particle	Quality factor
X-Rays, gamma rays, beta particles electrons or positrons	1
Thermal neutrons	5
Neutrons	20
Protons	10
Alpha particles	20

Adapted from Basic Radiation Protection Criteria, NCRP Reps. Nos. 39 and 91, National Council on Radiation Protection and Measurements, Bethesda, MD, 1980, 1987.

of ionization per unit of air (0.000258 coulomb of energy deposited per kilogram of air). Unfortunately, the roentgen is not applicable to high energy X-rays (3 MeV) or to particulate radiations. As with most units, when very small amounts of radiation are concerned, a milliroentgen (mR) is utilized. This is equal to 1/1000 of a roentgen. In the newer international system (SI), the unit of exposure is simply coulomb per kilogram of air. For conversion, 1 R equals 2.58×10^{-4} coul/kg. Certainly for most biologic purposes an associated temporal unit is also extremely useful; that is exposure per unit of time (e.g., R/min.)

The amount of ionization that occurs in air may not seem very germaine to biological discussions. Another unit was proposed in 1953 and was known as the *rad*. This is defined as deposition of 100 ergs of energy in 1 g of tissue. A new international unit is now in use, the *gray* (Gy). The gray is defined as 1 J of energy deposited in each kg of absorbing material and is equal to 100 rad. Thus 1 rad equals 10 mGy. For low-LET radiations, exposure of tissue to 1 R causes energy deposition of almost 1 rad.

Unfortunately, not all radiations are equally effective in causing biological damage, although they may cause the same energy deposition in tissue. For these purposes, a unit of *dose equivalence* was derived. A dose equivalent is obtained by multiplying the absorbed dose by a quality factor and a distribution factor. The distribution factor is really important only in the case of nonuniform internal deposition of a radionuclide. The quality factor takes into account the LET of the radiation. The unit previously utilized for dose equivalent has been the *rem* (acronym of roentgen equivalent man). The international unit now more widely in use is the *sievert* (Sv). One Sv equals 100 rem and 1 rem therefore equals 10 mSv. The quality factor for X-rays and gamma rays is one so that 1 Gy of X-ray is equivalent to 1 Sv. With alpha rays, protons, and fast neutrons, quality factors have been proposed that range between 10 and 20. Table 2 gives the quality factors of different radiations and energies.

One of the major problems in accident evaluation, patient management, and prognostic categorization concerns expression of absorbed dose. One might be informed that, in a given accident, a patient had received 200 rad (2 Gy). The medical implications of this are significant if this is the estimated absorbed dose at midline in the body. On the other hand, if the patient received 200 rad (2 Gy) only to the hand, the consequences are relatively minor. Thus, it is always important to express absorbed dose to a particular tissue or portion of the body as well as the time over which that dose was received. As we will see later, in almost all accidents, there is a very steep gradient of absorbed radiation doses across portions of the body.

IV. ATOMIC STRUCTURE

An atom can be thought of as a collection of protons, neutrons, and electrons. The protons and neutrons generally comprise the nucleus or central portion of the atom with a variable number of negatively charged electrons in various orbits about the nucleus. The number of neutrons in an atom is usually abbreviated by N and the number of protons is represented by Z (also called the atomic number). The mass number or total number of particles in the nucleus is represented by A and is simply the sum of N (neutrons) and Z (protons). The symbolism used to designate an atom is charcterized by the name of the element and the mass number (e.g., ^{238}U). When characterized in this fashion, the species is known as a nuclide. By definition, all isotopes of a given element have the same number of protons and a different number of neutrons. Thus all isotopes of iodine have 53 protons. Many isotopes are stable and it is a common misconception that an isotope is necessarily radioactive. For any given element, there may be many nuclides which have configurations of protons and neutrons that are unstable.

V. RADIOACTIVITY

When nuclides have an odd number of neutrons and protons, they are usually unstable and this instability may result either from proton or neutron excess. Nuclides attempting to reach stability by emitting radiation are known as *radionuclides*. When an unstable nuclide transforms spontaneously and emits radiation, the radionuclide is said to be *radioactive*. Nuclear decay in an attempt to reach stability may involve simply the release of energy from the nucleus or may result in a change in the number of protons and neutrons within the nucleus.

The amount of radioactivity present or the number of disintegrations that occur each second is referred to as *activity*. In the past, the unit of activity used was the curie (3.7×10^{10} disintegrations per second). This is a somewhat inconvenient unit, and it has recently been replaced by an international unit known as the becquerel (Bq). The bequerel corresponds to one disintegration of the radionuclide per second. Specific activity is the activity per unit mass of material (e.g., Bq/g).

Radionuclides decay in an exponential fashion and the term physical half-life (often simply referred to as half-life or T $^1/_2$) is used to characterize radionuclides. This term refers to the time taken for the activity of a radionuclide to lose one half of its value by decay. Each radionuclide has a unique and unalterable physical half-life. Half-lives of the different radionuclides range from hundredths of a second to millions of years. There is, in addition to physical half-life, a biological half-life. The biological half-life refers to the time it takes an organism to eliminate a compound or chemical on a biologic basis. Thus, if a stable compound were given to an individual and half of it were eliminated by the body (perhaps in urine) within 3 h, the biologic half-life would be 3 h.

The concept of effective half-life incorporates both the physical and biologic half-lives, and it is this term that is most important in dealing with patients and in assessing the absorbed radiation dose. The formula used to calculate effective half-life is as follows:

$$\frac{1}{\text{effective } T_{1/2}} = \frac{1}{\text{biological } T_{1/2}} + \frac{1}{\text{physical } T_{1/2}}$$

As a simple example, if the biological half-life of a radionuclide is 3 h and the physical half-life is 6 h, then the effective half-life is 2 h. Note that the effective half-life is always shorter than either the physical or the biological half-life. The importance of this concept can be seen in a situation in which there is ingestion of a long-lived insoluble radionuclide with a physical half-life of perhaps a thousand years. If there is no absorption by the body, the material will simply pass through the gastrointestinal tract and be eliminated within hours or days, and the fact that the radionuclide has such a long physical half-life will be of very little importance in calculation of absorbed dose to the individual.

VI. FACTORS AFFECTING BIOLOGICAL RESPONSE

All ionizing radiation has the potential to cause ionization with subsequent cell damage. The physical absorption of ionizing radiation in tissue results in a chemical reaction, free radical formation. A free radical is an atom or molecule that has a single unpaired electron. The two substances to the body that are most likely to be involved in this transformation following irradiation are oxygen and water. The free radicals formed are an extremely reactive chemical species, and biological effects occur when there is free radical interaction with various components of the cell. Free radicals may act either as oxidizing or reducing agents and may form peroxides when they react with water. They may inactivate cellular mechanisms directly or may interact with genetic material such as DNA and RNA.

Although radiochemical events may not immediately appear to have much clinical relevance, they form the basis of the effects which become later clinically apparent. Since oxygen and water are easily involved in free radical formation, they become modifiers of the radiation effect. Lack of oxygen or water in a tissue makes it relatively more resistant to radiation. The ability of oxygen to enhance radiation damage is occasionally referred to as the "oxygen effect". The induction of free radicals in the initial step of radiation damage has implications for development and use of both radioprotective and radiosensitizing agents. For the most part, radioprotective agents are free radical scavengers that keep free radicals from interacting with other cellular compounds and thus avert radiation injury. Essentially all radioprotective and radiosensitizing agents must be in the tissue cells at the time the radiation is absorbed. The introduction of protective or sensitizing agents even a short time after radiation exposure will not have a significant effect.

The sensitivity of various cells in the body to radiation depends upon a number of factors, one of which is the phase of the cell in the DNA synthetic cycle. Cells are most sensitive as they undergo mitosis. Rapidly dividing cells are more sensitive to radiation than cells which divide slowly. Table 3 shows the radiosensitivity of some normal tissues. Cellular death due to radiation rarely occurs at a dose less than 5 rad (0.05 Gy), although there may be some genetic damage. If there is genetic damage and it is repaired incorrectly, radiation carcinogenesis may result (Figure 3).

The radiosensitivity of a given organ and the pathological changes that may be identified following irradiation depend not only on the physical parameters of the exposure, but also on the radiosensitivity of the various organ components. In cases in which the functional or parenchymal cells of the organ are rapidly dividing, loss of the parenchymal function will be the initial critical factor in patient survival. An example of such tissue is the bone marrow. When there is radiation of an organ that has parenchymal cells with a very slow turnover rate, the controlling factor and ultimate clinical problems are the result of damage, not to the slowly dividing parenchymal cells, but to the more sensitive connective tissue and microcirculation. An example of such an organ is the brain.

TABLE 3
Radiosensitivity of Normal Cells

Radiosensitivity	Cell types
Very high	Lymphocytes
	Immature hematopoietic cells
	Intestinal epithelium
	Spermatogonia
	Ovarian follicular cells
High	Urinary bladder epithelium
	Esophageal epithelium
	Gastric mucosa
	Mucous membranes
	Epidermal epithelium
	Epithelium of optic lens
Intermediate	Endothelium
	Growing bone and cartilage
	Fibroblasts
	Glial cells
	Glandular epithelium of breast
	Pulmonary epithelium
	Renal epithelium
	Hepatic epithelium
	Pancreatic epithelium
	Thyroid epithelium
	Adrenal epithelium
Low	Mature hematopoietic cells
	Muscle cells
	Mature connective tissues
	Mature bone and cartilage
	Ganglion cells

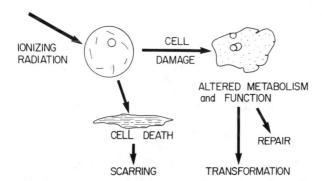

FIGURE 3. Possible cellular changes following exposure to ionizing radiation. If radiation exposure is high enough, cell death and ultimate tissue scarring may result if the organism survives. If the cell recovers on an acute basis, there remains a possibility of altered metabolism and function, which may be repaired, or there may be transformation to a carcinogenic cell. (From *Medical Effects of Ionizing Radiation,* Mettler, F. A. and Moseley, R. D., Eds., Grune & Stratton, New York, 1985. With permission.)

THE PENETRATING POWER OF RADIATION

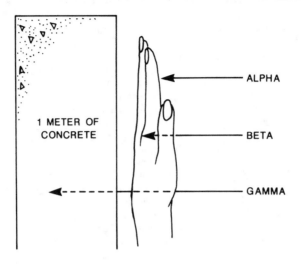

FIGURE 4.   Relative penetrating powers of alpha, beta, and gamma radiation.

TABLE 4
Half-Value Layer (HVL) for Photons

Photon energy (MeV)	Water (cm)	Concrete (cm)	Lead (cm)
0.1	4.2	1.7	0.015
0.2	5.0	2.3	0.065
0.4	6.5	3.0	0.27
0.6	7.8	3.6	0.5
0.8	8.8	4.0	0.7
1.0	9.6	5.0	0.9
2.0	14.0	7.0	1.3
5.0	23.0	11.0	1.5

From *Medical Effects of Ionizing Radiation*, Mettler, F. A. and Moseley, R. D., Eds., Grune & Stratton, New York, 1985. With permission.

Since the body is composed of many types of tissues with varying radiosensitivity, the response to total body irradiation is a spectrum of clinical symptoms that occurs as a function of damage to those systems which are affected. For whole-body irradiation, whole-body absorbed doses of 100 to 500 rad (1 to 5 Gy) predominantly affect the hematological and intestinal systems. If death of the individual occurs, it is due to failure of these systems with bleeding, infection, and electrolyte loss. In situations in which the whole-body absorbed doses are extremely high (>20 Gy), death may occur sooner, due to failure of other systems (such as the circulatory system) which are less rapidly dividing. This is discussed in more detail in Chapter 6. The amount of ionization (and hence cell damage) may vary significantly, depending upon the energy of the radiation. The energy of the incident radiation is also extremely important in terms of penetration into tissue (Figure 4). One measure of penetration is the thickness of absorber required to reduce the exposure rate to one half. This thickness is called the half-value layer (HVL). Once the energy of incident photons is known, the HVL can be found in Table 4 and then the absorbed dose to tissues at a certain depth can

TABLE 5
Particulate Radiation

Particle	Charge	Mass (AMU)	Comments
Proton	+1	1.008	
Neutron	0	1.009	
Electron	−1	0.0005	Also called *negatron* or *beta minus*
Positron	+1	0.00054	Also called *beta plus*
Deuteron	+2	2.015	Also called *heavy hydrogen:* consists of a proton and a neutron
Alpha	+2	4.034	Consists of two protons and two neutrons

From *Medical Effects of Ionizing Radiation,* Mettler, F. A. and Moseley, R. D., Eds., Grune & Stratton, New York, 1985. With permission.

TABLE 6
Range of Alpha Particles

Energy (MeV)	Mean Range in Air (cm)	Range in Water (μ)
0.5	0.25	—
1.0	0.5	7.2
2.0	1.0	—
3.0	1.5	—
4.0	2.5	—
5.0	3.5	45
6.0	4.6	—
7.0	6.0	60
8.0	7.4	80

Note: An alpha particle requires at least 7.5 MeV to pentrate the protective layer of skin (0.7 mm, or 70 μm).

From *Medical Effects of Ionizing Radiation,* Mettler, F. A. and Moseley, R. D., Eds., Grune & Stratton, New York, 1985. With permission.

be calculated. An example of the penetration of diagnostic X-ray is as follows: a 100 kVp beam is reduced to approximately 50% at 4 cm depth in tissue and to 3% at approximately 20 cm in tissue. From this, it can be seen that the midline dose in the body from 100 kVp gamma and X-rays entering the body from one side may be from 5 to 25% of the surface or skin dose.

In addition to X-rays and gamma rays, there are particulate radiations referred to earlier (Table 5). Alpha particles consist of two protons and two neutrons. They are relatively heavy, travel slowly, and carry a substantial electrical charge. Because of this, they do not penetrate tissues well. An alpha particle requires at least 7.5 MeV to penetrate the protective layer of skin (Table 6). Thus, for practical medical purposes, alpha particles only become important if there is internal contamination with an alpha-emitting radionuclide.

Beta minus particles (electrons) can penetrate up to several centimeters into tissue. A beta particle of at least 70 keV is required to penetrate the protective layer of skin. A useful rule of thumb is that the range in centimeters of beta particles in water (or tissue) is equal to the energy in MeV divided by two. Skin contamination with beta particles which are relatively energetic may cause skin burns. Table 7 indicates the range of beta particles in air and water.

Neutrons are uncharged and therefore they do not easily interact with tissue. They are much more penetrating than a proton of the same energy. Much of the absorption of neutrons

TABLE 7
Maximum Penetration of Beta
Radiation (cm)[a]

Beta energy (MeV)[b]	Air	Water[b]	Lead
0.1	15	0.015	0.001
0.2	40	0.05	0.004
0.3	65	0.08	0.006
0.4	94	0.12	0.009
0.5	130	0.16	0.013
0.7	200	0.24	0.021
1.0	315	0.40	0.034
2.0	790	0.96	0.081
3.0	1360	1.70	0.144
4.0	2020	2.30	0.210

[a]   Beta-emitting radionuclides emit a spectrum of energies. Average energy is about one third of the maximum energy.
[b]   A useful rule of thumb is that the range in centimeters in water or tissue is equal to the energy in MeV divided by 2.

From *Medical Effects of Ionizing Radiation,* Mettler, F. A. and Moseley, R. D., Eds., Grune & Stratton, New York, 1985. With permission.

takes place as a result of interaction between the neutrons and hydrogen nuclei. The HVL in water for 8 MeV neutrons is 9.25 cm.

The time of exposure in a radiation accident is another important factor to be considered.[2,3] If the accidental exposure has just occurred and the absorbed dose is high, clinical effects that may be evident include manifestations of cell death in rapidly dividing systems such as skin, bone marrow, and gastrointestinal tract. If the exposure occurred days or even months ago, clinical findings may include symptoms related to cellular death of the more slowly dividing systems and perhaps cellular death due to narrowing of a blood vessels with subsequent ischemia.

Rubin and Casarett[4] indicated three clinical phases in human biological response: (1) acute, (2) subacute, and (3) late clinical period. In the acute clinical period, there is an initial destructive process with various repair processes in any organ system. Survival of the patient during this time depends upon the dose received and the radiosensitivity and volume of tissue irradiated. Later, in the subacute period (6 to 12 months after exposure), underlying damage in parenchymal tissues may become manifest due to vascular deterioration, fibrosis, myointimal proliferation, and sclerosis of small arteries and arterioles. During the late clinical periods (12 months and later after irradiation) an organ system may demonstrate continued deterioration of the vascularity, decreased resistance to stress, and dense fibrosis. Several years after radiation, the major biological sequela identified is that of radiation carcinogenesis.

The time over which the radiation is received or its fractionation is also very important. In general, dividing a radiation dose or protracting the dose over a longer time period will result in less injury. As an example, a tissue which receives 2,000 rad (20 Gy) in an hour may not survive; whereas the same tissue having received a dose of 5,000 rad (50 Gy) over 6 to 8 weeks may well be able to tolerate this insult.

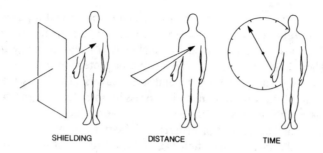

FIGURE 5. Three methods of radiation exposure reduction.

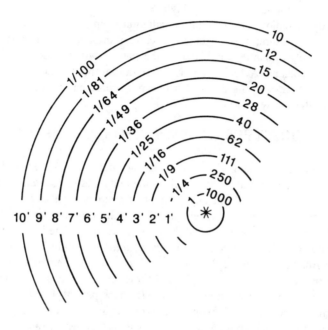

FIGURE 6. Effect of distance on radiation exposure.

VII. RADIATION PROTECTION PRINCIPLES

Whether dealing with a radioactive source or radioactive contamination, it is important to keep individual absorbed doses as low as possible, consistent with being able to provide good medical practice. The basic factors employed to reduce exposure to ionization radiation are reducing time and quantity while increasing distance and shielding (Figure 5).

The amount of radiation exposure received from a source is directly proportional to the amount of time spent in the radiation field. Doubling the amount of time spent at a fixed point in a radiation field will double the absorbed dose. Most radiation-monitoring instruments are rate meters that measure exposure in mR or R/h and sometimes in cpm. With these instruments, the absorbed dose to an individual can be estimated from the mR/h multiplied by the number of hours or fraction of an hour spent in the area.

Distance is probably the most effective way of reducing radiation exposure. The more distant one is from a source of radiation, the lower the radiation dose will be. The absorbed dose varies as the inverse square of the distance between the source and the person. If one doubles the distance from a radiation source, the absorbed dose would be 1 over 2 squared ($1/2^2 = 1/4$). If the distance is tripled, the dose is reduced to a value of $1/3^2$ or one ninth (Figure 6).

Interposing absorbing material between a radiation source and a person will decrease the absorbed dose to the person. The denser the material, the greater is its ability to stop radiation. Lead is most commonly used for shielding, although in many instances leaded glass or leaded acrylic is also utilized. The amount of protection provided by such objects can be calculated from tables of HVL or tenth-value layers (TVL). As mentioned earlier, HVL is the amount of the absorbing material necessary to reduce the radiation exposure to one half, and one-tenth value layer is the amount of material required to reduce the radiation exposure to one tenth. The amount of material necessary to attenuate the radiation depends upon the energy of the incident radiation (see Tables 4 to 7). In most radiation accidents (particularly industrial sources such as ^{192}Ir, ^{60}Co radiographic sources, or nuclear power plants), shielding is not very practical. The reason for this is that the energy of the radiation emitted from such radionuclides is very high.

The quantity of radioactive material or radiation from a source also clearly affects the magnitude of the exposure; e.g., if there is a certain amount of radioactive contamination present, removal of a quantity of this from the patient will reduce exposure to both the patient and the attendants. Actually, this is a variation of the distance factor since what one is really doing is increasing the distance between a source and an object by moving some of the source further away.

VIII. TYPES OF RADIATION ACCIDENTS

The two most general categories of radiation accidents are (1) external exposure (irradiation) from a source of radiation distant from the body and (2) contamination.[5-7] External radiation accidents may arise from any number of sources such as an X-ray machine, a radioactive source, or even a linear accelerator. Under these circumstances, there is no direct contact between the radiation source and the person involved. The individual is referred to as having been externally *exposed* or externally *irradiated* (Figure 7). Once the person has been removed from proximity of the radiation source or the source has been removed or turned off, no further irradiation takes place. At this point, persons assisting the patient are not in danger of receiving any radiation exposure from the patient. In other words, irradiation from an external source of beta, gamma or X-rays will not cause the patient to become radioactive. As a typical example, a patient who has had a chest X-ray or one who receives a radiotherapy treatment from a ^{60}Co source is not radioactive and poses no hazard to individuals nearby.

External radiation exposure may be subdivided into whole body exposure or local exposure. Obviously these are very simplistic categories, since it is very unusual that there would be a circumstance in which the whole body would be irradiated uniformly (front, back, head, feet, etc.). Local exposure or partial body irradiation in reality is a very steep gradient of absorbed doses from a particular body portion to much lower doses elsewhere on the body.

Accidents involving radioactive *contamination* are entirely different in terms of concept and treatment.[6,7] Contamination refers to unwanted radioactive material on the body surface or within the body (Figure 7). Simplistically, contamination may be thought of as radioactive dirt and may be in the form of radioactive liquid, particles, or even gases. A contaminated individual will continue to be irradiated by the radioactive material until such time as it is removed from the patient or it physically decays. The medical staff attending such a patient must be careful to prevent spread of the radioactive contamination to uncontaminated portions of the patient's body or to themselves. Contamination may be external (located on the skin), or it may be internal (located within the body). Internal contamination may result from inhalation, ingestion, direct absorption through the skin, or penetration of radioactive materials through open wounds.

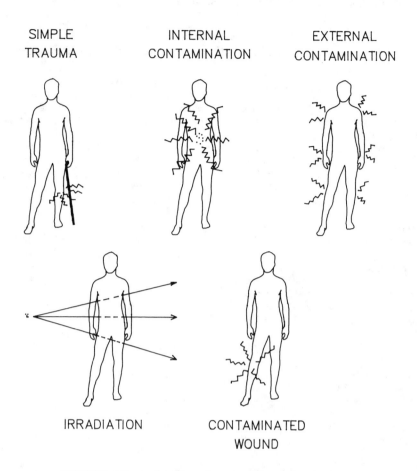

| SIMPLE TRAUMA | INTERNAL CONTAMINATION | EXTERNAL CONTAMINATION |

IRRADIATION   CONTAMINATED WOUND

FIGURE 7. Types of accidents that may occur in a nuclear facility.

IX. NONACCIDENTAL SOURCES OF RADIATION EXPOSURE

It is important to understand that radiation and radioactivity are an integral part of our environment, and have been for millions of years. There is radioactive material present in the air we breathe, the food we eat, and in most everything that is around us. The sources to which we are exposed in our everyday life are of three general types. Those of (1) natural origin, (2) enhanced natural sources (due to human activity increasing the level), and (3) man-made sources of radiation. Natural sources include cosmic radiation, terrestrial radiation, and radiation from radionuclides that are present in our bodies from inhaled and ingested materials. The absorbed radiation dose from natural sources is approximately 100 to 300 millirad (1 to 3 mGy) per year. Natural background radiation varies significantly, depending upon the altitude of the environment and the amount of radioactive materials present in the soil. There are a few areas in the world where the natural background is as high as 17,500 (175 mGy) mrad/year.

Exposure to medical uses of radiation contributes about 100 mrad (1 mGy) on the average to persons living in the U.S. This figure is somewhat misleading, since it averages all of the X-rays taken in the U.S. over all the people. Individual radiographic examinations vary substantially in the amount of radiation given. A skin dose from a chest X-ray is approximately 40 mrad (0.4 mGy), whereas from a cardiac catherization, studied skin doses may be as high as 30,000 mrad (300 Gy). A typical CT scan gives a skin dose of between 1,000 and 5,000 mrad (10 to 50 mGy). Radiation dose of the U.S. population from various sources is shown in Table 8.

TABLE 8
Sources and Magnitude of Radiation: Exposure of the U.S. Population

Source	Number of people exposed	Annual collective effective dose equivalent (person rem) in thousands	Annual effective dose equivalent[a] (mrem)[b]
Natural Sources			
Radon	230,000,000	46,000	200
Other	230,000,000	23,000	100
Occupational	930,000	200	0.9
Nuclear fuel cycle	—	14	0.05
Medical			
Diagnostic	c	9,100	39
Nuclear Medicine	c	3,200	14
Therapy	c	—	—
Consumer products			
Tobacco	50,000,000	65,000	280
Other	230,000,000	2,800	12
Miscellaneous Environmental sources	~25,000,000	16	0.07
Total	230,000,000	83,500	360

[a] To the U.S. population
[b] Divide by 100 for mSv
[c] Number of persons not known

From Ionizing Radiation Exposure of the Population of the United States, Rep. No. 93, National Council on Radiation Protection and Measurements, Bethesda, MD, 1987.

The average annual effective dose equivalent from all sources to the entire U.S. population is obtained by summing the annual collective effective dose equivalents and dividing by the number of U.S. population. The result is approximately 650 mrem (6.5 mSv) annually for all people in the U.S. from all sources. The contribution of tobacco products is very large and comes predominantly from ^{210}Po in the tobacco smoke. If the contribution from tobacco is excluded, the result is 365 mrem (3.6 mSv) annually for nonsmokers, or about 1 mrem (10 μSv) per day. It is important to be able to have a general feel for the naturally occurring radiation exposure level, as well as the magnitude of rather commonplace medical X-ray examinations. For example, for handling a radioactive contaminated patient, the exposure rate to the medical staff rarely would result in absorbed-dose rates in excess of 100 mrem/h. Thus, if one were to attend to such a patient for a period of 1 h, the dose would be approximately 25% of the natural background radiation that would incur during the course of a year and would be substantially less than the dose that would be received if one had a plain abdominal X-ray.

It is also instructive to review the occupational and recommended dose limits for various activities. These also provide some indication as to what levels of radiation are felt to be relatively safe for occupationally exposed persons. As can be seen from Tables 9 and 10, an absorbed whole body dose of 5 rad (50 mGy) in any one year is the maximum allowable dose. At the present time, the highest recorded dose to a medical person handling a radioactively contaminated and injured patient from a commercial nuclear power plant in the U.S. has been measured as 14 millirad (140 μGy). This is well below even the recommended dose limit for the general public (500 mrad or 5 mGy in one year). Note should be made that for non-lifesaving emergencies, a whole body dose limit of 25 rad (0.25 Gy) is the recommended dose limit. In situations in which emergency life-saving is involved, the whole

TABLE 9
Occupational Dose Limits

Limit for occupational whole body exposure: critical organs, gonads, lens of the eye, and bone marrow	1.25 rem/quarter-year 5 rem in any one year
Limit for occupational exposure of hands	18.75 rem/quarter-year
Limit for nonoccupational exposure (including exposure of minors)	0.125 rem/quarter-year
Single-tissue or organ limit, if not covered in separate recommendation	15 rem in any one year
Fertile women	0.5 rem to fetus during entire gestation

From *Medical Effects of Ionizing Radiation,* Mettler, F. A. and Moseley, R. D., Eds., Grune & Stratton, New York, 1985. With permission.

TABLE 10
Recommended Dose Limits (General Public)

Public (individual)	0.1 rem in any one year (continuous or frequent exposure) 0.5 rem in any one year (infrequent exposure)
Students (individual)	0.1 rem in any one year
Family of radioactive patients	0.5 rem in any one year (<45 yr old) 5 rem in any one year (45 or older)
Emergency	
Lifesaving	100 rem (whole body) 300 rem (hands and forearms)
Nonlifesaving	25 rem (whole body) 100 rem (hands and forearms)

From *Medical Effects of Ionizing Radiation,* Mettler, F. A. and Moseley, R. D., Eds., Grune & Stratton, New York, 1985. With permission.

body dose limit recommended by the National Council on Radiation Protection and Measurements is 100 rad (1 Gy) (Table 11).

TABLE 11
Guidelines for Emergency Actions

Life-Saving Actions

This applies to search for and removal of injured persons, or entry to prevent conditions that would probably injure numbers of people.

1. Rescue personnel should be volunteers or professional rescue personnel (e.g., firemen who "volunteer" by choice of employment).
2. Rescue personnel should be broadly familiar with the consequences of exposure.
3. Women capable of reproduction should not take part in these actions.
4. Other things being equal, volunteers above the age of 45 should be selected.[a]
5. Planned dose to the whole body shall not exceed 100 rem (1 Sv).[b]
6. Hands and forearms may receive additional dose of up to 200 rem (i.e., a total of 300 rem or 3 Sv).
7. Internal exposure should be minimized by the use of the best available respiratory protection, and contamination should be controlled by the use of available protective clothing.
8. Normally, exposure under these conditions shall be limited to once a lifetime.
9. Persons receiving exposures as indicated above should avoid procreation for a period up to a few months.

Actions in Less Urgent Emergencies

This applies under less stressful circumstances where it is still desirable to enter a hazardous area to protect facilities, eliminate further escape of effluents, or to control fires.

1. Persons performing the planned actions should be volunteers broadly familiar with exposure conseqeunces.
2. Women capable of reproduction shall not take part.
3. Planned whole body dose shall not exceed 25 rem (0.25 Sv).
4. Planned dose of hands and forearms shall not exceed 100 rem or 1 Sv (including the whole body component).
5. Internal exposure shall be minimized by respiratory protection, and contamination controlled by the use of protective clothing.
6. Normally, if the retrospective dose from these actions is a substantial fraction of the prospective limits, the actions should be limited to once in a lifetime.

[a] The purpose of this limit is to avoid unnecessary genetic effects whenever possible.
[b] With quality factors used in ordinary circumstances, this dose equivalent could represent exposure risk considerably above 20 times that for 5 rem (50 mSv) spread over a year because the recovery inherent in low dose and low dose rate for the low LET components may not be applicable. On the other hand, the risk may be considerably less than 20 times as great because the normal QF values do not apply to large acute exposures.

From Basic Radiation Protection Criteria, NCRP Rep. No. 39, National Council on Radiation Protection and Measurements, Bethesda, MD, 1980. (*Note*: NCRP Rep. No. 91, 1987, is less specific and only indicates that only actions involving life-saving justify acute doses in excess of 10 rem [100 mSv].)

REFERENCES

1. Protection of the public in the event of major radiation accidents: principles for planning, Ann. ICRP, 40, 2, 1984.
2. Manual on Early Medical Treatment of Possible Radiation Energy, Safety Ser. No. 47, International Atomic Energy Agency, Vienna, 1978.
3. **Mettler, F. A. and Moseley, R. D.,** *Medical Effects of Ionizing Radiation*, Grune & Stratton, New York, 1985.
4. **Rubin, P. and Casarett, G. W.,** *Clinical Radiation Pathology*, W.B. Saunders, Philadelphia, 1968.
5. Evaluation of Radiation Emergencies and Accidents, Selected Criteria and Data, Tech. Rep. Ser. No. 152, International Atomic Energy Agency, Vienna, 1974.
6. What the General Practitioner (M.D.) Should Know about Medical Handling of Overexposed Individuals, Tech. Doc. 366, International Atomic Energy Agency, Vienna, 1986.
7. **Shleien, B.,** Preparedness and Response in Radiation Accidents, Public Health Service HHS Pub. FDA 83-8211, U.S. Department of Health and Human Services, Rockville, MD, 1983.
8. Ionizing Radiation Exposure of the Population of the United States, Rep. No. 93, National Council on Radiation Protection and Measurements, Bethesda, MD, 1987.

Chapter 2

HISTORICAL ASPECTS OF RADIATION ACCIDENTS

Fred A. Mettler, Jr. and Robert C. Ricks

TABLE OF CONTENTS

I. INTRODUCTION

Radiation accidents are extremely rare events; however, the last two years have witnessed the largest radiation accidents in both the eastern and western hemispheres. It is the purpose of this chapter to review how radiation accidents are categorized, examine the temporal changes in frequency and severity, give illustrative examples of several types of radiation accidents, and, finally, to describe the various registries for radiation accidents.

II. CLASSIFICATION AND FREQUENCY OF RADIATION ACCIDENTS

The most widely known and most complete registry of radiation accidents is maintained at the Radiation Emergency Assistance Center/Training Site (REAC/TS) Registry of Oak Ridge Associates Universities in Oak Ridge, TN. As of January 1, 1988, the registry contained 190 significant events involving about 140,000 persons. A significant radiation accident is one in which an individual exceeds at least one of the following criteria:

1.   Whole body dose equal to or exceeding 25 rem (0.25 Sv).
2.   Skin dose equal to or exceeding 600 rem (6 Sv).
3.   Absorbed dose equal to or greater than 75 rem (0.75 Sv) to other tissues or organs from an external source.
4.   Internal contamination equal to or exceeding one half the maximum permissible body burden (MPBB) as defined by the International Commission on Radiological Protection.
5.   Medical misadministrations, provided they result in a dose or burden equal to or greater than the criteria 1) to 4) already listed.

There is an average, therefore, of approximately 20 significant radiation accidents per year which are identified. Of these, approximately 10 to 15 per year occur in the U.S. There may be additional unreported accidents in some countries. One can surmise that radiation is more widely utilized in the U.S. and, therefore, U.S. experience accounts for about half of the accidents. It is possible that the radiation accidents are more reliably reported in the U.S. Each year the REAC/TS group of Oak Ridge, TN receives 50 to 60 calls for assistance. Approximately two thirds of these calls request assistance for events which ultimately turn out *not* to have involved a significant exposure.

The number of accidents, as well as the number of fatalities, is shown in Table 1. Including the accident at Chernobyl, as well as the recent accident in Goiania, Brazil, there have been 66 acute fatalities due to radiation accidents. One the average, worldwide since 1944, there have been less than two deaths annually from radiation accidents. This can be contrasted to U.S. statistics of 50,000 deaths annually from traffic accidents and 8,000 fatalities annually from fire. The listing of accidents in which fatalities occur is shown in Table 2. It can be seen from this table that almost half of radiation accident deaths occurred as a result of the 1986 Chernobyl accident. In addition, the table indicates that the majority of injuries to others in accidents involving fatalities resulted in total body irradiation, and in fact total body irradiation is the predominant cause of death in radiation accidents. Only very few fatalities occur as a result of local irradiation or internal contamination. The number of fatalities by year is shown graphically in Figure 1. This indicates that two thirds of the fatalities have occurred in the last decade for a rate of almost five fatalities per year. It should be noted that there are several other fatalities which are known to be due to radiation exposure which were not listed either in Table 2 or in Figure 1. This is because they were not due to accidents, but to intentional exposure for purposes of suicide.

TABLE 1
Major Radiation Accidents
Worldwide (1944 —
November 1987)

Number of accidents	290
Persons involved	136,607
Significant exposures	24,845
Acute fatalities	65

TABLE 2
Radiation Accidents with Radiation Fatalities

Year	Site	Deaths	TBI[a]	Injuries of others in accident		
				Local	Internal	Combined
1945	Los Alamos, NM	1	1			
1946	Los Alamos, NM	1	7			
1954	Marshall Islands	1	22			
1958	Yugoslavia	1	5			
	Los Alamos, NM	1	2			
1960	U.S.S.R.	1				
1961	Germany	1		2		
1962	Mexico City	4	1			
1963	People's Republic of China	2				4
1964	Germany	1			3	
	Rhode Island	1	3			
1968	Wisconsin	1				
1972	Bulgaria	1				
1975	Brescia, Italy	1				
1978	Algeria	1	4	2		
1981	Oklahoma	1				
1982	Norway	1				
1983	Argentina	1				
1984	Morocco	8				3
1985	Canada	1				
1986	Georgia and Texas	1		1		1
	Chernobyl, U.S.S.R.	29	174			
1987	Goiania, Brazil	4				16
Total	23 accidents	65	219	5	3	24

[a] TBI, total body irradiation.

The classification of radiation accident by device for the period 1944 until January 1, 1988 is shown in Table 3. The frequency of accidents by time is shown in Figure 2. The figure demonstrates that the majority of major radiation accidents are due to radiation devices. A radiation device may be an X-ray machine or even an accelerator; however, most radiographic devices involved in accidents are encapsulated, highly radioactive sources used for industrial radiography. Examples of these types of accidents will be given later in this chapter. It should be pointed out that, with the exception of Chernobyl, radiation devices have been responsible for the majority of fatalities.

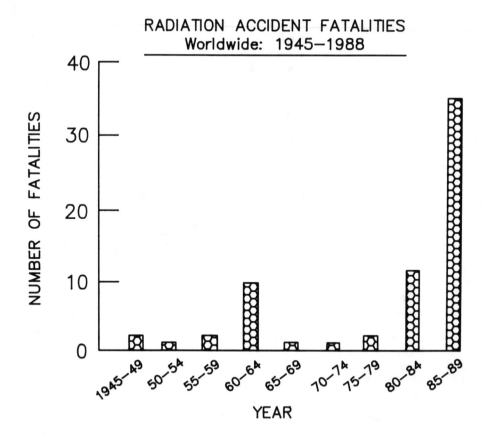

FIGURE 1.   Radiation accident fatalities worldwide by year.

TABLE 3
Major Radiation Accidents
Worldwide (1944 — January
1988) Classed by "Device"

Criticalities	
Critical assemblies	5
Reactors	8
Chemical operations	5
Radiation Devices	
Sealed sources	129
X-ray devices	63
Accelerators	14
Radar generators	1
Radioisotopes	
Transuranics	27
Tritium	3
Fission products	10
Radium spills	2
Diagnosis and therapy	19
Other	4
Total	290

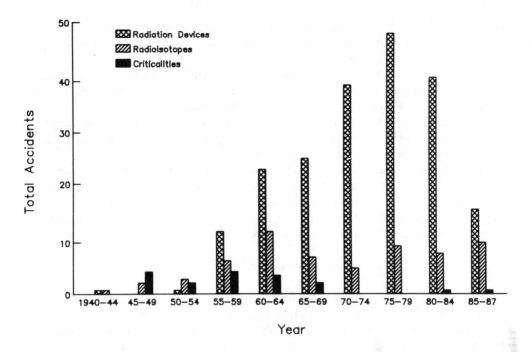

FIGURE 2.   Radiation accidents worldwide by year and device.

III. CRITICALITY ACCIDENTS

Criticality accidents occur when enough fissionable material, such as enriched uranium or ^{239}Pu is brought together. If the neutron flux is high enough, the material will undergo a nuclear reaction (become critical). All criticality accidents, with the exception of Chernobyl, occurred between the years of 1945 and 1965. There were 13 accidents during that period which resulted in five fatalities. Three of the early accidents will be described in the following paragraphs.

Two early criticality accidents occurred at Los Alamos Laboratories, which were then involved in the Manhattan Project. The accidents occurred during experiments which were designed to provide information about the fission characteristics of metallic plutonium. Neutron leakage from the plutonium sphere utilized was great enough so that a fission chain reaction could not be sustained. By placing neutron reflecting material around the sphere, it was possible to sustain criticality. The LA-1 accident occurred on August 21, 1945, at 9:55 p.m. Tungsten carbide bricks were to be stacked about a plutonium sphere. The experiment called for five bricks on each side; however, as the final brick was being placed, it slipped out of the hand of the worker and fell into the center of the assembly, causing enough reflection of neutrons so that criticality occurred. A LA-2 accident occurred on May 1, 1946. In this accident, a physicist was instructing his successor. Two concentric hemispherical shells of beryllium were placed about a neutron source. The shells would reflect enough neutrons to cause criticality and the physicist was holding these spheres apart with a screwdriver. The screwdriver slipped and the spheres came in contact, allowing enough neutron reflection to cause criticality. Eighty-five percent of the energy of both these chain reactions was dissipated as heat, but personnel in the area were exposed to large amounts of neutrons, gamma rays, very soft X-rays, and electrons. In the first accident, the experiment operator died in 24 d and in the second the physicist died in 9 d.

The Oak Ridge Y-12 criticality accident occurred in Oak Ridge, TN, on June 16, 1958. The criticality was triggered by an unplanned transfer of enriched uranium to a 55-gal drum and eight workers were exposed to a mixed neutron gamma field. No fatalities resulted, although five of the patients developed bone marrow depression. Absorbed doses ranged from 230 to 365 rad (2.3 to 3.65 Gy).

The accidents at Los Alamos are examples of criticality accidents as the result of manipulation of a critical assembly, while the accident at Y-12 demonstrates criticality as a result of a chemical operation. Criticalities can also happen as a result of an excursion in a nuclear reactor. There have been six such accidents to date. One occurred in Mol, Belgium, on December 30, 1965. In this accident there was a criticality excursion in a small experimental reactor. The one patient subsequently died from high but nonuniform exposure. Absorbed dose to the chest was estimated to be in the range of 600 rad (6.0 Gy) from gamma exposure and neutron exposure. The accident which occurred at Chernobyl also was the result of instability in a reactor. The accident was complicated by additional factors such as an explosion, loss of coolant, and fire. The Chernobyl accident as well as the accident at Three Mile Island are discussed in detail in Chapter 17.

IV. RADIOISOTOPES

Accidents involving radioisotopes usually refer to those radioactive materials which are unsealed. Radioisotopes which are sealed in capsules are usually classed under the heading of radiation devices and will be discussed later in this chapter. As mentioned earlier, the definition of a significant accident involving radioisotopes is one in which there is more than one half of a maximum permissible body burden of radioactive material within the body. There have been between 15 and 20 such accidents resulting in three fatalities. One fatality occurred in West Germany in 1961; however, there are few details of this accident. In 1968, there was a misadministration of ^{198}Au which was injected into the peritoneal cavity of a patient who had ovarian carcinoma. One thousand times more radioactivity was injected than was intended. The patient suffered significant bone marrow depression and ultimately died from a cerebral hemorrhage, probably as a result of radiation-induced thrombocytopenia. The third fatality as a result of internal radionuclides occurred in October 1987, Goiania, Brazil. A 6-year-old girl had ingested ^{137}Cs. The estimated dose from the ingested cesium was approximately 50 rad (0.5 Gy) per day. This accident is described in more detail later in this chapter.

In addition to radioisotopes causing significant exposure from internal deposition, they also can cause clinically significant external exposure, particularly when fresh fission products are involved. The major accident in this regard occurred on March 1, 1954, in which there was a test explosion of a thermonuclear weapon in the Bikini Atoll in the Pacific. The yield of the weapon was 17 megatons, which was significantly greater than expected, and there was an unpredicted shift in the winds which caused a radioactive cloud to drift over several inhabited atolls and a fishing boat. The fallout exposed 239 Marshallese on the Rongelap, Ailingae, and Utirik Atolls. On the Rongelap Atoll, which is 100 miles from Bikini, there were 67 people exposed to fallout which was described as being snow-like. The estimated gamma dose to 67 individuals was 175 rad (1.75 Gy). On the Ailingae Atoll, 110 miles from Bikini, there were 19 persons exposed to a mist-like fallout with an estimated gamma dose of 70 rad (0.7 Gy). There were 23 Japanese tuna fishermen on a boat called the *Lucky Dragon* which was approximately 100 miles from the detonation. The fishermen were exposed to white ashes which fell on the vessel for approximately 5 h. The ashes were noted to adhere to exposed skin and absorbed gamma doses were estimated to be in the range of 200 to 700 rad (2.0 to 7.0 Gy). One individual died as a result of this accident. Twenty-eight American servicemen were also exposed during the course of this accident; however, no fatalities resulted.

V. RADIATION DEVICES

Accidents involving radiation devices may be classified in two major categories: (1) those in which a radiation source is found or taken from a site by persons who are not aware that it is radioactive and (2) accidents in which there is exposure of the device operator secondary to carelessness or malfunction of the device. Six accidents will be described in the first category to point out that there are many similarities involved in the accidents.

In the People's Republic of China on January 11, 1963, a ^{60}Co gamma ray source of 10 Ci (3.7×10^{11} Bq) was taken by a child to his house. The source had been used for irradiation of seeds. Six persons were exposed to gamma doses ranging from 200 to 8,000 rad (2.0 to 80.0 Gy). Two of the patients died.

In Chiba, Japan on September 17, 1971, an ^{192}Ir source of 5 Ci (1.85×10^{11} Bq) was found by a construction worker who picked it up, put it between his belt and trousers, and took it home. The source remained in the room for 4 to 5 d, during which five men were in and out of the room several times. No fatalities resulted.

On May 5, 1978 an ^{192}Ir source of 25 Ci (9.25×10^{11} Bq) fell from a truck in Algeria. It was found by two young boys, 3 and 7 years old, who handled the metallic, pencil-like object for several hours and later took it home. The source remained in the kitchen for approximately 6 weeks. The source was found after 38 d. One of the patients died and the two children had significant local radiation burns.

There have been at least two accidents with inadvertant or unsuspected exposure to radioactive sources from radiation therapy machines. The first of these was an accident in Ciudad Juarez, Mexico. Through an unknown sequence of events, a ^{60}Co radiotherapy machine from a hospital was taken to a junkyard for scrap metal. The machine, with its cobalt source inside, was processed and made into a reinforcing bar to be used in concrete construction as well as restaurant furniture. Some of the reinforcing bars which had been manufactured were sent to Los Alamos National Laboratories in New Mexico to be used for a construction project. Since Los Alamos Laboratories is engaged in research with radioactive materials, there are site radiation monitoring devices and, as the truck delivered the radioactive construction materials, the radioactivity was identified. Subsequent investigation revealed that the material could be traced to the Yonke Fenix junkyard. Fortunately, no fatalities resulted.

A similar accident occurred in late September of 1987 in Goiania, Brazil. In this instance, a ^{137}Cs therapy machine was removed from a partly demolished cancer treatment center by junk scavengers and sold to a junkyard dealer. The machine contained approximately 1,400 Ci (5.18×10^{13} Bq) of ^{137}Cs. The junkyard dealer noted that the machine had a green glow at night, and broke open the capsule with a sledgehammer and exposed the ^{137}Cs source. The source was admired by friends and neighbors and was eventually broken into pieces, distributed, and even powdered. Fifty-four patients were initially hospitalized, eight of whom had the acute radiation syndrome. Four fatalities resulted from the accident, including a 6-year-old girl who ate approximately 27 mCi (1.0×10^9 Bq) of the powdered cesium. There were 244 persons involved in the accident with 20 receiving significant exposures.

The second type of accident involving radiation devices is concerned with overexposures due to operator error or defective radiation devices. Each year there are millions of industrial radiographs obtained in the U.S. These are done to evaluate the integrity of metallic objects such as pipewells and airplane propellers. Most of the industrial radiographic devices utilize an intensely radioactive gamma-emitting source such as ^{192}Ir or ^{60}Co. The sources range from 10 to 100 Ci ($3.7 - 37 \times 10^{11}$ Bq) in activity. Dose rates at contact often are in the range of 50,000 rad (50 Gy) /min. Over 90% of the accidents involve radiation burns of the hands, but if the sources are inadvertently placed in pockets, significant burns of the thighs and buttocks can result.

The number of overexposures of industrial radiographers equals the number of over-exposures from all other Nuclear Regulatory Commission (NRC) licensees, even though the industrial radiographers comprise only a small percentage of NRC licensees. The actual number of accidents is probably significantly greater than that identified in the REAC/TS registry, since many industrial radiography accidents are probably not reported. The following is an example of one accident of this type. In September 1985, an industrial radiographer was utilizing a 70-Ci (2.6×10^{12} Bq) ^{192}Ir source. Approximately 6 exposures were made. As the radiographer carried the instrument back to his truck, he noticed a loose object in the extension tubing. He correctly surmised that the source had become disconnected from the cable and had not been retracted into the shielding. He proceeded to empty the source out of the tube, extend the cable, pick up the source, and reattach it. The source was then retracted into the shielding. Approximately 15 d later, the radiographer noted blistering of the skin on his fingertips and loss of fingernails. Absorbed dose to the fingertips was estimated at 10,000 rad (100 Gy) and dose to the whole body in the range of 50 rad (0.5 Gy).

^{60}Co sources are also used for product sterilization. Typically, medical supplies, chemicals or other objects may be exposed to millions of rads for various purposes. Such stationary radiation units typically have stronger sources of activity and even a momentary malfunction or inadvertent exposure may cause significant medical sequelae. Example 1 occurred on June 13, 1974, in Parsippany, NJ, at a plant utilizing a radiation source to sterilize medical and chemical products; a 61-year-old man entered the hot cell thinking the cobalt source was in the "down" position. When he realized the source was in the "up" position, he turned around and left. The exposure was estimated to be between 5 and 10 s to a 120,000 Ci (4×10^{15} Bq) cobalt source. Significant bone marrow depression occurred; however, the patient survived. Almost a carbon-copy accident occurred on September 23, 1977, in Rockaway, NJ. A 32-year-old man was exposed for approximately 10 s to a 500,000 Ci ^{60}Co (1.85×10^{16} Bq) source. Construction at the facility caused alteration of the hot cell entry and the source-up warning sign was obscured from view and the electrical interlock on the door was not functional. In this case, significant bone marrow depression occurred; however, the individual recovered.

On February 4, 1971, a research technologist and control operator were performing seed irradiation experiments at the University of Tennessee. The technologist was exposed for approximately 40 s to a 7,700-Ci (2.9×10^{14} Bq) ^{60}Co source at a distance of approximately 50 cm. Ultimately, the midline dose was estimated to be approximately 130 rad (1.3 Gy). The cause of the accident was ascribed to several malfunctions, including inoperable warning lights, incomplete closing of door, a door limit switch having been tied in closed position and a door limit switch that was nonfunctional. Established procedures also were not followed, nor did the technologist observe the radiation monitors, which were functioning properly.

Failure to observe established safety procedures and technical malfunction also have been the cause of severe overexposures in electronic radiation devices. In fact, technical failures are more likely to result in accidents with sophisticated radiation devices such as accelerators than with industrial radiography devices. One accident of this type occurred on October 4, 1967 near Pittsburgh, PA. Three technicians were called to repair the cooling system of a Van de Graaff linear accelerator. In order to repair the system, they unlatched the control panel, removed a key from the private vault, unlocked the safety tunnel door, and opened the inside door to the target. Each of these four maneuvers had been put in place to automatically shut down the accelerator. The men were not aware that the safety interlock system had failed and that they were being exposed to a steady beam of X-rays while doing the repairs. No fatalities resulted; however, there were extensive local injuries (requiring amputation) as well as bone marrow depression.

There are a large number of devices in use throughout the U.S. for radiation therapy.

In the last several years, the application of computers for dose determination as well as machine operation has greatly added to the complexity of the devices, and thus increased the possibility for accidental overexposure. In 1986, there was at least one patient death reported as a result of a modified software program for a linear accelerator. The software program which controlled the dose delivered by the machine to the patient had a significant error (known as malfunction 54) when one tried to change the treatment protocol.

Computer software is also utilized to calculate the absorbed dose when therapeutic radioactive sources are placed in patients. Changes in these procedures also have resulted in errors with ensuing fatalities. In at least one circumstance, approximately 20 patients were given a dose to the tumor volume of 60,000 rad (600 Gy) when a dose of 15,000 rad (150 Gy) was intended. The number of accidental overexposures due to poorly calibrated and malfunctioning radiation therapy equipment is probably significantly underreported.

The last example presented is not really an accidental exposure, but rather a deliberate, bizarre exposure, and it is included as an example of what unlikely things actually do occur. In 1971, a petroleum engineer applied for a license for two sources of 2 Ci (7.4 × 10^{10} Bq), each of ^{137}Cs to be utilized for oil- and gas-well logging. The engineer was divorced from his wife, but had custody of two sons on two weekends a month and one month a year. Over a six-month period, one of the sons noted shiny silver pellets in the earphones of headphones that he was told to wear, in a pillow he was told to use, and ultimately in a sock he found in his bed. The youngster had multiple lesions which became ulcerated and only after a period of one year did physicians recognize the ulcerations as being radiation necrosis. This case of child abuse ultimately resulted in the child being effectively castrated. The child had to have the testes replaced with prostheses and had to undergo some 16 operations over the next four years for plastic repair and skin grafts.

The preceding descriptions represent a partial list of radiation accidents, but clearly demonstrate the most typical types and patterns of occurrence. The four most common causes of accidents appear to be (1) use of systems which are highly dangerous as well as being unstable, (2) loss of highly radioactive sources which are recovered by unsuspecting individuals, (3) human error and deliberate violation of safety procedures, and (4) use of complicated systems by personnel not familiar with the operational computer systems and ramifications of software changes.

VI. RADIATION ACCIDENT REGISTRIES

A registry of radiation accidents is maintained by REAC/TS at Oak Ridge Associated Universities on Oak Ridge, TN. It is funded by the U.S. Department of Energy (DOE). Each event is recorded in a registry log book and assigned a sequential four-digit registration number. There are four subcategories of registries within the central registry. These are the Diethylenetriaminepentaacetic acid (DTPA) registry, DOE study registry, U.S. radiation accident registry, and a foreign registry.

The DTPA registry includes all individuals who have had administrations of DTPA for treatment of suspected or actual internal contamination for actinides. The DOE study registry is also known as "the equal to or greater than 5 rem" study registry. It is intended as the basis for epidemiological evaluation of the health and mortality of persons who have exceeded permissible exposure limits in their employment with the U.S. DOE and its predecessors, such as the Atomic Energy Commission, the Energy Research and Development Administration, or civilians in the U.S. Navy Reactor Program.

The U.S. radiation accident registry was developed under the guidance of the U.S. Atomic Energy Commission and it includes those persons who have received significant doses as defined by REAC/TS (see earlier in this chapter). The most common radiation accident registered is that of high-dose local exposure, most commonly to the hands. The foreign registry is an incomplete list of generally anecdotal accidents from other countries around the world. Registrants in the U.S. radiation accident registry are requested to participate in programs designed for long-term followup. There is no monetary reward for participation in the program, and an individual can withdraw at any time. Usually there is an annual medical followup of these individuals by local physicians.

SELECTED BIBLIOGRAPHY

1. Accidental exposure involving X-ray spectrometer unit, Serious Accidents, Issue 338, December 6, Division of Operational Safety, U.S. Atomic Energy Commission, Washington, D.C., 1974.
2. Accidental radiation excursion at the Y-12 plant June 16, 1958, Unclassified report, Rep. Y 1234, U.S. Atomic Energy Commission, Washington, D.C., 1958.
3. **Allen, W. R.,** Radiation injury to the hand, *J. Kansas Med. Soc.,* 67, 447, 1966.
4. **Andrews, G. A.,** Criticality accidents in Vinca, Yugoslavia, and Oak Ridge, Tennessee. Comparison of radiation injuries and results of therapy, *JAMA,* 179, 191, 1962.
5. **Andrews, G. A., Sitterson, B. W., Kretchmar, A. L., and Brucer, M.,** Accidental radiation excursion at the Oak Ridge Y-12 Plant IV. Preliminary report on clinical and laboratory effects in the irradiated employees, *Health Phys.,* 2, 134, 1959.
6. **Andrews, G. A., Sitterson, B. W., Kretchmar, A. L., and Brucer, M.,** Criticality accident at the Y-12 plant, in *Proc. Sci. Meet. Diagnosis and Treatment of Acute Radiation Injury,* International Document Service, Division of Columbia University Press, New York, 1961, 27.
7. **Andrews, G. A., Hubner, K. F., and Fry, S. A.,** Report of 21-year medical follow-up of survivors of the Oak Ridge Y-12 accident, in *The Medical Basis for Radiation Accident Preparedness,* Hubner, K. F. and Fry, S. A., Eds., Elsevier/North Holland, New York, 1980, 59.
8. **Andrews, G. A.,** Mexican ^{60}Co radiation accident, *Isot. Radiat. Technol.,* 1, 200, Winter 1963.
9. **Auxier, J. A.,** Nuclear accident at Wood River Junction, *Nucl. Saf.,* 6, 298, 1965.
10. **Auxier, J. A., Berger, C. D., and Dunning, D. E.,** Americium-241 distribution and excretion in humans and the effects of chelation, in *Abstracts of Papers Presented at the 29th Annu. Meet. Health Physics Society,* Pergamon Press, New York, 1984, 72.
11. **Bailey, E. D. and Wukasch, M. D.,** A case of felonious use of radioactive materials, in *Proc. IV Int. Cong. Radiation Protection Association,* Vol. 3, International Radiation Protection Association, Paris, 1977, 987.
12. **Barlotta, F. M.,** The New Jersey radiation accidents of 1974 and 1977, in *The Medical Basis for Radiation Accident Preparedness,* Hubner, K. F. and Fry, S. A., Eds., Elsevier/North Holland, New York, 1980, 151.
13. **Baron, J. M., Yachnin, S., Polcyn, R., Fitch, F. W., and Sturner, W. Q.,** Accidental Radiogold (^{198}Au) Liver Scan Overdose with Fatal Outcome, in *Handling of Radiation Accidents,* Proc. Symp. Handling of Radiation Accidents organized by the International Atomic Energy Agency in collaboration with the World Health Organization, IAEA, Vienna, 1969, 399.
14. **Basson, J. K., Hanekom, A. P., Coetzee, F. C., et al.,** Health Physics evaluation of an acute overexposure to a radiography source, in *A Systematic Approach to Safety:* Proc. 5th Cong. IRPA, Pergamon Press, 1980, 64.
15. **Beninson, D., Placer, A., and Vander Elst, E.,** Estudio de un caso de irradiacion humana accidental, in *Handling of Radiation Accidents,* Proc. Symp. Handling of Radiation Accidents organized by the International Atomic Energy Agency in collaboration with the World Health Organization, IAEA, Vienna, 1969, 415.
16. **Bliss, S. P.,** Medical Aspects of an Accidental Exposure to a Van de Graaff Generator, Premier Colloq. Int. Protection Aupres des Granda Accelerateurs, Presses Universitaires de France, Paris, 1962, 35.
17. **Boulenger, R., Parmentier, N., Le Go, R., et al.,** Description et analyse de l'accident de criticite survenu au reactor Venus á Mol le 30 Decembre 1965, in *Les Irradiations Accidentelles en Milieu de Travail,* EUR-3666, 1967, 357.
18. **Brucer, M.,** The acute radiation syndrome: a medical report on the Y-12 accident June 16, 1958, Unclassified report, ORINS 25, U.S. Atomic Energy Commission, Washington, D.C.
19. **Callihan, D. and Thomas, J. T.,** Accidental radiation excursion at the Oak Ridge Y-12 Plant 1. Description — physics of the accident, *Health Phys.,* 1, 363, 1959.

20. Chernobyl: Health and Environmental Consequences of the Chernobyl Nuclear Power Plant Accident, Report to the US-DOE Office of Energy Research, from the Interlaboratory Task Group on Health and Environmental Aspects of the Soviet Nuclear Accident, Prepared by the Committee on the Assessment of Health Consequences in Exposed Populations, DOE/ER-0332, UC-41 and 48, U.S. Department of Energy, Washington, D.C., 1987.

21. Chernobyl; Summary Report on the Post-Accident Review Meeting on the Chernobyl Accident, IAEA Safety Ser. No. 75-INSAG-1, International Atomic Energy Agency, Vienna, 1987.

22. Chernobyl; Fry, the Chernobyl reactor accident: the impact on the United Kingdom (1987 Mayneord Lecture), *Br. J. Radiol.*, 60, 1147, 1987.

23. **Clarke, R. H.**, Reactor accidents in perspective, *Br. J. Radiol.*, 60, 1182, 1987.

24. **Cohen, N., Sasso, T. L., and Wrenn, McD.**, Metabolism of americium 241 in man; an unusual case of internal contamination of a child and his father, *Science,* 205(4414), 64, 1979.

25. **Collins, V. P. and Gaulden, M. E.**, A case of child abuse by radiation exposure, in *The Medical Basis for Radiation Accident Preparedness,* Hubner, K. F. and Fry, S. A., Eds., Elsevier/North Holland, New York, 1980, 197.

26. **Conard, R. A. et al.**, Review of medical findings in a Marshallese population twenty-six years after accidental exposure to radioactive fallout, BNL 51261, Brookhaven National Laboratory, Upton, NY, January, 1980.

27. **Cronkite, E. P. et al.**, Some effects of ionizing radiation on human beings: a report on the Marshallese and Americans accidentally exposed to radiation from fallout and a discussion of radiation injury in the human being, TID 5358, Washington, D.C., U.S. Government Printing Office, 1956.

28. **Degos, M. M., Gaultier, F., Fournier, F., Daniel, F., and Reboul, M.**, Radionecrose par l'iridium 192, Societe française de dermatologie et de symphiligraphie 76, 19, 1969 (in French).

29. **Dousset, M. and Jammet, H.**, Les accidents humains d'irradiation d'origine nucleaire, in *Proc. Symp. Irradiations Accidentelles et Centre International de Radiopathologie avec la Participation de la Societe Française de Radioprotection Creteil,* Galle, P., Masse, R., and Nenot, J. C., Eds.

30. **Elliott, G. A.**, Accidental acute irradiation from cobalt-60, *S. Afr. Med. J.,* 34, 524, 1960.

31. **Franger, H. and Lushbaugh, C. C.**, Radiation death from cardiovascular shock following a criticality accident. Report of a second death from a newly defined human radiation death syndrome, *Arch. Pathol.,* 83, 446, 1967.

32. **Fuqua, P. A., Norwood, W. D., and Marks, S.**, Biologic effects of human radiation exposure; report of a criticality accident, *J. Occup. Med.,* 7, 85, 1965.

33. **Gilberti, M. V.**, The 1967 radiation accident near Pittsburgh, Pennsylvania, and a follow-up report, in *The Medical Basis for Radiation Accident Preparedness,* Hubner, K. F. and Fry, S. A., Eds., Elsevier/North Holland, New York, 1980, 131.

34. **Guskova, A. K. and Baisogolov, G. D.**, Two cases of acute radiation disease in man, in *Int. Conf. Peaceful Uses of Atomic Energy,* Vol. 11, United Nations, New York, 1956, 35.

35. 1976 Hanford americium exposure incident, *Health Phys.,* 45, 4, 1983.

36. **Harrison, N. T., Escott, P. C., Dolphin, G. W., et al.**, The investigation and reconstruction of a severe radiation injury to an industrial radiographer in Scotland, in *Proc. Third Int. International Radiation Protection Association,* CONF-730907-P1., W.S. Snyder, Ed., U.S. Atomic Energy Commission, Washington, D.C., 1974, 760.

37. **Hasterlik, R. J. and Marinelli, L. D.**, Physical dosimetry and clinical observations on four human beings involved in an accidental critical assembly excursion, in *Proc. Int. Conf. Peaceful Uses of Atomic Energy,* Vol. 11, United Nations, New York, 1956, 25.

38. **Heid, K. R., Breitenstein, B. D., Palmer, H. E., et al.**, The 1976 Hanford Americium Accident, TID-28938 UC 48, Batelle Northwest Laboratories, Richland, WA, 1979.

39. **Heid, K. R., Brietenstein, B. D., Palmer, H. E., McMurray, B. J., and Wald, N.**, The 1976 Hanford Americium Accident, in *The Medical Basis for Radiation Accident Preparedness,* Hubner, K. F. and Fry, S. A., Eds., Elsevier/North Holland, New York, 1980, 345.

40. **Hempelmann, L. H., Lisco, H., and Hoffman, J. G.**, The acute radiation syndrome: a study of nine cases and a review of the problem, *Ann. Intern. Med.,* 36, 279, 1952.

41. **Hempelmann, L. H., Lushbaugh, C. C., and Voelz, G. L.**, What happened to the survivors of the early Los Alamos nuclear accidents? in *The Medical Basis for Radiation Accident Preparedness,* Hubner, K. F. and Fry, S. A., Eds., Elsevier/North Holland, New York, 1980, 18.

42. **Hirashima, K., Sugiyama, H., Ishihara, T., Kurisu, A., Hashizume, T., and Kumatori, T.**, The 1971 Chiba, Japan accident: exposure to iridium 192, in *The Medical Basis for Radiation Accident Preparedness,* Hubner, K. F. and Fry, S. A., Eds., Elsevier/North Holland, New York, 1980, 179.

43. Hot-cell operator received an estimated 400 rad dose, *Nucl. Saf.,* 17, 495, 1976.

44. **Horan, J. R. and Gammill, W. P.**, Health physics aspects of the SL-I accident, *Health Phys.,* 9, 177, 186, 1963.

45. **Howland, J. W., Ingram, M., Mermasen, H., and Hansen, C. L.,** The Lockport incident: accidental partial body exposure of humans to large doses of X-irradiation, in *Proc. Sci. Meet. Diagnosis and Treatment of Acute Radiation Injury,* International Document Service, Division of Columbia University Press, 1961, 11.

46. **Hurst, G. S., Ritchie, R. H., and Emerson, L. C.,** Accidental radiation excursion at the Oak Ridge Y-12 Plant. III. Determination of radiation doses, *Health Phys.,* 2, 121, 1959.

47. Industry's first radiation accident, studied by AEC firms, *Nucleonics,* 22(9), 21, 1964.

48. **Anon.,** Yugoslavian Criticality Accident, October 15, 1958, *Nucleonics,* 17(4), 106, 1959.

49. **Jacobson, A., Wilson, B. M., Banks, T. E., and Scott, R. M.,** ^{192}Ir over-exposure in industrial radiography, *Health Phys.,* 32, 291, 1977.

50. **Jammet, H. P.,** Treatment of victims of the zero-energy reactor accident at Vinca, in *Proc. Sci. Meet. Diagnosis and Treatment of Acute Radiation Injury,* International Document Service, Division of Columbia University Press, New York, 1961, 83.

51. **Jammet, H., Congora, R., Le Go, R., and Doloy, M. T.,** Clinical and biological comparison of two acute accidental irradiations: Mol (1965) and Brescia (1975) in *The Medical Basis for Radiation Accident Preparedness,* Hubner, K. F. and Fry, S. A., Eds., Elsevier/North Holland, New York, 1980, 91.

52. **Jammet, H., Gongora, R., Jockey, P., and Zucker, J. M.,** The 1978 Algerian accident: acute local exposure of two children, in *The Medical Basis for Radiation Accident Preparedness,* Hubner, K. F. and Fry, S. A., Eds., Elsevier/North Holland, New York, 1980, 229.

53. **Jammet, H., Gongora, R., Pouillard, P., Le Go, R., and Parmentier, N.,** The 1978 Algerian accident: four cases of protracted whole-body irradiation, in *The Medical Basis for Radiation Accident Preparedness,* Hubner, K. F. and Fry, S. A., Eds., Elsevier/North Holland, New York, 1980, 113.

54. **Jammet, H., Mathe, G., Pendic, B., Duplan, J. F., Maupin, B., Laterjet, R., Kalic, D., Schwarzenbeg, L., Djukic, Z., and Vigne, J.,** Etudes de six cas d'irradiation totale accidentelle, *Rev. Fr. Etud. Clin. Biol.,* 4, 210, 1959.

55. **Jammet, H., Strambi, E., Gongora, R., and Nenot, J. C.,** Interet de l'association des methodes physiques et biologiques pour l'evaluation de la dose et de sa repartition dans les cas d'irradiation globale aigue accidentelle, in *Proc. 4th Int. Cong. IRPA, Vol. 3, International Radiation Protection Association,* Paris, 1977, 961.

56. **Karas, J. S. and Stanbury, J. B.,** Fatal radiation syndrome from an accidental nuclear excursion, *N. Engl. J. Med.,* 272, 755, 1961.

57. **Knowlton, N. P., Jr., Leifer, E., Hogness, J. R., Hempelman, L., Blaney, L. F., Gill, D. C., Oakes, W. R., and Schafer, C. F.,** Beta ray burns of human skin, *JAMA,* 141, 239, 1949.

58. **Krizek, T. J. and Ariyan, S.,** Severe acute radiation injuries of the hands. Report of two cases, *Plas. Reconstr. Surg.,* 51, 14, 1973.

59. **Kumatori, T., Hirashima, K., Ishihara, T., Kurisu, A., Sugiyama, H., and Hashizume, T.,** Radiation accident caused by an Iridium-192 radiographic source, in *Handling Radiation Accidents: Proceedings of a Symposium,* International Atomic Energy Agency, 1977, 35.

60. **Kumatori, T., Ishihara, T., Hirashima, K., Sugiyama, H., Ishii, S., and Miyoshi, K.,** Follow-up studies over a 25-year period on the Japanese fishermen exposed to radioactive fallout in 1954, in *The Medical Basis for Radiation Accident Preparedness,* Hubner, K. F. and Fry, S. A., Eds., Elsevier/North Holland, New York, 1980, 33.

61. **Kurschakov, N. A.,** Sluchay ostroy luchevoy bolezni u cheloveka (A case of acute radiation sickness in man) (transl.), Gosudarstvennoe Izdatel'stro Meditsinskoy Literatury, Moscow, 1962, 150.

62. **Lanzl, L. H., Rozenfeld, M. L., and Tarlov, A. R.,** Injury due to accidental high dose exposure to 10 MeV electrons, *Health Phys.,* 13, 241, 1967.

63. **Littlefield, G., Joiner, E. et al.,** Six year cytogenetic follow-up study of an individual heavily contaminated with americium 241, in *Dosimetry, Radionuclides and Technology; Proc. 7th Int. Cong. Radiation Research,* Sect. E3-05, Barendsen, G. W., Kal, H. B., and Van der Kogel, A. J., Martinus Nijhoff, The Hague, 1983.

64. **Lloyd, D. C., Purrott, R. J., Prosser, J. S., et al.,** Doses in radiation accidents investigated by chromosome aberration analysis. VIII. A review of cases investigated: 1977, NRPB-R70, National Radiologic Protection Bureau, Oxford, U.K., 1978.

65. **Lubenau, J. O., Davis, J. S., McDonald, D. J., and Gerusky, T. M.,** Analytical X-ray hazards: a continuing problem, *Health Phys.,* 16, 739, 1969.

66. **Lushbaugh, C. C. et al.,** Clinical course of Case K, *J., Occup. Med.,* 3(Special Suppl.), 150, 1961.

67. **Lushbaugh, C. C., Fry, S. A., Ricks, R. C., Hubner, K. F., and Burr, W. W.,** Historical update of past and recent skin damage radiation accidents, *Br. J. Radiol.,* 7(Suppl. 19), 12, 1986.

68. **Lushbaugh, C. C., Fry, S. A., and Ricks, R. C.,** Medical and radiobiological basis of radiation accident management, *Br. J. Radiol.,* 60, 1159, 1987.

69. **Maxfield, W. S. and Porter, G. H.,** Accidental radiation exposure from Iridium^{192} camera, *Proc. IAEA Symp.* Handling Radiation Accidents, International Atomic Energy Agency, Vienna, 1969.

70. **McCandless, J. B.,** Accidental acute whole body gamma irradiation of seven clinically well persons, *JAMA,* 192, 185, 1965.

71. **Martinez, R. G., Cassab, G. H., Ganem, G. G., et al.,** Observation on the accidental exposure of a family to a source of cobalt-60, Revista Medica Inst. Mex. Seguro Social, 3(Suppl. 1), 4, 1964. (transl.).

72. **Marshall, E.,** Morocco reports lethal radiation accident, *Science,* 225, 395, 1984.

73. **Mettler, F. A., Jr. and Moseley, R. D., Jr.,** *Medical Effects of Ionizing Radiation,* Grune & Stratton, Orlando, 1985.

74. **Menoux, A. M.,** Etude Clinique des Radiolesions Provoquees par l'Exposition Localisée Accidentelle aux Rayonnements Ionisants, Doctoral thesis, Université René Descartes, Academie de Paris, 1977.

75. **Minder, W.,** Interne Kontamination mit Tritium, *Strahlentherpie,* 137, 700, 1969.

76. **Miyoshi, K. and Kumatori, T.,** Characteristics of hematological findings of the Japanese fisherman exposed to radioactive ashes in the Bikini area, Proc. 8th Int. Cong. Hematology, Pan Pacific Press, Tokyo, 1962, 29.

77. **Orlov, V. M., Petuskov, V. N., and Sych, L. I.,** Acute radiation injury of the hands, *Med. Radiol.,* 15(1), 53, 1970 (in Russian).

78. **Parmentier, N. C., Nenot, J. C., and Jammet, H. J.,** A dosimetric study of the Belgian (1965) and Italian (1975) accidents, in *The Medical Basis for Radiation Accident Preparedness,* Hubner, K. F. and Fry, S. A., Eds., Elsevier/North Holland, New York, 1980, 105.

79. **Paxton, H. C., Baker, R. D., Maraman, W. J., and Reider, R.** Los Alamos criticality December 30, 1958, *Nucleonics,* 17(4), 107, 1959.

80. **Pendic, B.,** The zero-energy reactor accident at Vinca, in *Proc. Sci. Meet. Diagnosis and Treatment of Acute Radiation Injury,* International Document Service, Division of Columbia University Press, New York, 1961, 67.

81. **Petersen, D. F.,** Neutron dose estimates in SL-I accident, *Health Phys.,* 9, 231, 1963.

82. **Peterson, D. F.,** Rapid estimation of fast neutron doses following radiation exposure in criticality accidents: the S^{32} (n, p) P^{32} reaction in body hair, in *Personnel Dosimetry for Radiation Accidents,* International Atomic Energy Agency, Vienna, 1965, 217.

83. **Preston, R. J., Brewen, J. G., and Gengozian, N.,** Persistence of radiation induced chromosome aberrations in marmoset and man, *Radiat. Res.,* 60, 516, 1974.

84. **Radojicic, B., Hajdukovic, S., and Antic, M.,** Follow-up studies of exposed persons in the zero energy reactor accident at Vinca, in *Proc. Sci. Meet. Diagnosis and Treatment of Acute Radiation Injury,* International Document Service, Division of Columbia University Press, New York, 1961, 105.

85. **Robbins, L. L., Aub, J. C., Cope, O., et al.,** Superficial "burns" of skin and eyes from scattered cathode rays, *Radiology,* 46, 1, 1946.

86. **Ross, J. P., Holly, F. E., Zarem, H. A., Rothman, C. M., and Shabo, A. L.,** The 1979 Los Angeles accident: exposure to iridium 192 industrial radiographic source, in *The Medical Basis for Radiation Accident Preparedness,* Hubner, K. F. and Fry, S. A., Eds., Elsevier/North Holland, New York, 1980, 205.

87. **Rossi, E. C., Thorngate, A. A., and Larson, F. C.,** Acute radiation syndrome caused by accidental exposure to cobalt-60, *J. Lab. Clin. Med.,* 59, 655, 1962.

88. **Rubin, L. S.,** The Riverside radiation tragedy, *Columbus Monthly,* p. 52, April 1978.

89. **REAC/TS** Radiation Accident Registries, personal communications and unpublished data and press reports.

90. **Saenger, E. L., Kereiakes, J. G., Wald, N., and Thoma, G. E.,** Clinical course and dosimetry of acute hand injuries to industrial radiographers from multicurie sealed gamma sources, in *Proc. 3rd Int. International Radiation Protection Association,* Vol. 1, Office of Information Services (Tech. Div.), U.S. Atomic Energy Commission, Washington, D.C., 1974, 773.

91. **Safronov, Ye. I.,** A case of radiation sickness from internal irradiation. Studies in medical radiology, USSR JPRS 24, 452, Office of Technical Services, Washington, D.C., May 4, 1964.

92. **Sagstuen, E., Theisen, H., and Henriksen, T.,** Dosimetry by ESR spectroscopy following a radiation accident, *Health Phys.,* 45, 961, 1983.

93. **Schenck, R. R. and Gilberti, M. V.,** Four-extremity radiation necrosis, *Arch. Surg.,* 100, 729, 1970.

94. **Schneider, G. J., Choné, B., and Blonnigen, T.,** Chromosomal aberrations in a radiation accident — dosimetric and hematological aspects, *Radiat. Res.,* 40, 613, 1969.

95. **Seelantag, W.,** Two cases of Tritium fatality, in *Tritium, Proc. Tritium Symp.,* Moghissi, A. and Carter, M. W., Eds., Messenger Graphics, Phoenix, Az, 1971.

96. **Shipman, T. L.,** A radiation fatality resulting from massive overexposure to neutrons and gamma rays, *Proc. Sci. Meet. Diagnosis and Treatment of Acute Radiation Injury,* International Document Service, Division of Columbia University Press, New York, 1961, 113.

97. **Shipman, T. L., Ed.,** Acute radiation death resulting from accidental nuclear critical excursion, *J. Occup. Med.,* Spec. Suppl., 3(2), 146, 1961.

98. **Stavem, P. et al.,** A radiation accident with lethal outcome, *J. Norw. Med. Assoc.,* 33(103), 2240, 1983 (in Norwegian; summary in English).

99. **Stavem, P., Brogger, A., et al.,** Lethal acute gamma radiation accident at Kjeller, Norway: report of a case, *Acta Radiol. Oncol.,* 24(1), 61, 1985.
100. **Steidley, K. D.,** A ^{60}Co hot cell accident, *Health Phys.,* 31, 382, 1976.
101. **Steidley, K. D., Zeik, G. S., and Ouellette, R.,** Another ^{60}Co hot cell accident, *Health Phys.,* 36, 437, 1979.
102. **Thoma, G. E., and Wald, N.,** The diagnosis of management of accidental radiation injury, *J. Occup. Med.,* 1, 421, 1959.
103. Ionizing radiation: sources — biological effects, U.N. Scientific Committee on the Effects of Atomic Radiation 1982 Report, United Nations, New York, 1982.
104. **Vassileva, B. and Kruschikov, I.,** Suizid mit caesium 137. *Psychiatr. Neurol. Med. Psychol. (Leipzig),* S116-119 30 February 2, 1978.
105. **Vodopick, H. and Andrews, G. A.,** Accidental radiation exposure, *Arch. Environ. Health,* 28, 53, 1974.
106. **Vodipick, H. and Andrews, G. A.,** The University of Tennessee Comparative Animal Research Laboratory Accident in 1971, in *The Medical Basis for Radiation Accident Preparedness,* Hubner, K. F. and Fry, S. A., Eds., Elsevier/North Holland, New York, 1980, 141.
107. **Weigensberg, I. J., Asbury, C. W., and Feldman, A.,** Injury due to accidental exposure to X-rays from an X-ray fluorescence spectrometer, *Health Phys.,* 39, 237, 1980.
108. **Ye, G. Y., Yong, L., Nue, T., et al.,** The People's Republic of China accident in 1963, in *The Medical Basis for Radiation Accident Preparedness,* Hubner, K. F. and Fry, S. A., Eds., Elsevier/North Holland, New York, 1980, 81.

Chapter 3

TRANSPORTING RADIOACTIVE MATERIALS AND POSSIBLE RADIOLOGICAL CONSEQUENCES FROM ACCIDENTS AS MIGHT BE SEEN BY MEDICAL INSTITUTIONS

Robert M. Jefferson

TABLE OF CONTENTS

I. INTRODUCTION

When considering the full range of possible consequences arising from the transportation of radioactive materials, there are two facts at work which together define the actual risk involved. The first of these facts is that there is already an enormous amount of radioactive material being moved within our society. Consideration of this fact alone would lead one to the conclusion that the number of accidents involving radioactive materials is already correspondingly high. The corollary conclusion is that the need to treat accident victims resulting from these movements is also already very real. This apparent need is compounded when one realizes that, as time goes on, the number of shipments will continue to increase. Thus, the exposure factor is already in existence and increasing as time goes on.

In contrast to this first fact is a second fact which is gained from a historical look at the transport of radioactive materials. In the 30 to 40 years during which we in the U.S. have been transporting substantial quantities of radioactive material, there has never been an accident severe enough to cause a major release of these materials. Experience thus reveals that there has never been anyone injured radiologically or much less killed as a result of exposure to radiation or contamination arising as the result of an accident involving radioactive materials during transportation. (There have been mechanical injuries and deaths associated with these accidents, but no involvement radiologically.) In order to gain the perspective necessary to understand these two facts, it is useful to go back and review some of the data surrounding the transport of radioactive materials within the U.S.

II. TRANSPORT OF RADIOACTIVE MATERIALS

As shown in Table 1, there are approximately 500,000,000,000 packages of all sorts of materials transported every year in the U.S. Of these, about 100,000,000 contain some form of hazardous materials. These include toxins and poisons, combustibles and flammables, caustics and acids, explosives and incendiaries, all of which people accept as a normal part of living in an advanced society. About $2\,^3/_4\%$ of these packages of hazardous materials being shipped are radioactive.

Perhaps more significant than the total numbers involved is the distribution by end use of those radioactive materials being shipped within our society. As can be seen from Table 2, approximately two thirds of all of the packages containing radioactive material find some use in the medical profession. Most of these shipments of radioactive material are of small quantities, although there are enough large quantity shipments to bring the total number of curies shipped for the medical profession to approximately one third of the total curies shipped. Thus, the preponderance of shipments of radioactive materials in our country involve radiopharmaceuticals, thermoelectric generators (pacemakers), diagnostic sources, and treatment sources.

The next largest category includes such things as waste from a broad range of activities and consumer products, such as luminous exit signs, watch dials, and smoke detectors. This miscellaneous category accounts for roughly one quarter of the number of packages involved, but only about 2% of the radioactive material involved.

The preponderance of the activity being shipped is involved with industrial applications and consists mainly of cobalt, cesium, and strontium. Application of these materials would include such things as field radiography, well logging, thickness gauging, catalytic applications, and product treatment such as sterilization. While these industrial applications account for approximately two thirds of the curies involved, they are responsible for less than 8% of the total number of packages involved.

Nuclear power, which in the mind of the public is the major contributor to radioactive material transportation, is involved in only about 4% of total number of packages and less than 1% of the total radioactivity involved.

TABLE 1
Annual Shipping Statistics

500 billion packages/year shipped in U.S. (all goods)
100 million packages/year hazardous materials
2.75 million packages/year radioactive materials

TABLE 2
Distribution of Radioactive Packages by
End Use

Use	Packages (%)	Curies (%)
Medical	62.2	34.3
Industrial	7.6	63.1
Misc (inc. waste)	26.1	1.9
Nuclear power	4.1	0.7

III. PACKAGING OF RADIOACTIVE MATERIALS

When reviewing these statistics, there is an obvious difference between such things as radiopharmaceuticals and spent fuel, for instance. A similar comparison could be made between the source for a smoke detector and one used for field radiography purposes. These differences are accommodated in transportation by requiring different levels of protection for varying levels of radioactivity. While there are several "protections" required by the regulations, two are of primary interest in our considerations. All packaging designs for radioactive material transport must provide for the containment of the radioactive material. Containment means that the packaging must prevent release of material under stated conditions. A second protection (if the material is of high enough radioactivity level) is the requirement that shielding be included in the packaging in order to reduce the external radiation dose to a level that is not considered harmful to those persons in the transport activity who will be handling or otherwise located adjacent to the package of radioactive material. However, even these protections vary according to the quantity of radioactive material to be carried within a package.

The varying levels of protection are specified in the regulations by defining four categories. Since almost all materials are somewhat radioactive, the first of these is an exempt category which defines a level below which it it not required to provide special packaging nor even to mark the package as radioactive. An example of an exempt material would be the mantle out of a Coleman lantern which, because of its thorium content, is radioactive, but is below that level required to provide special packaging. Exempt material can be packaged as the shipper sees fit and can in fact be sent through the U.S. mail. The second of the four categories is called *low-specific activity (LSA)* and covers primarily those materials wherein the activity is so dilute there is little if any risk to the public even in the case where an accident occurs and these materials are released. The regulations specify that LSA materials must be packaged in "strong tight" packages. Generally speaking, a strong tight container would be a cardboard box with a 250-lb rupture strength, a fiberboard drum, a wooden box, or any of a number of similar types of packaging. Packages of radioactive material in this category must be labeled, but the package itself is designed and certified by the user.

The next higher category is called *Type A* and defines a category in which the quantity of specific isotopes within the package is below a specified level. This specified level, known as an A_2 quantity, is that quantity of material, which if released to the public, is considered

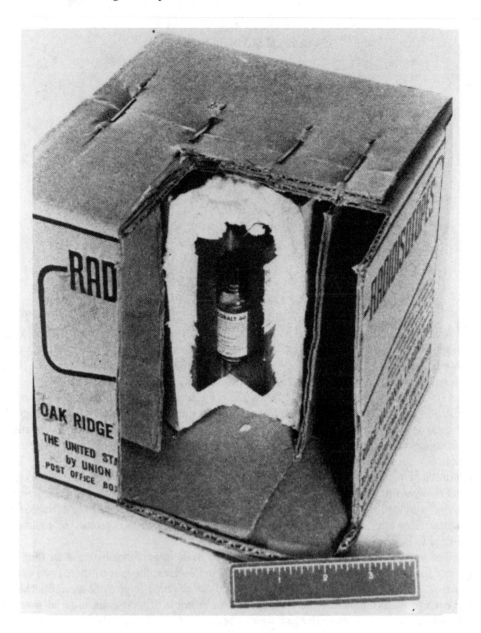

FIGURE 1.   Type A package for transporting radiopharmaceuticals showing internal construction.

as not capable of causing a public health hazard. These A_2 quantities for each radioisotope have been carefully developed by a consensus method involving both the International Commission on Radiologic Protection (ICRP) and the National Council on Radiation Protection and Measurements) (NCRP) committees. By far, the preponderance of nonexempt shipments of radioactive material are made in Type A packages. The bulk of these Type A packages being shipped are radiopharmaceuticals. Therefore, one of the most familiar radioactive materials packagings are the ones similar to that shown in Figures 1 and 2. These 1-ft cubic packages are designed to hold a vial of liquid radiopharmaceutical surrounded by absorbent material and any necessary shielding within a standard produce can. This can is held in the middle of the cardboard box by a set of interlocking spacers and the entire assembly is sealed with tape and labeled as shown in Figure 1.

35

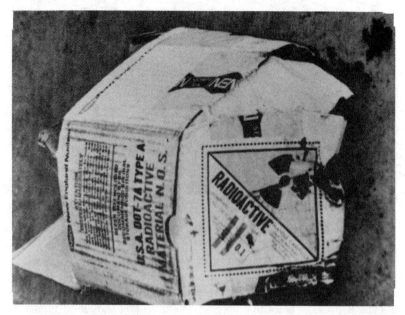

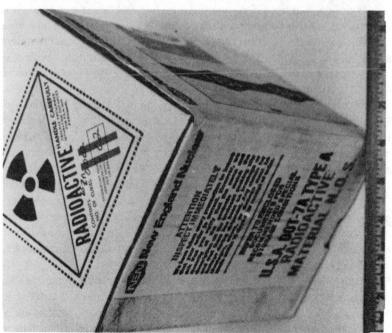

FIGURE 2.   Type A package before and after impact by a forklift on a loading dock.

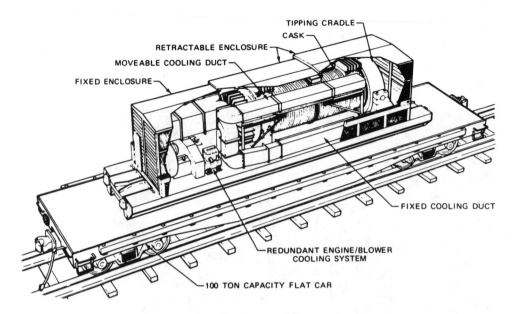

FIGURE 3.   Type B package.

Packages designed for more than an A_2 quantity are classified as *Type B* packages and must, in addition to the requirements for survival of normal handling conditions imposed on a Type A package, also be capable of surviving very severe accident conditions as well. The most common Type B package is a shipping cask similar to that shown on Figure 3. This 68-ton rail cask is designed to handle several spent fuel assemblies at one time. It is this Type B category packaging that concerns most people. These contain large quantities of radioactive material that, if released or if the shielding were compromised, could represent a rather sizable threat to public health. It is that very threat that dictated from the beginning that this category of packaging should be able to withstand not only the normal rigors of transport but very severe accidents as well.

The validity of this approach to regulating the transportation of large quantities of radioactive material is evident by the fact that there have been accidents, but there has been no radiological involvement of the public as the result of these accidents. Figure 4 shows the aftermath of an accident involving a spent fuel shipping cask which occurred in Tennessee in 1971. In this accident, the driver intentionally left the road to avoid a head-on collision. As a consequence, the truck rolled, with the cask on its frame coming to rest upside down in the ditch. The result of this accident was zero release of radioactive material. The cask was uprighted, cleaned, mounted on another vehicle, and transported to its final destination.

Figure 5 shows an air crash that occurred near Knoxville, Tennessee, in which an aircraft was carrying radioactive sources in Type B packages. There was no release of radioactive material into the environment as a result of this crash.

The Nuclear Regulatory Commission (NRC), which regulates these packagings, has for some time been concerned as to whether or not the regulations are sufficiently strict so as to provide adequate protection for the public. As a result, over the years, it has commissioned a number of studies designed to evaluate the adequacy of the regulations. Each of these studies has used progressively more refined techniques for evaluation. The results reported from these analytical evaluations have shown a consistent decrease in the projected risk involved in transporting these materials. The latest of these studies, published in 1987, concluded that the risk to the public of transporting radioactive materials was roughly one quarter of that previously determined by the study released in 1981.

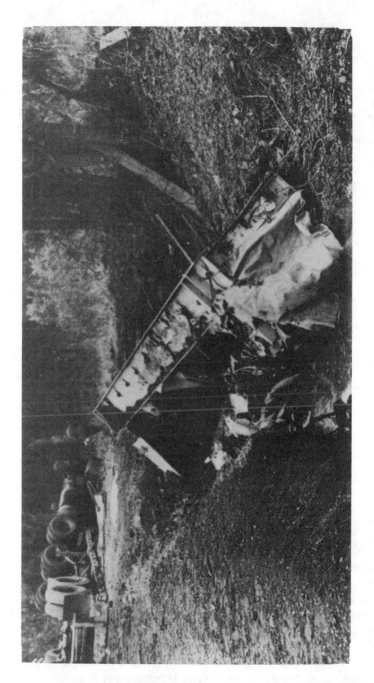

FIGURE 4. A spent fuel shipping cask accident (no release of material). The truck carrying a spent reactor fuel element overturned near Clinton, Tennessee, killing the driver. Maximum exposure measured at surface of the cask was 0.5 mR/h.

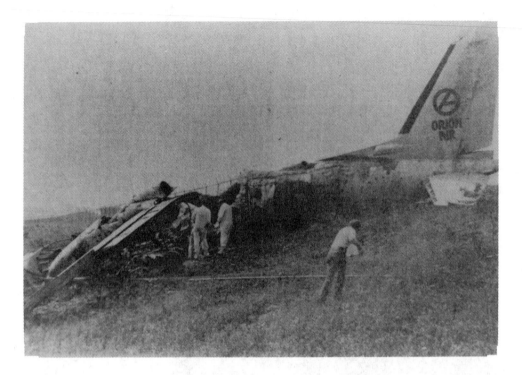

FIGURE 5.   Aircraft crash with radioactive cargo (no release of radioactive material into environment). The crash occured at Tri-Cities airport in Tennessee in July of 1983. The aircraft was carrying two Type B containers with 3900 Curies of ^{192}Ir in each and one type A package containing 4 mCi of ^{90}Y.

TABLE 3
Radioactive Material Accident Data

Package type	No. packages	No. releases	Survivability (%)
Strong	596	56	90.6
Type A	1,956	11	99.4
Type B	50	0	100.0
Total	2,602		

Note: There were 167 vehicular accidents from 1971 to March 1985 (about 1/ month) with 2602 packages involved (an average of 15.6 per accident).

While continued studies of the risk involved are reassuring, particularly since they continually predict lower and lower risks, the ultimate determinant of risk is experience. Since the beginning of 1971, the U.S. Department of Transportation (DOT) has collected statistics on the accident experience involving all hazardous materials transportation. Among the interesting information derived from these studies is the fact that, on a per mile basis, the transport of radioactive materials is much safer than the transport of other hazardous materials. That factor aside, it is also interesting to note the experiences with these various categories of radioactive material packaging, as they might indicate the relative safety of these shipments. Table 3 shows a breakdown of this experience. As was noted earlier, the Type A category handles the majority of shipments, therefore it is not surprising that the majority of accidents occur within that category as well. The thing that this figure reveals most clearly is that fact that the experience with these packagings is quite good. Even the industrial package or the strong tight package survives more than 90% of the accidents in which it is involved. The Type A package, designed to survive the normal rigors of transport, in fact, also survives the accident conditions as well. Over 99% of Type A packages involved in accidents continue to provide containment of their radioactive contents. The real sterling performer, though, is the Type B package, which has historically continued to provide protection even in the case of severe accidents. Not only has this protection been record perfect since 1971, but it has, in fact, been perfect since transportation of these materials began in the mid 1940s. It is of interest to note that the regulations convering Type B packaging are uniform worldwide and this perfect safety record stands throughout the western world (where statistics are available).

Perfect safety records are hard to believe, particularly when we continually see reports of chemical spills and other hazardous materials being routinely released as result of transportation accidents. The rational skeptic can thus logically ask, "How can this be?" The answer is simply that of all the hazardous materials routinely shipped within our society, only large quantity radioactive materials are required to be packaged in systems specifically designed to survive the rigors of accidents during transport. Furthermore, to assure the protection exists, Type B packagings must be certified by the NRC or the U.S. Department of Energy. Included in the specifications for these packages is a requirement that the package be designed to meet specific test requirements. While the regulations do not specifically require testing of every package, many of the packages in use today have been tested and shown to survive accidents far beyond the severity required by the regulations.

One such test program conducted in the mid-1970s consisted of staging accidents involving spent shipping fuel casks so as to expose them to "realistic" accident conditions. These tests included simulation of high speed impacts (up to 84 mph impact into a 20-ft cube of reinforced concrete) (see Figure 6) and hydrocarbon fires of extreme intensity (see Figure 7). These tests showed that the analytical tools then in use (and since improved) were quite capable of accurately predicting the physical results of these accident conditions. Thus, both experience and risk analysis reveal that the probability of creating some sort of radiological involvement as a consequence of an accident involving a package of radioactive material is indeed quite small. Furthermore, if there is a radiological involvement, it is in all likelihood going to be below clinically detectable levels.

IV. IDENTIFICATION OF RADIOACTIVE MATERIALS

One might be tempted then to conclude that medical emergency personnel could ignore the possibility that there could be someone brought to them who is radiologically involved as the consequence of an accident during the transport of radioactive materials. That is certainly not the conclusion I would recommend. While the probability of radiological involvement is exceedingly small, it is not zero and persons brought for treatment as a result of accidents involving the transportation of radioactive materials might be either contaminated or exposed. This is particularly true when you consider that contamination levels might be quite low, and that there are packages of radioactive materials which are not specifically designed to survive accident conditions. Thus, for the trained medical professional, it is most important to obtain certain information that would be very useful, were the patient contaminated or exposed. It would be useful to know, for example, what radioactive material is involved and in what form. These two pieces of information are available from the shipping manifest, which is required to be carried in the door pocket of the cab of the truck. Other information contained on that manifest that might be of interest is the name and telephone number of the shipper, from whom additional information might be obtained. Unfortunately, in many cases the DOT specification for the material will contain the letters *NOS* meaning "not otherwise specified". When this appears on the manifest, the material in the package

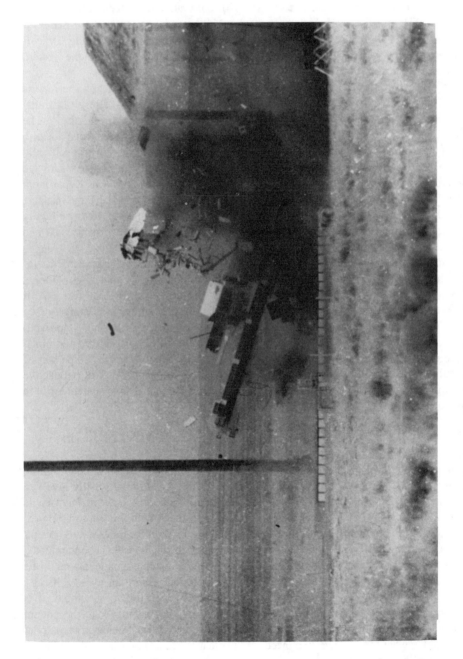

FIGURE 6. Truck-mounted spent fuel cask impacting 20-foot-thick concrete wall at 84 mph.

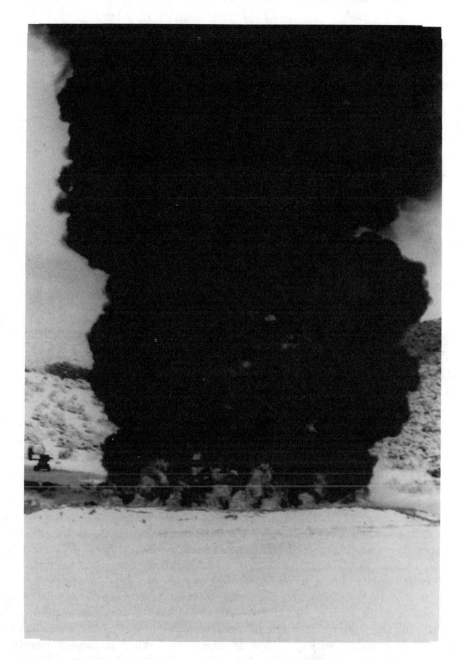

FIGURE 7. Rail cask for spent fuel during prolonged burn using kerosene.

is generally low-level material, although not uniformly so. In this case, the name and phone number of the shipper becomes more important, since a telephone contact might produce the needed information.

The next best source of information is the label on the package itself. There are three different labels which specify three different quantity levels of radioactive material within the package. The lowest level requiring labeling is specified by a white diamond, 4 in. on a side with the word *Radioactive I* (see Figure 8) across the middle and the familiar trefoil sign on the top. In the bottom half of this "white label", there should be information on the material contained in the package. Intermediate quantities of material are designated by

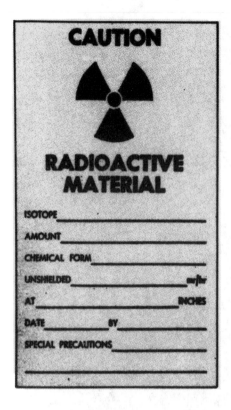

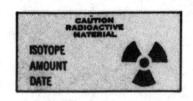

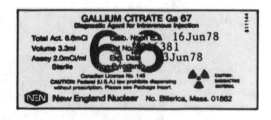

A

FIGURE 8.   Labels for radioactive materials package.

label of the same general layout as previously described, but with the top half yellow. In addition, the lower half will have two red bars in it (see Figure 8). This is known as a *yellow-II* label and it also should have a description of the material in the package written on the label. In addition, it will have information as to the quantity of material involved. The highest level materials are contained in packages with what are called *yellow-III* labels which are identical to yellow-II, but instead of having two red bars, there are three. This label likewise has information on the material and quantity contain within the package.

The least useful information, but the easiest to obtain, is information from the placard on the outside of the vehicle. Not all radioactive materials shipments are required to be placarded, but any shipment in which the entire contents of the vehicle are radioactive materials or in which any package within the vehicle has a yellow-III label is required to carry external placards on all four sides of the vehicle. The placard, by itself, contains no useful information from a medical standpoint. If the shipment is also displaying an orange card with a four digit black United Nations number on it, that can be of some limited use. The four-digit number on the orange card defines the various categories into which that particular shipment might fall. Numbers denoting radioactive materials include 2908 through 2918 and 2974 through 2982. Definitions of the meaning of those numbers can be found in the Department of Transportation Emergency Response handbook on hazardous materials.

A final source of information, albeit somewhat unreliable under some accident circumstances, is the driver of the vehicle. He is required by law to know the contents of his load and, if he is coherent, should be able to provide accurate information. No matter how it is obtained, information concerning the possible exposure is of utmost importance.

There are several facts which can be derived from all this information which would be

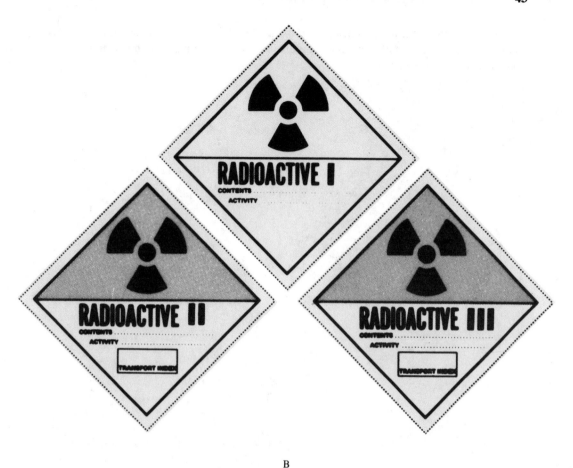

B

useful in the treatment of possible accident victims. One of these is that if there is an accident and if there is a release and if there is, as a consequence of that, an exposed or contaminated victim, the most likely route of exposure is uptake through ingestion or inhalation instead of direct whole-body external exposure. Further, if this occurs, in all likelihood, what has been the source of such exposure or uptake has been either a radiopharmaceutical or a material called *yellow cake*, the milled product from uranium mining (U_3O_8). Again this reemphasizes the importance of information on the possible exposure material and pathway. If the manifest, for example, indicates sealed sources of cesium or cobalt, it is highly unlikely that the pathway is ingestion and medical personnel should look for the effects of direct whole-body exposure. If, on the other hand, the manifest shows the material to be yellow cake or some other LSA material shipped as a finely divided powder, direct whole-body exposure is unlikely and ingestion is the route that should be suspected. Again, it should be reiterated that the most reliable source of information concerning the radioactive material itself would be the shipper whose name and phone number are to appear on the manifest carried in the driver's door pocket in the cab of the vehicle.

V. SUMMARY

In summary, medical personnel faced with treating victims of an accident involving radioactive material should be suspicious concerning possible radiological involvement. At the same time, they should be careful to obtain the necessary information in order to make a rational decision as to the likelihood of such involvement. Having made that decision, it is entirely possible then to approach the problem from a medical standpoint in such a way as to determine the extent of radiological involvement and to apply proper medical treatment consistent with that exposure.

Chapter 4

MILITARY RADIATION ACCIDENTS

Fred A. Mettler, Jr. and Steve N. Allen

TABLE OF CONTENTS

I. INTRODUCTION

Since 1945, there have been approximately 50 accidents in which nuclear weapons were involved (Table 1). Many of the details of these remain classified, however, several have been sufficiently declassified to be examined in some detail. In the broadest terms, nuclear weapons accidents may be classified in three categories. The first category is an accident in which a nuclear weapon was being carried and in which the carrier (often an aircraft) suffered the consequences of a fire or explosion. In most such accidents, the weapon is recovered essentially intact, without having detonated either the high explosives or undergone a nuclear yield. Nuclear yield refers to energy released in the detonation of a nuclear weapon from either nuclear fusion or fission. The second broad category of accidents are those in which the high explosives in the nuclear weapon detonate upon impact with resulting dispersion of plutonium in the environment. The third broad category of military accidents is that in which a significant nuclear yield results from the weapon. No accidents in this third category have as yet occurred.

Although there have been several accidents in which the high explosives in the weapon have detonated upon impact, actual nuclear yield is extremely unlikely, due to the construction design of U.S. weapons. In a simplistic fashion, weapon design involves a central core of plutonium which needs to be compressed instantaneously and equally from all sides for nuclear criticality to occur. The U.S. weapon design is often referred to as "one-point safe". The criterion for design safety of these weapons is that there must be less than one chance in a million of producing a nuclear yield equivalent to more than four pounds of TNT when the high explosive is initiated and detonated at any single point. This weapon design feature is responsible for lack of significant nuclear yield in U.S. weapons accidents.

In this chapter, nuclear weapon accident response procedures of the Department of Defense (DOD) will be examined, as will three specific accidents in which nuclear weapons were involved.

II. RESPONSE PROCEDURES

There are two phases of response to any nuclear weapons accident. The first "initial phase" includes accident notification procedures and immediate emergency measures in order to provide a federal presence and support. Actions during this phase include establishing command and control on site, fire suppression, reconnaissance, rescue, treatment of casualties and assessment of hazards.[1] (Figures 1 and 2.)

The second phase, or "follow-on phase" of the response, is led by a flag officer (admiral or general) as well as specialized teams within the DOD and the Department of Energy (DOE). In addition to continuing actions of the initial phase, other responsibilities include recovery of the weapon, detailed radiation monitoring, documenting of the accident, establishment of a claims processing facility, and finally, decontamination and site restoration. In all the phases, three primary areas of concern which need to be addressed are radiological health and safety, weapon recovery, and public affairs. Logistical support to accomplish these aims involve specialized communication, radiological, security, medical logistics, and legal teams.

The DOD has assigned responsibility for nuclear accident weapon response to the service in charge of the installation, naval ship, or geographic area where the incident or accident occurred. Should the accident occur beyond the boundaries described above (e.g., in a foreign country) the service having custody of the weapon at the time of the accident is assigned responsibility.

If the accident occurs within United States territory and the area is non-federal land, establishment of a National Defense Area (NDA) is undertaken. Establishment of an NDA

TABLE 1
Summary of Military Nuclear Weapon Accidents

Date	Vehicle	Location
Feb. 13, 1950	B-36	Off coast British Columbia[b]
April 11, 1950	B-29	Monzano Base, New Mexico[b]
July 13, 1950	B-50	Lebanon, Ohio[b]
August 5, 1950	B-29	Fairfield, California[b]
Nov. 10, 1950	B-50	Over water, outside U.S.[a]
March 10, 1956	B-47	Mediterranean Sea[a]
July 27, 1956	B-47	Overseas base
May 22, 1957	B-36	Kirtland AFB, New Mexico[b]
July 28, 1957	C-124	Atlantic Ocean[a]
October 11, 1957	B-47	Homestead AFB, Florida[b]
January 31, 1958	B-47	Overseas base
February 5, 1958	B-47	Savannah River, Georgia[a]
March 11, 1958	B-47	Florence, South Carolina[b]
November 4, 1958	B-47	Dyess AFB, Texas[b]
November 26, 1958	B-47	Chennault AFB, Louisana[b]
January 18, 1959	F-100	Pacific base
July 6, 1959	C-124	Barksdale AFB, Louisiana
September 25, 1959	P-5M	Off Whidbey Island, Washington[a]
October 15, 1959	B-52/KC-135	Hardinsburg, Kentucky
June 7, 1960	BOMARC missile	McGuire AFB, New Jersey
January 24, 1961	B-52	Goldsboro, North Carolina
March 14, 1961	B-52	Yuba City, California
November 13, 1963	Storage Igloo	Medina Base, Texas[b]
January 13, 1964	B-52	Cumberland, Maryland
December 5, 1964	Minutemen ICBM	Ellsworth AFB, South Dakota
December 8, 1964	B-58	Grissom AFB, Indiana
October 11, 1965	C-124	Wright-Patterson AFB, Ohio
December 5, 1965	A-4	Pacific Ocean[a]
January 17, 1966	B-52/KC-135	Palomares, Spain[c]
January 21, 1968	B-52	Thule, Greenland[c]
Spring 1968	Classified	Classified
September 19, 1980	Titan II ICBM	Damascus, Arkansas

[a]   One or more weapons not recovered.
[b]   Detonation of high explosive portion without significant plutonium dispersal.
[c]   Extensive plutonium dispersal.

temporarily places non-federal lands under control of the DOD and results only from an emergency event which involves classified defense material. The purpose of the NDA is to protect this classified material, therefore the NDA boundary is not determined by the size of the contaminated area, which may be much larger. The DOD defines the boundary and marks it with a physical barrier as well as with posted warning signs. The owner's consent and cooperation will be obtained whenever possible; however, military necessity often dictates a final decision regarding location, shape and size of the NDA without owner's consent. A similar area for a security zone can be established by the DOE in which case it is referred to a National Security Area (NSA).

Often, several agencies outside the DOD will also have a role in nuclear weapon accident response. The DOE has teams of scientists and technical specialities with sophisticated equipment ready for dispatch to the scene of a nuclear accident. The Federal Emergency Management Agency (FEMA) has a primary role in coordinating requests for federal agencies' assistance, as well as assuring that state and local off-site response actions are mutually supportive and coordinated. Primary off-site authority at the scene of a weapons accident rests with state and local officials.

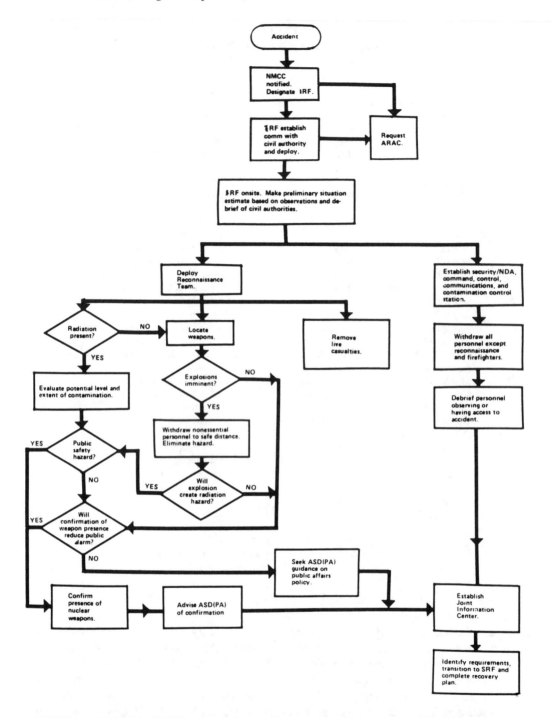

FIGURE 1.   Relationship of initial actions during a nuclear weapon accident response — ARAC (Atmospheric Release Advisory Capability), IRF (Initial Response Force), SRF (Service Response Force), NDA (National Defense Area), NMCC (National Military Command Center), ASD (Assistant Secretary of Defense for Public Affairs).

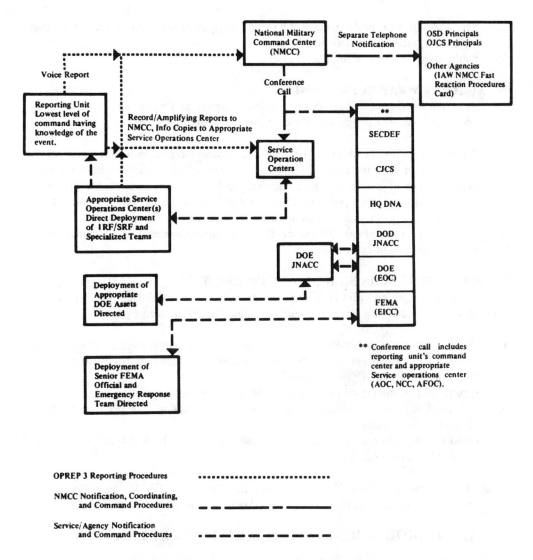

FIGURE 2. Nuclear weapons accident notification flow: DNA (Defense Nuclear Agency), CJCS (Chairman, Joint Chiefs of Staff), DOE (Department of Defense), JNACC (Joint Nuclear Accident Coordinating Center), OJCS (Office of Joint Chiefs of Staff), OSD (Office of Secretary of Defense), SEC DEF (Secretary of Defense).

There are three definitions utilized regarding unexpected events which involve nuclear weapons. These are as follows:

A. NUCLEAR WEAPON ACCIDENT

These are unexpected events involving nuclear weapons or radiological nuclear weapon components that result in any of the following:

1. Accidental or unauthorized launching, firing, or use by U.S. forces or U.S.-supported allied forces of a nuclear-capable weapon system which could create the risk of an outbreak of war
2. Nuclear detonation
3. Non-nuclear detonation or burning of a nuclear weapon or radiological nuclear weapon component
4. Radioactive contamination

5.   Seizure, theft, loss, or destruction of a nuclear weapon or radiological nuclear weapon component including jettisoning
6.   Public hazard, actual or implied

B. NUCLEAR WEAPON INCIDENT

This is an unexpected event involving a nuclear weapon, facility, or component resulting in any of the following, but not constituting a nuclear weapons accident:

1.   An increase in the possibility of explosion or radioactive contamination
2.   Errors committed in the assembly, testing, loading, or transportation and/or the malfunctioning of equipment and material which could lead to an unintentional operation of all or part of the weapon arming and/or firing sequence, or which could lead to substantial change in yield or increased dud probability
3.   Any act of God, unfavorable environment, or condition resulting in damage to a weapon, facility, or component

C. NUCLEAR WEAPON SIGNIFICANT INCIDENT

This is an unexpected event involving nuclear weapons or radiological nuclear weapon components which does not fall in the nuclear weapon accident category but

1.   results in evident damage to a nuclear weapon or radiological nuclear weapon component to the extent that the major rework, complete replacement, or examination or recertification by the DOE is required,
2.   requires immediate action in the interest of safety or nuclear weapon security,
3.   may result in adverse public reaction (national or international) or premature release of classified information, or
4.   could lead to a nuclear weapon accident and warrant that high officials or agencies be informed or take action.

In addition to these definitions, there are terms utilized by the DOD. The term *Bent Spear* refers to a nuclear weapon incident and *Broken Arrow* to a nuclear weapon accident.

III. RADIOLOGICAL AND HEALTH CONSIDERATIONS

The greatest hazard in weapons accidents to date has occurred following detonation of the weapons by explosives with subsequent dispersal or radioactive contamination (usually plutonium). This gradually dissipates and settles from the air as it moves downwind. If a weapon burns, contamination can be carried into the air by smoke and thermals from the fire. Most contamination has settled or disbursed approximately 2 h after the explosion or fire is over: consequently, inhalation hazard is markedly reduced, but internal contamination could still result from utilization of food or materials upon which airborne contamination has settled. The general accident site organization is shown in Figure 3.

Measurement of the quantity of radioactive material present depends upon the instrument utilized. The quantity of interest in general is the amount of plutonium in $\mu Ci/m^2$ and $\mu Ci/m^3$ of air. Unfortunately, field measurements are expressed in cpm or cps and the appropriate conversion for the instrument utilized and the surface monitored must be known in order to arrive at a meaningful number. Protective devices for emergency workers as a function of surface contamination are shown in Table 2.

A 17 cm² detector probe for assessment of alpha contamination can be utilized to determine requirements for bioassay sampling. Skin or clothing contamination above 75,000 cpm indicates a high priority, 12,500 to 75,000 cpm medium, and below 12,500 cpm low

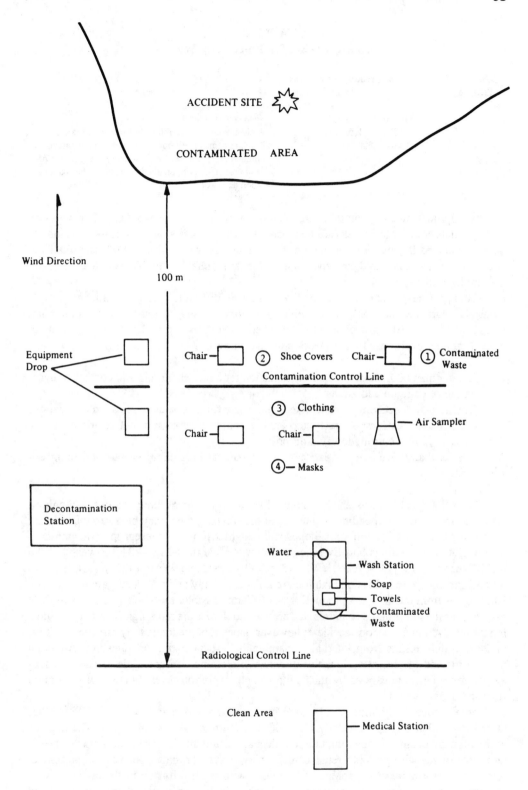

FIGURE 3.   U.S. Department of Defense example of contamination control station.

TABLE 2
Protective Devices for Emergency Workers

Contamination (μCi/m²)	Alpha reading cpm probe (60 cm²)	Protection
4.5	10,000	Shoe covers, gloves
4.5 — 450	10,000 — 1,000,000	Anticontamination clothing, full-face respirator
Above 450	Above 1,000,000	Pressure demand self-contained breathing apparatus or limited entry to essential personnel with full-face respirator: source of contamination should be fixed as soon as possible

priority. Optimal time for sampling for plutonium in bioassay is two days after exposure for fecal analysis and 2 to 3 weeks after exposure for urine analysis. Nasal smears occasionally may be obtained if plutonium inhalation is suspected; however, due to biological half-life of the nasal mucus and rapid clearance, a nasal smear is reliable only if it is collected within the first hour of exposure.

Although resuspension of deposited plutonium is difficult, it can be achieved by mechanical disturbance such as passing vehicles or wind. Resuspension factors of plutonium vary from 10^{-5} to 10^{-7} for plutonium deposited on soil and up to 10^{-3} on pavement. In general, action levels based on deposition are as follows:

1. Greater than 600μCi/m² — immediate action required: sheltering and controlled evacuation of children and adults.
2. Greater than 60μCi/m² — supervised area, sheltering, consider controlled evacuation.
3. Greater than 6μCi/m² — restricted area, respiratory protection not required, access on need only, controlled evauation possible.
4. Greater than 0.2μCi/m² — exceeds Environmental Protection Agency screening criteria.

The radiological hazards and contamination can come from three sources: plutonium, uranium, and tritium. Depending on the age of the weapon, there may be a variable amount of [241]Am present. The plutonium isotopes and daughter products present in a weapon containing plutonium, with its half-lives, are as follows: [239]Pu (half-life — 24,100 years), [240]Pu (6,570 years), [241]Pu (14.4 years), [242]Pu (376,000 years), and [241]Am (432 years). The detectable radiations from this combination are a 17-keV X-ray and a 60-keV gamma ray. The latter comes from the daughter product, [241]Am. When possible, the 17-keV X-ray is utilized to determine the limits of the contaminated area. Plutonium is the most significant radiological hazard involved in a weapons accident; however, since it is predominantly an alpha emitter, the hazard only results from internal contamination via inhalation or ingestion. Although the best method of protection is anticontamination clothing, it is possible to use chelating agents either intravenously or by inhalation to help excretion or elimination of plutonium from the body.

Three isotopes of uranium can be used in a nuclear weapon and include [234,235, and 238]U. Over 99% of that present is usually [238]U with a half-life of 4.5×10^9 years. The hazards of uranium are chemical rather than radiological and if uranium is ingested, a type of heavy metal poisoning with possible renal damage may occur. Tritium also may be present in weapons. It is a radioactive isotope of hydrogen with rapid diffusion in the air, and, subsequently, is very chemically reactive. Accidents which have occurred in rain, snow, or water or in an enclosed space, may cause a tritium hazard. Tritium is absorbed through the skin, and it mixes rapidly with the water in the body. It has an effective half-life in the body of only 8 to 12 d.

If a weapon detonation occurs with subsequent nuclear yield, a severe radiologic hazard may exist with fission products being present. These are beta and gamma emitters and special care must be taken when these are present.

In addition to their radiological hazards there are also other weapons components which are present which can cause difficulty, including beryllium, lithium, and lead. Any fire or explosion involving beryllium will liberate toxic fumes and smoke, and if it is known to be present, it should be handled with rubber gloves and anticontamination clothing, and a respirator (self-contained) should be utilized. Lithium is extremely reactive, and upon its exposure to water there is a violent chemical reaction. Reaction of lithium with the skin and the water in the skin will cause severe chemical burns. Respiratory, eye, and skin protection are required in the firefighting activities in which lithium is involved.

IV. THE PALOMARES ACCIDENT[2]

On the morning of January 17, 1966, two Strategic Air Command B-52G aircraft carrying nuclear weapons rendezvoused for an air refueling operation with two KC-135As. During refueling at 31,000 feet (Figure 4), a B-52 and a KC-135A tanker collided in the final stages of hook-up. There were four survivors of the accident, all from the B-52 crew. Three other crew members of the B-52 and all four crew members of the KC-135 perished in the accident. The accident resulted in burning wreckage in the village of Palomares, along the beach and possibly in the Mediterranean Sea (Figures 5 and 6). The village of Palomares is located on the southeastern coast of Spain with an estimated population of approximately 2,000. Notification by the Air Force to the Joint Nuclear Accident Coordinating Center (JNACC) and the Department of Defense was made. The B-52 was known to be carrying four nuclear weapons.

Notification of the U.S. embassy and the Spanish Foreign Office was also made. The Spanish *Guardia Civil* were the first governmental representatives on the scene and they immediately secured the area. By the evening of the accident, President Lyndon Johnson had been notified, and 49 U.S. personnel had arrived at Palomares. This number increased to more than 775 over the next several weeks.

Initial surveys indicated that there had been no nuclear explosion. The Spaniards indicated that some of them had seen parachutes with projectiles attached. The first weapon was found 900 ft from the beach and southeast of the village on the evening of the accident and it was only minimally damaged. Radiation checks were negative. Weapon number two was located at 09:30 hours the following morning; however, the weapon's high explosive had detonated and portions of the weapon were in a crater 20 feet in diameter and 6 feet in depth, although parts of the weapon assembly were found as far away as a hundred yards. Radiation detection equipment detected substantial alpha contamination in the area. At 10:30 hours weapon number three was found within the limits of the village of Palomares and, like weapon number two, its high explosive had also detonated. No nuclear yield had occurred. Parts of the weapon were spread over 500 yards with significant plutonium contamination at the site as well. The location and recovery of weapon number four did not occur until April 7, 1966. This weapon was recovered from the ocean and it was essentially intact.

Logistical considerations for both determination of the location of weapon number four, as well as decontamination and debris removal from weapons two and three were substantial. By January 31, 1966, 650 people were involved, with two thirds of these involved in either hunting for the weapon or cleaning up debris. The remaining were air police, communications, medical, claims, and other support personnel.

Radiological monitoring proved to be a significant problem. The PAC-1S was the only alpha detector available. Since the alpha particle of plutonium has a very short range in air (3 to 4 cm) the alpha detector had to be placed very close to the ground, and surface

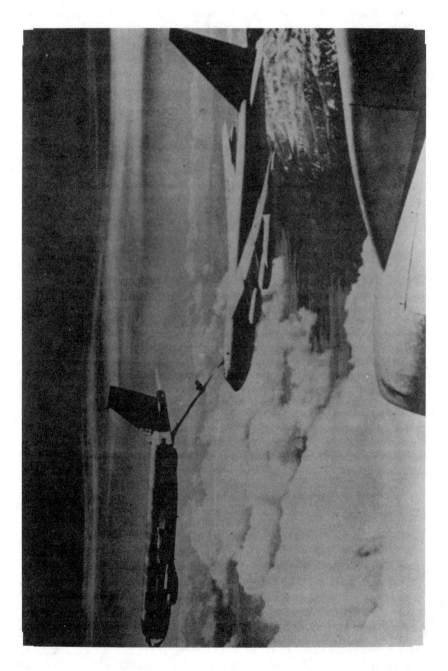

FIGURE 4.   KC-135 refueling a B-52.

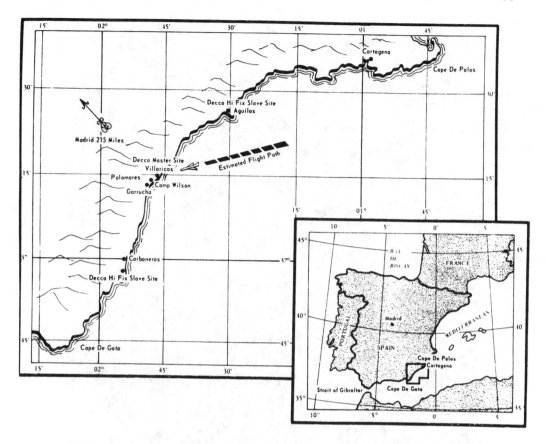

FIGURE 5.   Southeast Spanish coast and estimated flight path of aircraft in Palomares accident.

irregularities, such as grass, rock, etc., often penetrated the detector's extremely thin window, causing it to be inoperable. PAC-1S detectors were flown in from eight European locations, 14 U.S. sites, and one African site. One significant lesson that was learned from the Palomares accident was that a new instrumentation system had to be developed to locate contamination such as this in a hostile environment. A system was subsequently developed and used in the next accident discussed in this chapter. That instrument, however, was not used to detect alpha radiation, but the more penetrating gamma and X-rays present in weapons-grade plutonium. At Palomares with the PAC-1S 100,000 cpm was equivalent to 770 μgm/m^2. Readings obtained utilizing this instrument near the tail section of weapon number two read in excess of 2,000,000 cpm. Initial surveys were few, due to limitation in numbers of monitoring instruments, as well as a shift in the contamination pattern due to wind. In spite of the wind, negligible resuspension of plutonium occurred in the air. In fact, surgical masks were utilized for comfort as well as for psychological reassurance of the surrounding Spanish population. The following is a summary of the amended agreements concerning decontamination levels and methods employed at Palomares:

1.   Soil above 462 μgm/m^2 (32 μCi/m^2) would be scraped up and removed from Spain.
2.   Soil between 5.4 and 462 μgm/m^2 would be watered and plowed.
3.   Soil below 5.4 μgm/m^2 would be watered and the permissible level of contamination would be 10,000 cpm as measured on a PAC-1S instrument. Note: conversion factors are as follows: to convert μg/m^2 to μCi/m^2, divide by 13, thus all soil above 36 μCi/ m^2 was to be removed from Spain.

For the PAC-1S, 13,000 cpm corresponded to contamination levels of 100 μgm/m^2.

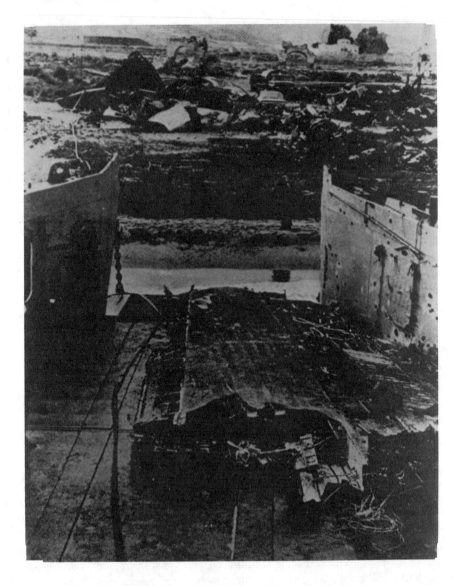

FIGURE 6.   Aircraft debris on Palomares beach.

Total area contaminated by the two weapons in which plutonium dispersal occurred were 630 acres initially and 650 acres after the wind had spread the contamination. Five hundred acres were located within the 700 cpm line, 41.5 acres in the 7,000 to 60,000 cpm lines, and 5.5 acres above 60,000 cpm. As a result of the negotiations therefore, approximately 5.5 acres had to be scraped, placed in barrels, and removed from Spain. In addition, all vegetation measuring greater than 400 cpm was also to be removed from Spain. Approximately 1500 cubic yards of contaminated soil and vegetation were removed from Spain in 4,810 55-gal drums (Figure 7). The acceptable level for cleanup at this accident site was eventually negotiated to be 5.4 μg/m (app. 0.4 μCi). Environmental Protection Agency (EPA) guidelines for cleanup in a similar accident today in the U.S. is 0.2 μg/m^2. In addition, due to some extremely rugged terrain, it became apparent that certain areas could not be decontaminated to the agreed level. Therefore, in these areas the standard was set at 60 μg/m^2, much higher than would be acceptable today. Aircraft debris which was not contaminated was stacked on the beach and dumped at sea by the Navy. The soil was shipped to Charleston,

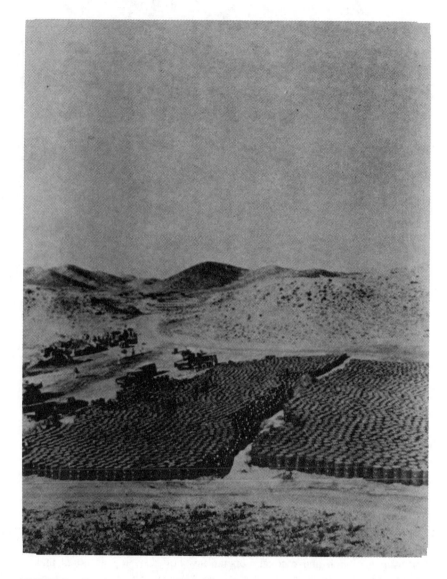

FIGURE 7.   Barrel storage area at Palomares for contaminated soil being removed to the U.S.

South Carolina, and then taken to the Savannah River Facility in Aiken, South Carolina, for burial.

One of the most interesting points regarding this accident concerns the subsequent examination of the residents of Palomares for possible plutonium inhalation, especially since a portion of the village was contaminated and the residents were not evacuated. One hunderd of the most likely exposed residents of Palomares were taken to Madrid and counted in the lung counter. Detection limit was 16 nCi and no positive lung counts were obtained. Urine samples were also obtained and no significant plutonium contamination was identified.

The location of the fourth nuclear weapon posed a significant problem. An extensive land search was conducted even though several Spanish citizens reported observing the splashdown of an object with a white parachute in the ocean. At least one Spanish fisherman indicated that at the time of the accident he had attempted to pull on board a very heavy object which was attached to a parachute, but was unable to do so and, for fear of damaging his boat, he released the parachute and its weight to sink into the water. Whether this is a

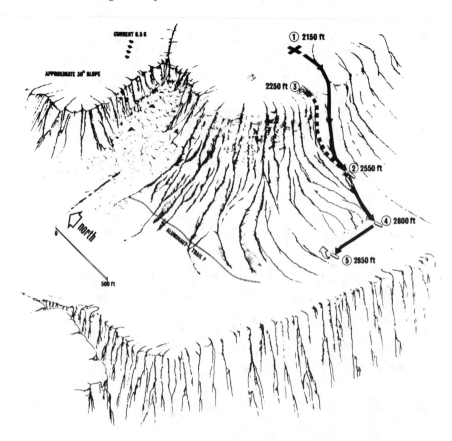

FIGURE 8.   Underwater canyon off Palomares coast showing path and depth of weapon.

true incident or not was never confirmed. The ground search was continued until March 3, 1966, at which point over 232 soil depressions, mineshafts, wells, and reservoirs had been examined in the search for the missing weapon.

The ocean search was initially limited by inaccuracies in navigation and effectiveness of available equipment. Spanish patrol craft secured the area and kept the local fishing fleet from interfering in search and recovery operations; however, it was noted that a Soviet ELINT trawler observed the operation for almost 2 weeks. The prime source of data was sonar equipment. Unfortunately, it detected items of all size and composition, from rocks and pebbles to aircraft debris. In addition, in water over 200 ft in depth, artificial light was required. The rough underwater terrain in much of the area limited the usefulness of the sonar system. Overall, 450 sonar contacts were made. Of these, 201 were identified as aircraft debris and recovered. The weapon itself was located on March 15th. Apparently the weapon initially, while suspended from its parachute, descended to a depth of 355 fathoms, touching down on the rim of an underwater ridge (Figure 8). It was subsequently dragged over the edge by the forces of current on the parachute and slid into a deep submarine canyon to a depth of 425 fathoms. The furrow created in the slide was discovered by the submarine ALVIN on March 1st. On March 15th, ALVIN successfully discovered a parachute-en-shrouded object at a depth of 2550 ft lying on a 70° slope. On March 26th an attempt was made to raise the weapon, but a line was severed and the weapon was dropped and landed even deeper at a depth of 2,800 ft. Ultimately, the weapon was raised with a grapel attached to a line of sufficient strength to lift the weapon (Figure 9).

Management of this accident led to significant political and public relations problems.

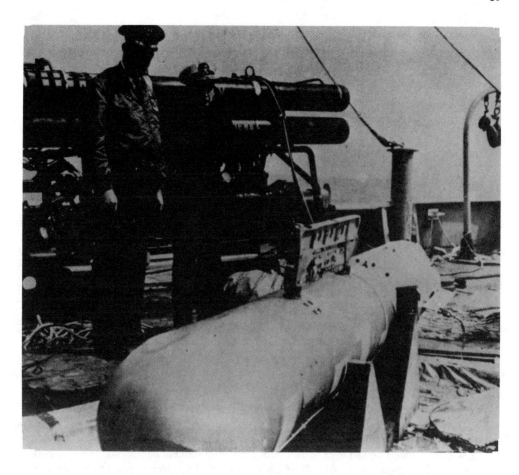

FIGURE 9. Recovered weapon aboard the Petrel.

Having such an accident on foreign soil limited the options available for security and decontamination. The Spanish government itself was quite concerned about assuring the local populace that no significant danger existed, and insisted that the U.S. government not evacuate the area or institute strict health physics protection measures. Ultimately, the U.S. government searched for a way to give some consideration to the people of Palomares for their help in management of the accident. This included help, not only with initial rescue of survivors, but in the subsequent cleanup operations and significant disturbance of their daily existence. Ultimately, partial funding for a desalination plant to treat the area's plentiful but saline groundwater was provided, in spite of the fact that some U.S. agencies opposed the project. They were concerned that funding such a plant would imply that the accident contamination had affected the local water supply which now required some treatment. Eventually the project was funded, but was plagued by a number of technical problems.

There has been continued monitoring of the area over the last 20 years. The potential dose to the bone marrow, bone surface, and lungs of individuals residing in the area has been estimated[3] and found to be less than the annual limits for each organ (as recommended by the International Commission on Radiologic Protection).

V. THE THULE, GREENLAND, ACCIDENT

Two years and four days after the Palomares accident, a B-52 bomber (HOBO-28) was flying an extended mission over the coast of Greenland. One hour after an aerial refueling,

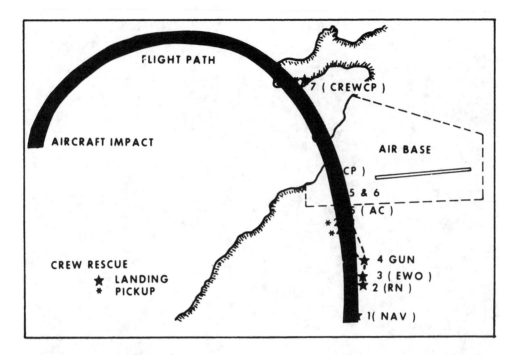

Crash path prior to impact on the ice.

FIGURE 10.   The flight path of Hobo-28 (a B-52 aircraft) prior to impact on the ice in Thule, Greenland.

a fire began which the crew was unable to extinguish. The pilot immediately began a descent for an emergency landing at Thule Air Base. Shortly after descent began, all electrical power was lost and a bail-out order was given and executed. The aircraft continued down in a steep left bank, struck the ice (Figure 10) and disintegrated from impact, explosion and fire. Speed at impact was approximately 500 knots, with a gross weight of 410,000 pounds, including 225,000 pounds of JP-4 jet fuel. Seven persons were aboard the aircraft and six survived. Several of the crew managed to land on the air base and walk to the hangars.

The aircraft crashed at 4:39 p.m. and, since it was known to be carrying nuclear weapons, a Broken Arrow sequence was initiated. The local environmental conditions were some of the most inhospitable one could imagine for accident management. January is the depth of polar darkness and the temperature was −24°F with a wind chill factor of −50°F. (In such environmental conditions, exposed human flesh would freeze in approximately 2 min.) The crash site was approximately 8 mi west of Thule on the open sea ice of North Star Bay. Initial helicopter reconnaissance reported only a blackened area approximately 500 × 2100 ft with no large pieces of debris in sight except the aircraft engines. Over the next 3 d several storms occurred with the equivalent temperature at times dropping below −100°F. The blowing wind created problems of visibility and aggravated the problem of spreading contamination with the blowing snow. The ice at the site was 2 to 4 ft thick.

Management and decontamination of the site and the accident were referred to as Project Crested Ice.[3] The Strategic Air Command Group arrived at 2:52 in the morning of January 21st. Notification was also made to the Danish government. It was clear that management would require construction of buildings on the ice and establishment of a functional facility. The first building was completed on January 24th and the second on January 25th. Vehicular traffic was allowed on the ice, although vehicles had to be adequately spaced while driving and parking so as not to overstress the ice. The harsh environment made it necessary to spend at least one shift out of every 24 h simply repairing equipment. The intense cold

61

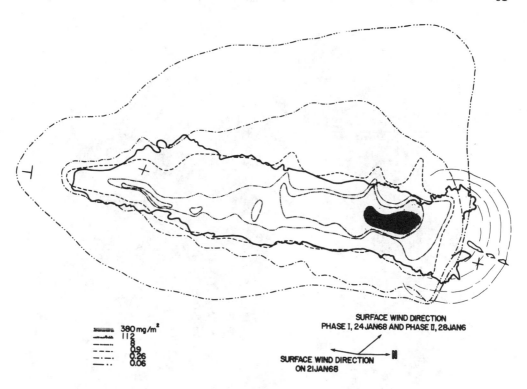

FIGURE 11. Plutonium contamination levels observed during Project Crested Ice.

caused flashlight batteries to last only a few minutes and engines had to be kept running, as they could not be started again if they were stopped.

The radiation monitoring found the greatest percentage of radioactive material being in the blackened area where the explosion and fire had occurred. It was apparent that removal of the black crust of the snow and ice would remove almost all the plutonium contamination. The explosion which had completely disintegrated the aircraft also resulted in thousands of small pieces and it was difficult to locate the four weapons. However, they were all accounted for by January 29th. The proximity of the location to the north pole made accurate mapping of the location with compasses nearly impossible. The surface winds were high enough that small lightweight aluminum parts were blown around and, therefore, as they were recovered they were stacked into piles and covered with chickenwire.

Ultimate integration of the contours at the crash site suggested that the amount of plutonium on the surface was 3,150 ± 630 g of which 99% was confined to the blackened pattern on the snow and ice (Figure 11). This was predominantly in the form of oxide particles, but was also associated with larger particles of low-density inert material resulting from the unburned JP-4 fuel from the plane. Tritium contamination in the form of tritium oxide was also found with the amount estimated at 1,350 Ci, ±50%. Approximately 150 g of plutonium were felt to be trapped in the ice, as well as 35 Ci of tritium.

Radiation monitoring was not only hindered by the short life of the batteries, but also by the fact that wires and electrical cable became very stiff and brittle and extreme care was necessary to prevent breakage (Figure 12). Initial monitoring was done with a standard low-range beta gamma survey meter. Alpha monitoring was done using the PAC-1S. No beta or gamma radiation was detected since there was no nuclear yield. However, widespread alpha contamination was detected on the surface of the snow, ice, and aircraft debris. An experimental instrument from Lawrence Radiation Laboratory at Livermore, CA was heavily utilized. This instrument was known as the FIDLER — an acronym for Field Instrument

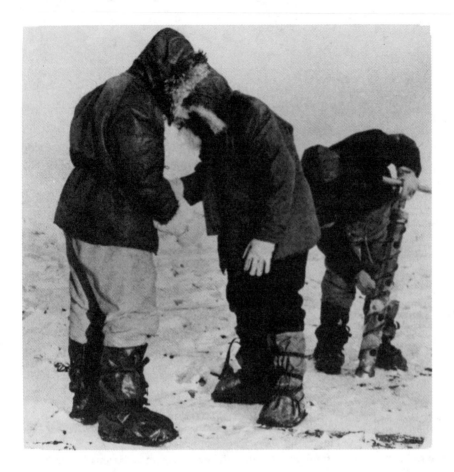

FIGURE 12.   Drilling for an ice core to monitor for plutonium dispersion (Project Crested Ice).

for Detection of Low Energy Radiation. This instrument consists of a small single-channel analyzer and scintillation detector with a 1/16 in. sodium iodide crystal coupled to a 5 in. photomultiplier tube. This was used for detection of the 60-keV photons associated with the americium present in the plutonium. Attenuation experience showed that 6 in. of snow would reduce the 60-keV gamma ray intensity by a factor of 2.

Most of the plutonium was at a depth of no more than a half inch. Because of the variable thickness of the overburden of ice and snow, it was necessary to apply different calibration factors in various areas. For example, where more fuel had burned and the contamination level was highest, the snow had melted and refrozen. Microscopic studies indicated the plutonium to be in oxide particles of a very wide size distribution. The median diameter was 2 μm , with a standard deviation of 1.7. The calculated mass median diameter was about 4 μm. The particles often adhered to pieces of debris of all kinds, including metal, glass, fiber, rubber, plastic, etc. The mass median diameter of the inert particles with which the plutonium was associated were 4 to 5 times larger than the plutonium particles themselves. Up to 80% of the plutonium was associated with low specific gravity debris that remained suspended in the jet fuel. Contamination levels of plutonium were as high as 380 mg/m^2.

In the first few days over 700 military personnel as well as American and Danish scientists came to Thule to help in the operation. Seventy-eight flights carrying almost 2,000,000 lbs. of cargo were required. At the site, Air Force personnel driving road graders took the black crusted snow in mechanized loaders and poured it into 10-ft-long wooden boxes which were covered to keep the snow from blowing. The snow was then put into specially constructed 25,000 gallon modified fuel tanks (Figure 13). Sixty-seven such tanks were filled. Once melting had occurred, the water was pumped into smaller containers for shipping to the U.S. All contaminated residue was finally cleared on September 17th, 1968. Residue was taken to Charleston, South Carolina and then moved to the Savannah River Plant near Aiken, South Carolina, for burial.

Examination of the water samples the following summer after the ice had melted did not indicate any significant contamination by plutonium. The total amount of ^{239}Pu contamination in the Bylot Sound area outside the crash site was estimated to be 1 to 5 Ci.

In fact, it was estimated that if the plutonium in all of the weapons had sunk into the bay, there was enough sea water that only one km^3 of seawater would have been more than sufficient to dilute all the plutonium oxide from the weapons to drinking water standards.

The contamination levels in both this accident and Palomares indicate that the highest levels were at least in the range of 1 mg/m^2 of contamination with plutonium. This corresponds to approximately 13 μCi/m^2.

VI. THE TITAN II ACCIDENT, DAMASCUS, ARKANSAS

The previous two accidents, that at Thule, Greenland, and at Palomares, Spain, both had high explosive detonation in some of the nuclear warheads which were involved in the accident. This last example of a nuclear accident is included since it is one of the more representative nuclear weapon accidents, i.e., a significant explosion or accident, but without detonation of high explosives or nuclear yield. It is an excellent demonstration of how the current design of nuclear weapons is such that they can withstand a substantial accident or explosion without detonation of either the high explosives or the nuclear device.

The Titan II accident occurred at the missile complex 374-7 located near Damascus, Arkansas, on December 18th to 19th, 1980. The accident was initiated by dropping a socket from a socket wrench during maintenance of the Titan II rocket. A subsequent fuel leak occurred. The leak was monitored at the site until the morning of September 19th, 1980. It was hoped that the fuel leak would stabilize. In the early morning hours it became apparent that the leak rate was increasing and a team of technicians was sent into the missile silo to take readings and to turn on the ventilation system. Following activation of the ventilation system, an explosion occurred. The explosion was caused by the collapse of the first stage. As fuel leaked from the first stage, it began to lose its structural integrity, eventually the weight of the second stage and warhead became too much and the first stage was crushed, initiating the explosion. The flame deflectors and silo doors, as well as a large amount of debris, came out of the silo causing immediate local evacuation. Two individuals were in the access portion of the silo at the time of the explosion. One individual died and the other survived after being blown to the area of the surrounding fence.

Initial surveys for radioactivity were made with the PAC-1S for alpha radiation and the AN/PDR-27 for beta and gamma detection. The actual warhead was found Saturday morning; however, monitoring for contamination did not reveal any evidence of plutonium dispersion and, in fact, the warhead itself was surprisingly intact. Personnel returning from the accident site were also monitored with PAC-1S instruments. Utilization of these instruments yielded some positive readings initially which were apparently due to faulty equipment, since later measurements did not reveal any evidence of contamination on the individuals. This particular accident underlines both the fragility of alpha detection equipment as well as the fact that these instruments were still in use in 1980, even though the Palomares accident in 1966 clearly indicated that better instrumentation was very desirable.

The cleanup effort was fairly extensive, with metal and concrete debris left on farmland nearby. Damage to surrounding trees was also observed. About a hundred people were

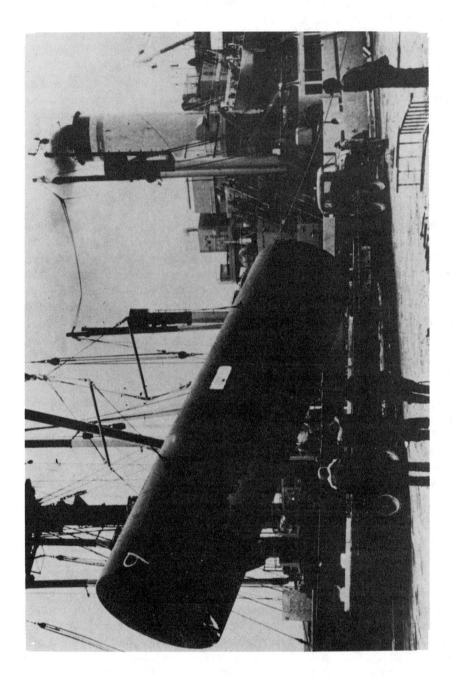

FIGURE 13.   25,000-gal modified fuel tank used to melt snow and ice (Project Crested Ice).

involved in the cleanup effort. However, as of one month after the accident, the silo door, several flame deflectors, and other debris approximately a quarter of a mile from the site had yet to be removed. Additional cutting torches and external contractors were necessary because of the weight of the debris. In addition, there were approximately 200,000 gal water and fuel which had to be removed from the inside of the silo in a pumping operation.

VII. SUMMARY

There have been approximately 50 accidents in which nuclear weapons have been involved. In the majority of accidents, there has not been a high explosive detonation and there has never been a nuclear yield. There have been at least two accidents in which six of the eight warheads involved suffered high explosive detonation and plutonium dispersion. These accidents have required massive logistical support for a period of months to facilitate decontamination, removal, and subsequent burial of the plutonium. To date, the U.S. government has not had a single weapons accident in which the plutonium has undergone criticality with subsequent nuclear yield. Such an accident is possible, but it is felt to have a probability of less than one in a million for having a nuclear yield in excess of 4 lb of TNT.

REFERENCES

1. Nuclear Weapon Accident Response Procedures (NARP) Manual, DNA5100.1, Defense Nuclear Agency, Department of Defense, Washington, D.C., January 1984.
2. Palomares Summary Report, Field Command, Defense Nuclear Agency, Technology and Analysis Directorate, Kirtland Air Force Base, N.M.
3. **Iranzo, E., Salvador, S., and Iranzo, C. E.,** Air concentrations of ^{239}Pu and ^{240}Pu and potential radiation doses to persons living near Pu-contaminated areas in Palomares, Spain, *Health Phys.,* 52, 453, 1987.
4. U.S. Air Force Nuclear Safety, Vol. 65 (Part II), Spec. Ed., AFRP 122-1, January-February, March 1970.

Chapter 5

EVALUATION OF EXTENT OF INJURY

Eugene L. Saenger

TABLE OF CONTENTS

I. INTRODUCTION

The purpose of this chapter is to describe some ways of determining whether or not radiation injury has occurred, and then to establish the extent of the injury so as to improve the management of the patient. Even among persons who are well-educated scientifically and knowledgeable about radiation effects, there is a disproportionate fear of radiation when it is encountered under unusual circumstances. For many years, I have advocated that if radiation is suspected, one should proceed as if the accident had occurred until the relevant facts can be established. Although my experience has borne out the value of this axiom, nevertheless it can be considered to cause some heightening of tension among those who are suspected of being injured and who are in the process of being evaluated.

As can be readily seen in the other chapters in this book, there is often a clearly recognized pattern and consistency in the symptoms and signs, particularly the time sequence of events following acute exposure and resulting in some form of the acute radiation syndrome (ARS). If the changes seem disproportionate, either occurring too early or too late, or persisting for too long a time, one must suspect some other etiology as possibly producing the observed changes. As an example of this type of disproportionate effect is the case of a patient presenting with a history of being exposed to radioactive fallout resulting in loss of hair, but without any other manifestations of radiation injury. Epilation is well known to be produced by radiation at levels of 300 to 400 rad (3 to 4 Gy). Experience in this regard has been gained over the years from many thousands of therapeutic epilations done for ringworm of the scalp. After therapeutic exposures at these doses, all of the scalp hair fell out between the 18th and 21st day as regularly as clockwork and regrowth started about 2 to 4 weeks afterwards. Within a period of 2 to 3 months after the treatment, the patient had a full head of hair. In contrast, in the patient with presumed exposure to radioactive fallout, the patient stated that the hair had fallen out over a period of the next 2 to 3 years and had not regrown. There were no stigmata of late radiation damage to the skin of the scalp such as fibrosis, atrophy, or telangiectasia. The exact circumstances of the radiation exposure were never clarified, but the amount of radiation encountered by this patient as shown by hematological examinations and other symptoms and signs demonstrated clearly that the permanent loss of hair was not associated with exposure to radiation.

My interest in radiation accidents began in about 1950 when the widespread uses of radioactive materials in nuclear medicine, industry, and nuclear power as known today were in their infancy. In 1951, a radium capsule containing 50 mg of radium sulfate — a very insoluble salt — ruptured at a local plant which, in those days, manufactured detection instruments for the many new uses of radiation, especially radioisotopes.[1] In its intact form, the capsule would give a dose of about 40 mR/h at a distance of 1 m (about 3 ft) when not shielded. After the source had broken, radium was dispersed all over the plant, into the street, into taxis, and the local YMCA. We obtained some advice from "experts" which demonstrated that few people understood how to evaluate either the extent of the problem or of the possible injury. One expert from out of town said that employees might get enough radiation to produce the acute radiation syndrome (about 150 to 450 rad). This would have required the employees to remain for about 3,750 h or more at 1 m from this source to acquire such dose levels. Based on this "expert advice", complete blood counts were done once as a baseline and again in 2 weeks on about 200 employees. Also, we were instructed to collect 24-h urine and stool specimens on the employees for three days. This part of the problem evaluation produced an aesthetic and storage impact all its own. In fact, the specimens ultimately were not assayed, but were discarded rather quickly. A number of additional mistakes in decontamination were made; as a result of our efforts, Cincinnati lost an industry employing 200 people. There has not been detectable human injury after a 33-year follow-up for those persons who inhaled radium. The first of these radium accidents was handled somewhat badly, not from the viewpoint of excessive exposure to workers and the public, but principally because of much unnecessary expense due to inexperience with radiation accidents. In the second similar accident, there was a rupture of a 12.5-mg radium capsule. This episode, due to previous experience, was handled far more efficiently.[2]

II. THE ACUTE RADIATION SYNDROME (ARS)

The effects of acute whole- and partial-body irradiation have received intensive study over the past decade largely because of interest in organ transplantation, especially bone marrow in the treatment of leukemia, lymphomas and aplastic anemia.

The major guidance for classification of the ARS and the tables are derived from several papers by Dr. Niel Wald of the University of Pittsburgh and Dr. George Thoma of St. Louis University who analyzed 31 cases of the ARS in 1959.[3] The guides which they developed from their very careful work have proven to be the single most useful source for diagnosis and prognosis and for planning of medical care of this syndrome. Excellent short summaries together with long-term followup of a great many cases of whole- and partial- body irradiation are given (see Chapters 6 and 7).[4]

The effect of external irradiation can be considered in two ways. The ARS manifests itself as a characteristic set of clinical pictures when either most of the body or large segments of the body are exposed in a relatively uniform way to ionizing radiation. Radiation doses sufficient to initiate the ARS come from external sources and consist of the more penetrating gamma rays, X-rays, neutrons, or combinations thereof. There have been occasional instances in which radioactive contamination has produced effects as seen in the ARS, but these cases are much less frequent than those resulting from external sources.[5,6,7]

Since neutrons induce radioactivity in the body, their presence can be determined relatively easily by the presence of ^{24}Na, ^{32}P, or ^{36}Cl. The induced radioactivity from neutron exposure is not hazardous to hospital personnel. In the ARS, it is the immediate effects of neutrons that are of concern, not their potential for induction of later cancer. In these circumstances, the neutrons have a relative biological effectiveness (RBE) and therefore a quality factor (Q) of 1 for the ARS.

In understanding the clinical and laboratory findings, several fundamental radiobiological principles are important. First, the greater the percentage of the body exposed, the greater the effect. Rarely will an accident victim have received completely uniform radiation exposure. Usually the radiation from an accidental exposure is irregularly distributed, perhaps moderating the typical clinical course. Thus, exposure is described as total-body irradiation (TB I), partial-body irradiation (PBR), or localized irradiation (LI). During an accident, the shielding of a relatively small portion of the body, for example the spleen, will give significant degrees of protection. Even the shielding of a proximal extremity helps by protecting bone marrow. Other important factors in determining the effects of exposure are the total dose and dose rate. The higher the dose, the greater the effect and the more rapid the onset of symptoms. The dose rate effect is observed when a dose which might be of lethal proportions if delivered within a very brief period of time — minutes or hours — is better tolerated if spread over days or weeks.

Estimates of the $LD_{50/60}$ are usually expressed as the median dose leading to death in 30 to 60 d. The estimate is useful for planning. In an individual case, it is the guide to the need for supportive or aggressive therapy. Three values are usually cited. For minimal therapy (essentially basic first aid), a value of 250 to 300 rad (2.5 to 3.0 Gy), median 340 rad (3.4 Gy) is given. With supportive therapy — antibiotics, blood derivatives, reverse isolation — the number rises to about 450 rad (4.5 Gy). With intensive treatment, assuming bone marrow transplantation is possible and necessary, the $LD_{50/60}$ is estimated to be 1100 rad (11.0 Gy).[8]

TABLE 1
Clinical Radiation Injury Groups

Group no.	Clinical manifestations (without treatment)	Approximate dose (rad)	Clinical classification
I	Mostly asymptomatic. Occasional minimal prodromal symptoms and subtle laboratory changes.	150	
II	Mild form of the ARS. Transient prodromal nausea and vomiting. Mild laboratory and clinical evidence of hematopoietic derangement.	400	Hematopoietic
III	A serious course. Hematopoietic complications severe, and some evidence of gastroenteric damage present in upper portion of group.	400—600	Hematopoietic
IV	An accelerated version of the ARS. Gastro-enteric complications dominate the clinical picture. Severity of hematopoietic compli-cations is related to survival time after exposure.	600—1500	Gastrointestinal
V	A fulminating course with marked cardio-vascular and/or CNS impairment.	5000+	Neurovascular, cardio-vascular, cerebral

TABLE 2
Clinical Course of the ARS as Compared to Clinical Pattern of Viral Disease

Viral infection	ARS	Approximate duration (for hematopoietic syndrome)
Inoculation or exposure	Exposure	
Delay	Delay	Minutes/hours
Prodromal stage (nonspecific systemic reaction)	Prodromal stage (cf. motion sickness)	1—4 days
Incubation period	Latent stage	2—3 weeks
Manifest illness (typical clinical picture)	Manifest illness (specific)	2nd or 3rd to 6th week
Convalescence	Recovery	8—15 weeks

Table 1 provides a well-tested classification of the changes that occur at acute dose levels of the ARS. This classification, developed by Thoma and Wald,[3] has been modified somewhat over the years, particularly in regard to Group V. In this category, the recorded deaths are now attributed to cardiovascular injury rather than to central nervous system (CNS). The approximate dose values can vary as much as ± 50%, depending on the factors mentioned above. The terms hematopoietic, gastrointestinal, etc., simply correspond to those used elsewhere in the literature on the ARS.

The clinical course of the ARS is shown in Table 2. Here it is compared in its clinical progression to a typical viral disease. The most common symptoms and signs of the prodromal stage and manifest illness are listed in Tables 3 and 4. Usually in the ARS, the time between exposure and development of prodromal changes is relatively short, on the order of hours to one or two days. The more rapidly these changes begin, the greater their degree of severity and the longer the symptoms and signs persist, the higher is the dose and the greater is the involvement of the body. Since accurate estimates of dose and dose distribution are usually not available in this early period, careful clinical observation will provide guidance as to the level of care needed for the exposed individual. In regard to the classification of ARS used in the U.S.S.R. at Chernobyl, four degrees of severity were considered, I being the mildest (Table 5). These correspond approximately to Injury Groups I to IV in Table 1.

TABLE 3
Signs and Symptoms Found in Prodromal
Stage of Acute Radiation Syndrome

Anorexia	Prostration
Nausea	Diarrhea
Vomiting	Abdominal pain
Weakness and fatigue	
	Sweating
Conjunctivitis	Oliguria
Erythema	
Fever	Paresthesia
Hyperesthesia	Coma
	Death
Ataxia	
Disorientation	
Shock	

Note: Symptoms are grouped and listed in increasing order of severity.

TABLE 4
Signs and Symptoms Found in Manifest
Illness Stage of Acute Radiation Syndrome

Anorexia	Sweating
Nausea	Oliguria
Vomiting	Weakness and fatigue
Diarrhea	Prostration
Abdominal pain	Weight loss
Abdominal distention	Hyperesthesia
Conjunctivitis	Paresthesia
Erythema	Ataxia
Jaundice	Disorientation
Fever	Shock
Infection	Coma
Purpura	Death
Hemorrhage	
Scalp pain	
Epilation	

Note: Symptoms are grouped and listed in increasing order of severity.

Inspection of these latter tables clearly indicates the importance of clinical observation in the prodromal period and the correlation with hematological changes.

In Injury Groups I to III, the prodromata will usually persist no longer than 48 h and will be followed by a latent period of about 18 to 21 d. The onset of the period of manifest illness begins at that time and in Groups I to III may last for 4 to 6 weeks with gradual recovery. In Group IV, the onset of manifest illness will be sooner, perhaps as early as 7 to 14 d after exposure, and death may well ensue in 2 to 4 weeks. For Group V, survival has been no more than 2 d, as described in a few carefully studied cases.

Historically, the classification of the ARS has been divided into the hematological, gastroenteric, and CNS phases. Subsequently, the CNS syndrome was subdivided into the

TABLE 5
U.S.S.R. Classification of Chernobyl Victims

	4th degree	3rd degree
Prodrome (onset) (h)	0.5 (vomiting @ 30 min, headache, fever)	0.5—1 (vomiting, headache, subfebrile); transient hyperemia of skin
Latent period (d)	6—8	8—17
Lymphocytes cells/μl (3—6 d)	<100	100—200
Granulocytes/μl	<500 (7—9 d)	<1,000 (8—20 d)
Platelets/μl	<40,000 (8—10 d)	<40,000 (10—16 d)
Skin burns	40—90%	6 severe, death in all
Enteritis	7—9 d	
TBR dose (Gy)	>6—12, 16	4.2—6.3
Deaths/patients	17/20(at Moscow 10 to 50d) (2 at Kiev 4 & 10 d)	7/23 at 2 to 7 weeks
Clinical findings	General intoxication, fever, oral & salivary lesions, beta burns severe enough to cause death, >8—10 Gy severe intestinal syndrome	High fever, infection, hemorrhage, severe skin injury
Estimate of survival	Unlikely	Probable with treatment

	2nd degree	1st degree
Prodrome (onset) (h)	1—2 (vomiting)	2 h+ (general reaction)
Latent period (d)	15—25	>30
Lymphocytes cells/μl (3—6 d)	300—500	600—1000
Granulocytes/μl	>1000 (20—300) in 15—20 d	3000—4000 (8—9 d)
Platelets/μl	40,000 (17—24 d)	60,000—40,000 (25—28 d)
Skin burns	Slight	Slight
TBR dose (Gy)	2—4	1—2
Deaths/patients	0/53	N.A.
Clinical findings	Infections, slight hemorrhage, elevated ESR	No severe skin change, moderate elevation of ESR
Estimate of survival	Possible without treatment	Probable without treatment

REFERENCES

The Accident at the Chernobyl Nuclear Power Plant and Its Consequences, Part II, Annexes 2,7, compiled by the U.S.S.R. State Committee on the Utilization of Atomic Energy for the International Atomic Energy Agency Experts Meeting, August 25 to 29, 1986, Vienna.

Summary Report on the Post-Accident Review Meeting on the Chernobyl Accident, IAEA Saf. Ser. No. 75-INSAG-1, International Atomic Energy Agency, Vienna, September 1986.

Barabanova, A. V., Baranov, A. V., Guskova, A. K., Keirim-Markus, I. B., Moiseev, A. A., Piatkin, E. K., Redkin, V. V., and Suvarova, L. A., Acute Radiation Effects in Man, Atominform-OH.3, Atominform, Moscow, 1986 (English transl. by the International Atomic Energy Agency, Vienna, September 1986).

cardiovascular phase and the CNS. In the two human cases surviving for 36 h[9] and 48 h,[10] both died due to collapse of the circulatory system and showed necrosis of cardiac muscle at autopsy. The true CNS syndrome characterized by the immediate onset of severe neurological changes with convulsions and death within minutes to a few hours following massive exposures (100,000 + rad) has been produced in animals, but has not been observed in man.

Most of the clinical findings during the manifest illness phase induced by total-body irradiation are from injuries in specific organs.[8] After very high doses, >2,000 rad (>20

Gy) in a short period of time, the predominant signs are those of hypotensive shock followed by anoxic convulsion, coma, and early death. Death will typically occur in less than 8 h without antishock therapy and within 30 to 48 h when antishock therapy is given. These effects are related to injury of the nervous and cardiovascular systems. At lower doses, 600 to 2,000 rad (6 to 20 Gy), the predominant symptoms are those of overwhelming sepsis and toxemia. Nausea, vomiting, diarrhea, dehydration, and death may also occur. At even lower doses, 200 to 600 rad (2 to 6 Gy), signs of infection and anemia may occur, and both are related to bone marrow depression with resulting decrease of blood cell formation. There is considerable overlap in the symptoms and mechanisms of death in these three dose ranges. However, the median lethal dose for total-body irradiation is in the dose range that causes death related to bone marrow depression. Death due to infection and toxemia is secondary to agranulocytosis and immune depression.

A group of symptoms of acute gastrointestinal and neuromuscular effects, designated the prodromal syndrome, may occur within minutes or hours after irradiation. However, the prodromal syndrome is not the result of gastrointestinal tract irradiation. It is an autonomic neurogenic response and is not secondary to gastrointestinal damage. It can be prevented experimentally by ablation of the CNS vomiting center.

Laboratory observations were made in the course of treating patients with metastatic cancer with total and partial body irradiation.[11] Although the prodromal symptoms were dose dependent and independent of volume of tissue exposed, the degree of hematological changes was quite different. Total-body irradiation showed the characteristic fall of formed elements with a nadir at 25 to 30 d and recovery. With the same dose for partial body irradiation, hematological changes were minimal.

The importance of dose rate as a factor affecting the severity of the ARS was realized over the past several years in preparing patients for marrow transplants. Either with or without pretreatment with cyclophosphamide, the use of a single exposure of 1,000 rad (10 Gy) midline dose at rates greater than 5 to 10 rad (0.05 to 0.10 Gy)/min resulted in a high incidence of radiation pneumonitis. Only when the exposures were fractionated to 165 to 200 rad (1.65 to 2.0 Gy) twice daily for 3 d or more was this complication minimized. The success of transplants was also improved.

III. LABORATORY TESTS

Table 6 gives a suggested pattern for obtaining laboratory tests for various stages of the acute radiation syndrome. It is important to realize that, with the exception of cultures of peripheral lymphocytes for chromosome changes, it is not necessary to take any large samples of blood in the early phase and that the routine blood counts, which are easily obtainable in any hospital, will provide all the necessary information. These changes have been reviewed repeatedly in the literature and will not be detailed here. The major changes of the formed elements are shown in Figures 1, 2, and 3. Special attention is directed to the use of the absolute lymphocyte count in evaluating the severity of injury within the first 48 h. This particular technique, originally derived from Dr. Gould Andrews, has been invaluable to me in separating very quickly what was occasionally thought to be a very severe injury from a circumstance which has turned out to be mild. At Chernobyl, patient classification in the first few days was done primarily on the basis of the absolute lymphocyte count and careful recording of clinical symptoms and signs.

There are two other useful diagnostic tests to relate the extent of exposure to degree of injury. The first is that of culture of the peripheral lymphocytes of the circulating blood. Radiation will induce changes — usually the formation of dicentrics or ring chromosomes or production of fragments. Cultures of chromosomes should be done as they will provide an estimate of the magnitude of the biological insult to the patient. There will be more

TABLE 6
Pattern for Laboratory Testing in the Clinical Management of Radiation Injury

Groups	I-II-III-IV			I	II		III		IV		V
Time (d)	1	2	3	STT	STT	18—48	STT	4—48	STT	4	1
Type A Procedures											
History											
Symptoms (onset)	x	x	x	x	x	D	x	D	x	D	D
Signs (duration)	x	x	x	x	x	D	x	D	x	D	D
Past medical	x										
Physical examination											
General						21 d	3 mo+	15—30 d	6 mo+	6 d	D
Body weight	x			x	x	D	x	D	x	D	D
Urinary output	x	x	x		x	D		D		D	6 h
Laboratory tests											
Hematology											
Hematocrit	x	x	x	x	x	D	x	STT	x	D	6 h
Leukocytes	x	x	x	x	x	D	x	D	x	D	6 h
Differential count	x	x	x	x	x	D	x	D	x	D	6 h
Calculation of total neutrophils and lymphocytes	x	x	x	x	x	D	x	D	x	D	6 h
Platelets	x	x	x	x	x	D	x	STT	x	D	6 h
Bone marrow aspiration		30 d	14 d			14 d	6 mo	14 d	6 mo	7 d	1 d
Chromosome	x	60 d				30 d	6 mo	30 d	6 mo	7 d	
Radioassay											
Blood ^{24}Na	x	x									
Whole-body counting	x	x									
Type B Procedures											
Laboratory tests											
Hematology											
Sedimentation rate	x	x	x	x	x	D	x	D	x	D	6 h
Reticulocytes	x	x	x	x	x	D	x	STT	x	D	6 h
Bleeding and Clotting time	x					STT		STT	— 75 d	3 d	6 h
Biochemistry											
Blood											
Non-protein nitrogen	x	prn	prn				prn			STT	6 h
Sodium	x	prn	prn				prn			prn	1 d
Chloride	x	prn	prn				prn			prn	1 d
Potassium	x	prn	prn				prn			prn	1 d
pH or CO$_2$	x	prn	prn				prn			prn	1 d
Serum bilirubin	x	x	x		x	STT	STT		— 30 d	D	6 h
Urine											
Routine analysis	x	x	x		x	D	x	D	x	D	6 h
Stool											
Occult blood	x					D		12d+		D	All
Ophthalmology											
Slit lamp		x		6 mo+			6 mo+		6 mo+		

Note: Recommended frequency of performance: STT: standard testing times: 6, 9, 12, 15, 18, 21, 24, 27, 30, 33, 36, 40, 48, 60, 75, 90, 105, and 120 days; 6 months, 1 year, and annually; x: at times indicated in column heading; d: day(s); D: daily during time indicated in column heading; prn: as indicated by clinical source; — D: STT up to indicated day.

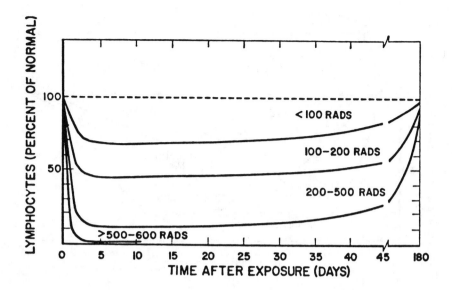

FIGURE 1. Smoothed average time-course of lymphocyte changes in human cases from accidental radiation exposure as a function of dose. (From Langham, W. H., *Radiobiological Factors in Manned Space Flight*, National Academy of Sciences, National Research Council, Washington, D.C., 1967).

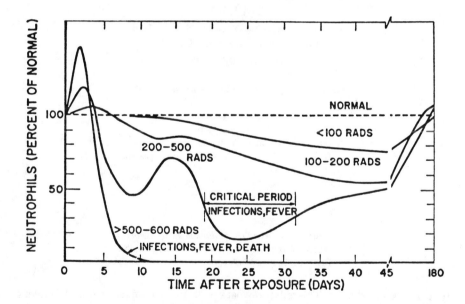

FIGURE 2. Smoothed average time-course of neutrophil changes in human cases from accidental radiation exposure as a function of dose. (From Langham, W. H., *Radiobiological Factors in Manned Space Flight*, National Academy of Sciences, National Research Council, Washington, D.C., 1967).

damaged chromosomes early than will be seen after some months following exposure. The ordering of these cultures can be guided from Table 6. It is also possible to utilize chromosome analysis to estimate the degree of nonuniform or partial body irradiation. Techniques and methods of calculations are given in an excellent publication by the International Atomic Energy Agency[12] and summarized in Chapter 8.

The other useful technique is sperm analysis. It has been shown by Heller et al.[13] that the changes in sperm counts are extremely sensitive indicators of radiation damage at rel-

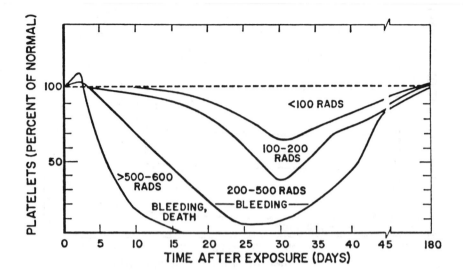

FIGURE 3. Smoothed average time-course of platelet changes in human cases from accidental radiation exposure as a function of dose. (From Langham, W. H., *Radiobiological Factors in Manned Space Flight,* National Academy of Sciences, National Research Council, Washington, D.C., 1967).

TABLE 7
Summary of Observations of Effects of
High-Intensity Doses of X-rays on
Spermatogenesis

Dose (rads)	Observed effect on sperm count
15	Moderate oligospermia
20	Moderate oligospermia
50	Pronounced oligospermia
100	Marked oligospermia and azoospermia
200	Azoospermia
300	Azoospermia
400	Azoopsermia
600	Azoospermia

From Langham, W. H., Ed., *Radiobiological Factors in Manned Space Flight*, National Academy of Sciences, National Research Council Washington, D.C., 1967.

atively low doses (Table 7). The only drawback with this technique is that it is necessary to obtain a sperm count within the first 40 d after exposure and a subsequent count sometime after the 60th d. Assuming that the testes have been exposed, this test will serve as a good biological dosimeter, being sensitive to doses as low as 15 rad (0.15 Gy). Also it will be helpful in determining whether or not the exposure was to the whole body and/or to the lower portion. If the sperm level does not decrease, then either the subject was not exposed or there was no exposure to the testes. In other words, if the blood counts show either a slight or more characteristic depression and the sperm counts do not change or change only slightly in comparison to the deviations in the blood counts and lymphocytes, one can assume that there was partial body irradiation. Similarly, if the sperm count drops but the blood counts show only a slight change, the radiation exposure was confined to the lower portion of the body. If all of the tests are of the same order of magnitude in their change, then the exposure was more likely a uniform whole body exposure. Estimates of dose distribution can be made after the 18th d by noting patterns of epilation, assuming regional doses of about 300 rad (3 Gy) or more.

IV. CONTAMINATION

The most important considerations in contamination are the radionuclides involved and their physical and chemical forms. These properties determine how the substance is metabolized. Many compounds encountered in industry are oxides and are very insoluble. Usually they are of large particle size, $>1\mu m$, so that, if inhaled, they are removed from the lung by ciliary action and swallowed or expectorated. Thus, many contaminants encountered in industry and in the environment rarely are retained in the body, but pass through the respiratory and gastroenteric tract unchanged. It is often difficult to determine the level of effort needed for decontamination of the skin. If too little contamination is removed, serious skin injury can occur as well as absorption of the offending materials into the body. If treatment is too vigorous, the protective barrier afforded by the skin can be impaired, thus facilitating absorption.

After superficial decontamination and cleansing of exposed portions of the body, an estimate of the level of contamination is desirable. At the hospital, this measurement can often be done by the usual gamma camera available in even a small nuclear medicine service. Methods of calibration have been published.[14] At the time of the accident, environmental samples of the contaminants should be taken to a radiochemical laboratory immediately. Identification of the offending nuclides can be obtained rapidly by pulse height analysis, by measuring decay rates or by carrying out absorption measurements of beta and/or gamma energy. Comparison with secondary standards will give further information as to energy. Simple tests of solubility in various decontaminants will be helpful. If no laboratory facilities are available at the accident site, these measurements can often be carried out in the hospital nuclear medicine laboratory. These steps will help to guide the rational decontamination program, keeping in mind the maxim *primum non nocere* — primarily, do no harm.

The extent of contamination varies greatly, depending on the nature and level of work at the site of the accidental release. The principal points to be considered in developing a medical program are outlined as follows:

1. Type of contamination — one or several nuclides: are they identified?
2. Forms of contaminant — physical and chemical state
3. Elapsed time since contamination
4. Number of individuals contaminated — male, female
5. Extent of body area involved
6. Contamination in presence of wound, burns, shock, ability to move, extent
7. Entrance routes: inhalation, ingestion, injection, percutaneous absorption, contamination of wound
8. Factors determining effects from radionuclides: (1) quantity entering body; (2) metabolic pattern; (3) radiation characteristics — types, decay scheme, and half-life, tissue and organ susceptibility
9. Radiation effects to be anticipated — early and late
10. Personnel available to aid in decontamination: (1) experience and training, (2) protective covering for decontamination personnel; (3) instrumentation
11. Physical facilities and equipment: (1) location — in plant, at hospital, (2) water — availability, disposal of effluents, (3) airborne contamination, (4) floor covering, (5) medical supplies, (6) protective coverings — plastic sheets, plastic pillow covers, paper, shoe covers, large paper or plastic bags, crayons, pencils, labels, tags

The most important clinical sign of radiation injury to the skin is erythema, which often occurs in waves. The earliest redness can occur within a few h to one-or two d and suggests serious injury. A second wave may develop at some interval of 7 to 21 d, both as a function of dose and energy. This erythema and the subsequent development of dry epidermitis, wet epidermitis, bulla formation, and ulceration has a progressive timetable of 2 to 4 weeks.

Some dose estimation can be made from the clinical evidence alone. Erythema as the only sign suggests doses of 250 to 600 rad (2.5 to 6.0 Gy) depending on the energy. Dry epidermitis will occur with doses of 600 to 1500 rad (6.0 to 15.0 Gy) and wet reactions and bulla formation with doses of 100 to 2500 rad (1 to 25 Gy) (see Chapter 9). Ulceration and necrosis suggest doses of 2000 to 3000 rad or greater.

These skin changes, although described in episodes of contamination, occur frequently with external radiation, especially after contact with highly radioactive sealed sources used in industrial radiography and with industrial X-ray units as employed in nondestructive testing.[15]

REFERENCES

1. **Saenger, E. L., Gallaghar, R. G., Anthony, D. S., and Valaer, P. J.,** Emergency measures and precautions in radium accidents, *JAMA*, 149, 813, 1952.
2. **Saenger, E. L. and Gallaghar, R. G.,** Radium capsules and their associated hazards, *Am. J. Roentgen Rad Therapy Nucl. Med*, 77, 511, 1957.
3. **Thoma, G. E. and Wald, N.,** The diagnosis and management of accidental radiation injury, *J. Occup. Med.,* 1, 421, 1959.
4. **Lushbaugh, C. C., Fry, S. A., Hubner, K. F., and Ricks, R. C.,** Total-body irradiation: a historical review and follow-up, in *The Medical Basis for Radiation Accident Preparedness,* Hubner, K. F. and Fry, S. A., Eds., Elsevier/North Holland, New York, 1980.
5. **Thompson, R. C.,** 1976 Hanford Americium exposure incident: overview and perspective, *Health Phys.,* 45, 837, 1983.
6. **Gale, R. P.,** Immediate medical consequences of nuclear accidents: lessons from Chernobyl, *JAMA,* 258, 625, 1987.
7. **Linneman, R. E.,** Soviet medical response to the Chernobyl nuclear accident, *JAMA,* 258, 637, 1987.
8. **Abrahamson, S., Bender, M., Book, S., et al.,** Health effects models for nuclear power plant accident consequence analysis. Low LET radiation. II. Scientific bases for health effects models (NUREG/CR-4214), rev. 1, part II, U.S. Nuclear Regulatory Commission, Washington, D.C., 1989, II-10.
9. **Shipman, T. L., Lushbaugh, C. C., Peterson, D. F., et al.,** Acute radiation death resulting from an accidental nuclear critical excursion, *J. Occup. Med.,* 1 (Special Suppl.), 421, 1959.
10. **Fanger, H. and Lushbaugh, C. C.,** Radiation death from cardiovascular shock following a criticality accident, *Arch. Pathol.,* 83, 446, 1967.
11. **Saenger, E. L., Silberstein, E. B., Aron, B. et al.,** Whole and partial body radiotherapy of advanced cancer, *Am. J. Roentgen Rad. Therapy. Nucl. Med.,* 117, 670, 1973.
12. Biological Dosimetry: Chromosomal Aberration Analysis for Dose Assessment, Tech. Rep. Ser. No. 260, International Atomic Energy Agency, Vienna, 1986.
13. **Heller, C. G., and Clermont, Y.,** Spermatogenesis in man: an estimate of its duration, *Science,* 140, 184, 1963.
14. **Nishiyama, H. Lukes, S. J., and Saenger, E. L.,** Low-level radionuclide contamination: use of gamma camera for detection, *Radiology,* 150, 235, 1984.
15. **Saenger, E. L., Kereiakes, J. G., Wald, N., and Thoma, G. E.,** Clinical course and dosimetry of acute hand injuries of industrial radiographers from multi-curie sealed gamma sources, in *The Medical Basis for Radiation Accident Preparedness,* Hubner, K. F. and Fry, S. A., Eds., Elsevier/North Holland, New York, 1980, 169.

Chapter 6

EFFECTS OF WHOLE-BODY IRRADIATION

Fred A. Mettler, Jr.,

TABLE OF CONTENTS

I. INTRODUCTION

Whole-body radiation exposure has been the etiology of death in over 80% of fatal radiation accidents. Acute high-level whole-body absorbed doses result in a complex clinical entity known as the acute radiation syndrome (ARS). This syndrome is a manifestation of the varying radiosensitivity of different organ systems in the body.[1] Human data is limited but comes from three major sources: (1) accidental exposures, (2) deliberate exposures, such as Hiroshima and Nagasaki, and (3) planned exposures, such as radiation therapy prior to bone marrow transplantation.

Some of the classification schemes used in patient evaluation have been presented in Chapter 5. The present chapter deals more with the pathogenesis and intricacies of the ARS.

II. DOSIMETRY AND DOSE RATE EFFECTS

One of the first problems encountered as one examines the available literature is that it is difficult to ascertain what the authors of various articles mean by *absorbed dose*. Some are referring to the dose in air or skin, some do not specify the site, some are referring to the mean bone marrow dose, and still others refer to the midline tissue dose (MTD). The most commonly quoted dose is probably the absorbed dose in air at the skin surface. For most accidental circumstances involving penetrating gamma rays, the absorbed dose value in air can be multiplied by a factor of 0.66 to obtain the MTD. Thus a dose in air of 1,000 rad (10 Gy) is equivalent to a MTD of about 660 rad (6.6 Gy) for the average adult.

III. THE LETHAL DOSE

The total body absorbed dose required to cause death is generally characterized by a median lethal dose (LD_{50}). This abbreviation refers to a dose required to kill 50% of the persons irradiated and it assumes no medical intervention. It is necessary to establish a temporal relationship with regard to mortality (Table 1). The most commonly used terms are the $LD_{50/30}$ and the $LD_{50/60}$. These are the doses which, if given, might be expected to result in death in half of the irradiated individuals within 30 and 60 d, respectively. The $LD_{50/30}$ air or surface dose for adults is estimated to be 350 to 400 rad (3.5 to 4.0 Gy).[2] Occasionally fatalities may result from penetrating radiation with surface doses as low as 200 rad (2 Gy). Generally, such fatalities occur in people who are more susceptible than the average person because of concurrent illness, age, etc. With whole-body acute surface doses in excess of 700 rad (7 Gy), essentially 100% of irradiated individuals will die without medical intervention. It is possible that, with appropriate supportive therapy, individuals may survive whole-body doses as high as 1200 rad (12 Gy). It is difficult to use any of the data from Chernobyl to evaluate the effect of medical treatment on the LD_{50}. The distribution of patients and their outcome is shown in Table 2. Although medical treatment was provided, most of the patients who died had extensive skin burns as well as whole-body irradiation and the former was felt to be the major cause of death in two thirds (19) of the patients with fatal outcomes. Other causes of death in Chernobyl patients were sepsis as well as hepatic and renal insufficiency.

Determination of the prognosis of irradiated individuals who suffer from the ARS is extremely difficult solely from an estimate of the absorbed skin dose. This is because of the uncertainty in dose-response curves, including the actual value of the $LD_{50/60}$ for man. Other factors, such as the presence of intercurrent disease in the individual, the quality of radiation, and the effect of shielding cause additional difficulties. When small portions of the body that contain active marrow are shielded, the value of the LD_{50} is markedly increased. Shielding as little as 10% of the active bone marrow in man may result in no deaths after

TABLE 1
Expected Temporal Distribution of Symptoms Following Whole-Body Irradiation

Midline tissue dose	Symptom	Percentage	Time postexposure
0.5—1.0 Gy (50—100 rads)	Anorexia	15—50	3—18 h
	Nausea	5—30	3—20 h
	Vomiting	15—20	4—16 h
1—2 Gy (100—200 rads)	Anorexia	50—90	1—48 h
	Nausea	30—70	4—30 h
	Vomiting	20—50	6—24 h
	Fatigue	25—60	3—72 h[a]
	Weakness	25—50	3—48 h
	Bleeding (mild)	10	1—5 weeks
	Fever	10—60	2 d—5 weeks
	Infection	10—50	1—5 week
	Death	<5	5—6 week
2—3.5 Gy (200—350 rads)	Anorexia	90—100	1—48 h
	Nausea	70—90	1—48 h
	Vomiting	50—80	3—24 h
	Diarrhea	10	4—8 h
	Fatigue (moderate)	60—90	2 h—6 weeks
	Weakness (moderate)	50—80	2 h—6 weeks
	Bleeding	10—50	1—5 week
	Fever	10—80	1—5 week
	Infection	10—80	2—5 week
	Ulceration	30	3—5 week
	Death	5—50	4—6 week
3.5—5.5 Gy (350—550 rads)	Anorexia[b]	100	1—72 h
	Nausea[b]	90—100	1—72 h
	Vomiting[b]	80—100	3—24 h
	Diarrhea[b]	10	3—8 h
	Fatigue	90—100	1 h—6 weeks
	Weakness	90—100	1 h—6 weeks
	Headache	50	4—24 h
	Bleeding	50—100	6 d—6 weeks
	Fever and infection	80—100	6 d—6 weeks
	Death	50—99	3.5—6 weeks
5.5—7.5 Gy (550—750 rads)	Anorexia	100	1—72 h
	Nausea	100	1—72 h
	Vomiting	100	1—48 h
	Diarrhea	10	4—6 h
	Fatigue and weakness (severe)		1 h—2 weeks
	Dizziness and disorientation	100	4—48 h
	Headache	80	4—30 h
	Bleeding, fever, infection, hypotension	100	10—14 d
	Death	100	2—3 weeks

[a] Possibly up to 6 wk.
[b] Symptom occurs in 60—100% of those exposed at 3—6 weeks.

Courtesy of James Conklin. From *Medical Effects of Ionizing Radiation*, Mettler, F. A. and Moseley, R. D., Eds., Grune & Stratton, New York, 1985. With permission.

doses in the region of the LD_{50}. The $LD_{50/30}$ is also related to body weight. When various animal species are considered, the $LD_{50/30}$ increases with a reduction in body weight. For example, the $LD_{50/30}$ in mice and rats is about 800 to 1200 rad (8 to 12 Gy), whereas in burros, pigs, and man it is about 200 to 400 rad (2 to 4 Gy).

Geometry of exposure and depth-dose distribution all affect the estimated or calculated

TABLE 2
Relationship between Absorbed Dose and Outcome in Chernobyl Patients

Number of patients	Bone marrow dose in rad (Gy)		Deaths	Time to death in days
31	80—200	(0.8—2.0)	0	—
43	200—400	(2.0—4.0)	1	96
21	420—630	(4.2—6.3)	7	16—48
20	600—1600	(6.0—16.0)	19	14—91

LD_{50}. In animal experiments, the values obtained for unilateral irradiation are about 20% higher than when the irradiation is bilateral. In addition, the value obtained when the irradiation is dorsal is about two thirds the value obtained when the irradiation is from the ventral surface. There are also some biological variables that should be considered. The LD_{50} for very young children is probably lower than that of adults by a factor of 2 or more. The highest value is probably obtained about puberty with a gradual decrease as one gets older. There may be some sex difference in the value of the lethal dose but this has not been shown with certainty in humans.

The effect of dose protraction or fractionation on the LD_{50} has been studied after several accidents. Data from accidents in China,[3] Algeria,[4] Mexico,[5] and Morocco[6] indicate that individuals have survived approximate marrow doses as follows:

Exposure time (d)	Marrow dose
5—9	800 rad (8 Gy)
38	1400 rad (14 Gy)
106	980—1700 rad (9.8—17 Gy)

The data also indicate that for the exposure times of 5 to 40 d individuals have died with marrow doses of 4000 rad (40 Gy) and for exposure times of about 100 d marrow doses in excess of 1500 rad (15 Gy) usually cause death.

These values suggest the maximum survivable protracted marrows doses assuming reasonable medical care.

IV. THE ACUTE RADIATION SYNDROME

The ARS usually occurs following total-body irradiation with absorbed doses in excess of 100 rad (1 Gy). "Total body radiation" carries the connotation of homogeneous uniform dose, although this is very rarely the circumstance in most radiation accidents. Usually the dose is delivered in a fashion that irradiates one part of the body substantially more than the others. The ARS can occur even when the dose is not homogeneous (e.g., if only the torso was irradiated). In addition, there have been at least two fatalities due to the ARS following internal contamination. One was due to a misadministration of ^{198}Au into the peritoneal cavity of a patient with ovarian cancer, and the other occurred to a young girl who ingested ^{137}Cs in the Goinias, Brazil, accident of 1987.

For purposes of convenience, some rather arbitrary delineations of the temporal sequence of clinical events after whole-body radiation exposure have been used. These are as follows: (1) prodromal period, (2) latent period, (3) period of illness, and (4) period of recovery or death.

A. PRODROMAL PERIOD

The prodromal period may occur 1 to 6 h after the radiation exposure and it is a period of transitory symptoms. The time of onset, type, and number of symptoms depend on the radiation dose. Some of the symptoms, particularly nausea and vomiting, are difficult to evaluate from the clinical viewpoint since they may be psychogenic in origin. Regardless of this, reasonably accurate estimates were made utilizing the onset, duration, and incidence of these symptoms in the Chernobyl accident. Prognostic evaluation generally depends on severity and duration of prodromal symptoms, presence of and extent of erythema, lymphocyte count, and the time of occurrence of the lowest number of various blood cell types. The appearance and persistence of immature cells in the peripheral blood is a favorable prognostic indicator (see Chapter 5). Data from various accidents have been used to obtain estimates for the effective dose that will produce prodromal response in 50% of irradiated persons (ED_{50}). From these data[7,8] the following values have been obtained:

- Anorexia   60—130 rad (0.6 — 1.3 Gy)
- Nausea   120—170 rad (1.2—1.7 Gy)
- Vomiting   170—270 rad (1.7—2.7 Gy)
- Diarrhea   240—300 rad (2.4—3.0 Gy)

A more detailed list is presented in Table 1. After superlethal doses of several thousands of rads (10s of Gy), all individuals will begin to show all prodromal symptoms within 5 to 15 min.

The mechanism of the prodromal syndrome is not well understood, but it appears that abnormalities in the autonomic nervous system are responsible for the early gastrointestinal symptoms.[9] The gastrointestinal symptoms are anorexia, nausea, vomiting, diarrhea, intestinal cramps, salivation, and dehydration. Prodromal responses can be prevented by shielding the abdomen, unless there are large absorbed doses to the head. Under such circumstances, associated neuromuscular symptoms are fever, headache, hypotension, apathy, sweating, and fatigue, and the reaction is usually maximal within 30 min. The portions of the brain responsible for radiation-induced nausea and vomiting appear to be the chemoreceptor trigger zone (CTZ) and the vomiting center. In animals, ablation of the CTZ eliminates prodromal vomiting.[10] Analysis of prodromal symptoms in sick patients undergoing radiation therapy suggests that concurrent illness does not cause a greater incidence of prodromal symptoms for a given absorbed dose.

The effect of dose protraction upon the prodromal response is not very well known; however, there is some data from accidents. In the Mexican radiation accident[5] one individual received 300 rad (3 Gy)/d for 7 d and 25 rad (0.25 Gy) for the next 17 d. This individual had anorexia and vomiting only after 7 d. Another person involved in the same accident who received about 100 rad (1.0 Gy) over 106 d only experienced fatigue about day 40. In general, absorbed doses of about 10 to 20 rad (0.1 to 0.2 Gy)/d to the abdomen rarely produce nausea.

B. LATENT PERIOD

The latent period is the time between the prodromal phase and the symptomatic changes that will occur later due to bone marrow, gastrointestinal, or neurovascular abnormalities. If the whole-body absorbed dose at the skin surface is less than 400 rad (4 Gy) the prodromal symptoms usually subside in 48 h and the patient may remain free of symptoms for 1 to 3 weeks. After this time, hematologic abnormalities will become obvious. With higher absorbed doses (in the range of 600 to 800 rad or 6 to 8 Gy) the latent period usually is <7d, after which time sepsis and gastrointestinal abnormalities predominate. With very high absorbed doses (in excess of 1500, or 15 Gy) the latent period may only last a few hours before vascular abnormalities become evident.

C. MANIFEST ILLNESS PERIOD

The ARS is generally divided into three or four clinical subgroups. These are (1)

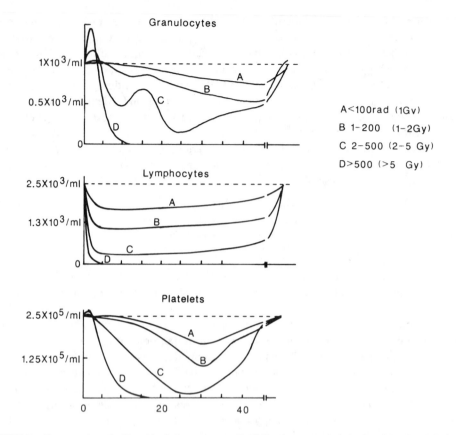

A<100rad (1Gv)

B 1-200 (1-2Gy)

C 2-500 (2-5 Gy)

D>500 (>5 Gy)

FIGURE 1. Concentration of various blood elements up to 40 d following acute whole-body-penetrating radiation.

hematopoietic syndrome, (2) gastrointestinal syndrome, (3) cardiovascular syndrome, and (4) central nervous syndrome. The hematopoietic syndrome refers to the prognostic groups II and III of Thoma and Wald[11] (as outlined in Chapter 5). The absorbed skin dose to produce this syndrome is usually in excess of 200 rad (2 Gy) and may range as high as 700 rad (2 to 7 Gy). The duration of the latent period is 1 to 3 weeks, with subsequent signs and symptoms related to damage of stem cells in the bone marrow and lymphatic organs, as well as decreased immune response. In the hematopoietic syndrome there is rapid reduction in the lymphocytes (usually within 48 h). The lymphocyte counts at days 4 to 7 postexposure at Chernobyl yielded the following correlation:

Lymphocyte count	Mean whole-body dose in rad (Gy)
950	100 (1.0)
600	200 (2.0)
375	300 (3.0)
225	400 (4.0)
170	500 (5.0)
90	600 (6.0)

There may be a transient rise in granulocytes, but after several days these will decrease, as will platelets, reaching a nadir at approximately 30 d after exposure (Figure 1). The abortive rise of granulocytes is probably due to mobilization of cells from the marrow or extramedullary sites and possibly by accelerated maturation of precursor cells. At day 10, after whole-body doses between 200 and 500 rad (2 to 5 Gy), there is a beginning of a second abortive rise. There is then a second decline (about day 25 to 30) due to lack of recovery in the stem cell population. The absence of the second abortive rise indicates doses in excess of 500 rad (5 Gy). There is a dose dependence of the white cell count and after about 600 rad (6 Gy) the granulocyte level is reduced to 10% in 12 to 14 d. The time between day 15 to 30 postirradiation is crucial with regard to fever and infection. The onset of fever is better correlated with the minimum number of granulocytes rather than the absolute number.

The time course of thrombocytopenia is broadly similar to that for granulocytopenia, but there is no abortive rise. After about 100 rad (1 Gy) a decrease in platelets to 100,000/ml is observed by day 30. The higher the dose, the earlier is the decline, and after doses greater than 600 rad (6 Gy) a minimum level of 10,000/cmm is observed by day 10 to 15. Hemorrhage is likely to occur at platelet levels below 30,000/cmm, causing anemia and possibly requiring transfusion. Some anemia does occur on the basis of red cell precursor depletion, but this is less marked than with the granulocytes due to longer lifespan of the red cells in the circulation. The granulocytopenia and the thrombocytopenia lead to hemorrhage and infection and this is the usual cause of death. Dose protraction will cause less hematologic response than acute doses; however, if the doses are delivered in <2 days, not much difference is detected from an acute single dose. As the protraction is extended, significant differences can be ascertained. In the Mexican accident,[5] one survivor received an estimated marrow dose of 900 to 1700 rad (9.0 to 17 Gy) over about 100 d; the lowest recorded white count was 2000/ml and the lowest platelet level was 70,000/ml.[5]

The gastrointestinal syndrome usually occurs when absorbed skin doses on the trunk exceed 700 rad (7 (Gy) of penetrating radiation. In most circumstances after the prodromal period there is a latent period of 1 to 4 d. If the absorbed skin dose does not exceed approximately 1200 rad (12 Gy), regeneration of the bowel epithelium is possible. With higher doses, initial loss of the intestinal stem cells at the base of the mucosal crypt occurs with subsequent denudation of the mucosa. As the intestinal/vascular barrier is broken, there is fluid and electrolyte loss into the intestinal lumen and sepsis caused by the normal bacterial flora in the intestine which now have access to the bloodstream. The sepsis is usually markedly aggravated by the decrease in granulocytes occurring simultaneously as a result of depressed bone marrow. Fluid loss is exacerbated by diarrhea and failure of absorbtion of fluid in the colon. The presence of bile in the intestine appears to be one of the main factors in the production of the radiation-induced diarrhea. Treatment with antibiotics may be expected to increase survival time, although there are very limited human data in this regard. Death resulting from the gastrointestinal syndrome usually occurs at 3 to 14 d postexposure. Accidental deaths involving the gastrointestinal syndrome have been rare. There was one person in the 1946 Los Alamos criticality accident who died on the 9th day postexposure. The granulocyte count was below 500/cmm on day 6 and remained low until death.[12] At Chernobyl there were 10 patients who were felt to have the gastrointestinal syndrome. These patients all developed diarrhea from day 4 to 8 postexposure and all died within 3 weeks.

As was pointed out in Chapter 5, there has been a lot of debate and not much data concerning the existence of either a cardiovascular syndrome or neurovascular syndrome in man. In monkeys, irradiation of the head alone can produce the central nervous system syndrome. In one accident a man receiving inhomogeneous total-body irradiation with a total dose to the front of the head of about 10,000 rad (100 Gy) of mixed gamma and neutron radiation died after 35 hours. The main pathological finding in the brain of this individual was severe edema. In this particular case, the heart received a dose of about 12,000 rad (120 Gy) and showed interstitial myocarditis, which was felt to be the primary cause of death.[13] It is clear that from the few accidents which have happened in which the dose range has exceeded 1,500 rad (15 Gy), changes of hypotension, vascular damage, and cerebral edema have occurred. Usually, these individuals die within 48 h regardless of treatment. Identification of this level of absorbed dose usually can be done by the almost immediate onset of severe projectile vomiting and nausea, as well as confusion, ataxia, and diarrhea. In this patient group there is almost total lymphocyte depletion within 24 h and an extremely early abortive rise of the granulocytes (sometimes exceeding 30,000/cmm). High radiation doses also can cause sensory changes such as a reduction in tactile sensitivity.

D. OTHER ASSOCIATED CHANGES

Changes in the oral mucosa can been seen following whole-body irradiation. In the atomic bomb survivors, mucosal lesions occurred on the tonsils, pharynx, nasal passages, and tongue. The lesions occurred during a time span that ranged from a few days to five weeks. The mean time of occurrence was 20 to 25 d and this was also the time that epilation and purpura (hemorrhage) were also noted. With absorbed doses of 1000 rad (10 Gy), the latent period is only a few days and edema is seen to extend at least as far as the larynx. This is accompanied by initial symptoms of swelling and pain in the gums and throat. With lower doses of 500 to 1000 rad (5 to 10 Gy) there is hyperemia of the oral and nasal cavities. By day 4 to 5 there is edema of the soft palate and posterior pharynx. These changes may be followed by bleeding, ulceration, and necrosis. Healing occurs slowly, but is improved with the use of antibiotics. The lymphoid areas are generally most affected and the last to heal.[14] Oropharyngeal changes were seen in 80 patients from Chernobyl. Mild abnormalities occurred from days 8 to 25 and included desquamation and edema of the tongue and cheeks as well as tenderness of the gums. In some other patients, a more severe form was seen beginning at day 3 postexposure and reaching a maximum by day 10. In this form, there were erosions and ulceration of the oral mucosa, thick mucous, and intense pain. In those patients who were also suffering from the hematopoeitic syndrome, herpes-like rashes occurred on the face and lips and there also was a pronounced radiation parotitis.

Pulmonary changes have been important in accidental exposures. The lung is the most radiosensitive organ in the thorax. At Chernobyl, there were seven patients who died after receiving very high whole-body doses and had a terminal event or period that was marked by respiratory insufficiency and pneumonitis. Death occurred in these patients from 14 to 30 d postexposure. Autopsies revealed interstitial edema, but without destruction of the epithelium of the trachea or bronchi. At this time the etiology of this pneumonitis is not well understood, but it appears likely that it was due to a combination of factors including vascular permeability, fluid imbalance, sepsis, inhalation of smoke, fumes, and radioactive materials. It should be noted here that there is a separate entity known as "radiation pneumonitis"; however this is usually seen about 1 to 3 months after radiation therapy. The threshold for development of the entity is about 600 to 700 rad (6 to 7 Gy) for a single acute exposure and the incidence is about 30% for a single dose of 800 rad (8 Gy).

V. INTERNAL CONTAMINATION

Accidental exposures involving internal contamination of medically significant proportions are rare, although there have been several in which the resultant absorbed doses were high enough to cause bone marrow depression and other findings that one normally only associates with whole-body external irradiation. As a result, it is prudent to review those circumstances which might be encountered accidentally.

There are various therapeutic regimens used in medicine which involve the administration of large activities of radioactive colloids. Radioactive colloidal ^{198}Au is used to irradiate serosal and peritoneal surfaces for treatment of malignancies such as carcinoma of the ovary. In one accident, a misadministration of about 200 mCi (7400 MBq) of ^{198}Au was injected into the peritoneal cavity of a patient in Wisconsin and resulted in estimated doses to the liver and spleen of 7300 rad (73 Gy) and 440 rad (4.4 Gy) to the bone marrow.[15] Death occurred at day 69 from cerebral hemorrhage due to thrombocytopenia. Similar overdosages have been reported in patients treated with ^{32}P for polycythemia vera.[16] An administered activity of 4 to 6 mCi (148 to 210 MBq) delivers a marrow dose of about 140 rad (1.4 Gy). Administered activities in the range of 60 mCi (2100 MBq) give marrow doses in excess of 1000 rad (10 Gy) and will cause severe pancytopenia and thrombocytopenia.

^{131}I is commonly administered to patients for treatment of hyperthyroidism and thyroid carcinoma. Thyroid ablation is common with administered activities in excess of 20 mCi (740 MBq),[17] although hematologic depression is rarely noted unless administered activities exceed 300 mCi (11,000 MBq). Treatment of chondrosarcoma is sometimes done through administration of ^{35}S. This treatment form is limited by the hemotoxicity which is seen following administered total activities in the range of 6 mCi (200 MBq) per kilogram of body weight.[18]

In addition to medical misadventures with internal emitters, there are reported occupational circumstances in which internal contamination resulted in somatic effects. At least two fatalities have occurred as the result of internal contamination with large and continuous exposure to tritium (^{3}H).[19] These exposures resulted in slow but progressive hyperplastic anemias.

VI. SUMMARY

The ARS is due to the varying cellular kinetics and radiosensitivity of organ systems within the body. There is a fair amount of human data from accidents with regard to the hematopoeitic form, but very few accidents have ever been described in which the gastrointestinal form predominates, and perhaps only one or two accidents in which cardiovascular changes were seen. The neurological syndrome has so far only been documented in animal models. Complete expression of the acute radiation syndrome may occur only hours after extremely high doses (>4000 rad or 40 Gy), or it may occur weeks after lower absorbed doses (100 to 1000 rad or 1 to 10 Gy). The ARS has a period of prodromal symptoms, a latent period, and a period of manifest illness, the duration and severity of which is related to absorbed dose. The ARS is not seen at absorbed whole-body doses of less than 100 rad (1 Gy) and is essentially always fatal if the absorbed dose exceeds 1500 rad (15 Gy).

REFERENCES

1. **Mettler, F. A. and Moseley, R. D.,** *Medical Effects of Ionizing Radiation,* Grune & Stratton, Orlando, 1985.
2. United Nations Scientific Committee on the Effects of Atomic Radiation (UNSCEAR), *Ionizing Radiation: Sources and Biological Effects,* Vienna, 1982.
3. **Ye, G., Liu, Y., Tien, N., et al.,** The People's Republic of China accident in 1963, in *The Medical Basis for Radiation Accident Preparedness,* Hubner, K. F. and Fry, S. A., Ed., Elsevier/North Holland, New York, 1980, 81.
4. **Jammet, H., Gongova, R., Poullard, T., et al.,** The 1978 Algerian accident: four cases of protracted whole body irradiation, in *The Medical Basis for Radiation Accident Preparedness* Hubner, K. F., and Fry, S. A., Eds., Elsevier/North Holland, New York, 1980, 113.
5. **Martinez, G. R., Cassab, H. G., Ganem, G. G., et al.,** Observations on the accidental exposure of a family to a source of cobalt-60, *Rev. Med. Inst. Mex. Seguro Soc.,* 3(Suppl. 1), 14, 1964.
6. **Nenot, J. C.,** Surexposition accidentelle prolongée, in *Problems, Diagnostique et Prognostique: Proc. Sem. Medical Treatment Applicable to Cases of Radiation Overexposure,* Commonwealth of European Communities, 1986.
7. **Lushbaugh, C. C.,** Reflections on some recent progress in human radiobiology, *Adv. Radiat. Biol.,* 3, 277, 1969.

8. **Lushbaugh, C. C., Fry, S. A., Hubner, K., et al.,** Total body irradiation: a historical review and followup, in *The Medical Basis for Radiation Accident Preparedness,* Hubner, K. F. and Fry, S. A., Eds., Elsevier/ North Holland, New York, 1980, 3.

9. **Harding, R. K. and Davis, C. J.,** Progress in the elucidation of the mechanisms of radiation-induced vomiting, *Int. J. Radiat. Biol.* 50, 947, 1986.

10. **Borison, H. K. and Wang, S. C.,** Physiology and pharmacology of vomiting, *Pharmacol. Rev.,* 5, 193, 1953.

11. **Thoma, G. E. and Wald, N.,** The diagnosis and management of accidental radiation injury, *J. Occup. Med.,* 1, 421, 1959.

12. **Hemplemann, L. H., Lisco, H., and Hoffman, J. G.,** The acute radiation syndrome: a study of nine cases and a review of the problem, *Ann. Inter. Med.,* 36, 279, 1952.

13. **Shipman, T. L.,** A radiation fatality resulting from massive over-exposure to neutrons and gamma rays, in *Diagnosis and Treatment of Acute Radiation Injury,* World Health Organization, Geneva, 1961, 113.

14. **Oughterson, A. W. and Warren, S.,** *Medical Effects of the Atomic Bomb in Japan,* McGraw-Hill, New York, 1956.

15. **Baron, J. M., Bachnin, S., Polcyn, R., et al.,** Accidental radio-gold (gold-198) liver scan overdose with a fatal outcome, in *Handling of Radiation Accidents,* International Atomic Energy Agency, Vienna, 1969, 399.

16. **Gmur, J., Bishoff, B., Coninx, S., et al.,** Spontaneous hematologic recovery from bone marrow aplasia after accidental 10-fold overdosage with radio-phosphorus, *Blood,* 61, 746, 1983.

17. **Halnan, K. E. and Pochin, E. E.,** Symposium on the thyroid. II. Aspects of the radio-iodide treatment of thyroid carcinoma, *Metabolism,* 6, 49, 1957.

18. **Mayer, K. M., Pentlow, K. S., Marcov, R. C., et al.,** Sulfur-35 therapy for chondrosarcoma and chordoma, in *Therapy in Nuclear Medicine* Spencer, R. P., Ed., Grune & Stratton, New York, 1978, 185.

19. **Minder, W.,** Interne kontamination mit tritium, *strahlentherapie,* 137, 700, 1969.

Chapter 7

TREATMENT OF WHOLE-BODY RADIATION ACCIDENT VICTIMS

David E. Drum and Joel M. Rappeport

TABLE OF CONTENTS

I. INTRODUCTION

Whole-body radiation exposure incidents present a number of unique challenges. The acute, nonstochastic effects of high doses of radiation over 25 rads (0.25 Gy) delivered to humans is generally manifest in rather categorical fashion; depending on the dose, either the patient is largely unharmed functionally or he is seriously injured. Radiation initiates microchemical changes within a nanosecond time frame; there exists no specific therapy to stop or reverse the sequence of events that follow. Thus, the range for effective therapeutic intervention is rather small, between 150 to 1500 rad (1.5 to 15 Gy) for humans. Nevertheless, it is likely that a large uncomplicated exposure to as much as 750 rad (7.5 Gy) might be survivable without dramatic measures such as bone marrow transplantation.

Review of the available information about past accidents shows that the majority of radiation accidents are mixed injuries.[1] Very severe local irradiation or internal contamination is also involved, together with other physical injuries. As extreme safety measures are put in place around the world, it is even more likely that most symptomatic whole-body exposures also will involve serious injuries from burns, inhalation, chemicals, or heat stress. These injuries alone engender substantial morbidity and mortality, and their massive patient care needs become an integral part of managing the whole-body exposure.

Because high-dose exposures leave no unique trace of their encounter with the body, it is possible that these mixed injuries have contributed to deaths after radiation accidents more often than is generally believed.

The best pure analogy to accidental severe whole-body overexposure to radiation is that used as part of conditioning regimens for human bone marrow transplantation. Although the range of dose rates employed for these procedures, from approximately 3 to 50 rad (30 to 500 mGy) per minute is limited, and the patients often are far more ill than would be a healthy worker, the lessons learned from the short- and long-term management of over 10,000 procedures done around the world provide a valuable and reassuring background for supportive treatment.[2-5]

At lower dose rates, the whole-body equivalent effects of our long-standing and widespread use of ^{131}I for treatment of thyroid cancer afford yet another unappreciated reservoir of information and experience.

TABLE 1
General Treatment Outline

1. Secure ABCs (airway, breathing, circulation) and physiologic monitoring as appropriate.
2. Treat major trauma, burns, and respiratory injury.
3. Obtain blood samples adequate for trauma, plus cell and HLA typing.
4. Treat contamination as needed.
5. Interrogate and give reassurance to the patient.
6. Administer symptomatic treatment — e.g., for nausea, fever, diarrhea, and apprehension.

The ultimate therapeutic needs after whole-body exposures depend not only on total dose, but upon dose rate, nature of the radiation, volume or mass of the sensitive organs irradiated, the prior health status of the individual, and upon the homogeneity of the radiation field,[6-8] and other accident conditions.

II. PRACTICAL TREATMENT CONSIDERATIONS

Given the severe limitations in medical characterization plus the complexity of the few serious and/or fatal radiation overexposures that have occurred, any planning for the details of treatment must be done in a very practical way, anticipating that most therapeutic needs must be met as they occur.

A. TREATMENT PRINCIPLES

A general treatment outline is summarized in Table 1. These principles apply to any severe mixed-trauma injury. Adequacy of airway, breathing, and circulatory function must be secured, and appropriate monitoring of large vessel pressures, blood gases, electrolytes, and urine output *must* be established as appropriate at the earliest point. Because the major problems related to any survivable exposure will, for the most part, occur remote from the immediate accident event, major life-threatening trauma must be treated first.

The usual blood analyses and cell typing activities should be completed promptly and, in the event of a radiation accident, appropriate heparinized blood samples be drawn for later cytogenetic analyses and for HLA typing. This is an important and unique feature; a severe radiation overexposure may so rapidly deplete peripheral lymphocytes that none remain to serve as a basis for donor identification.

Much useful information may be gained by interrogating the patient, by documenting an objective assessment of mental state, and by offering warm personalized support and reassurance. Radiation workers usually have received instruction about the adverse effects of radiation, hence their apprehensiveness may be of a different nature yet equally as profound as that experienced by a person without such training. Symptomatic treatment for the mild nausea, fever, diarrhea, and anxiety may be required, using whatever pharmaceuticals are comfortably used at the treatment facility. In many instances, these symptoms may not need specific treatment if the reassurance serves to mitigate apprehension and the symptoms are not inordinate.[9-11]

B. DOSIMETRIC OVEREXPOSURE CATEGORIES

It has been customary to classify overexposures arbitrarily according to the estimated absorbed dose. This is a major simplification, because few accidental overexposures will involve homogeneous whole-body radiation, and both the symptoms and therapeutic needs are dependent on many variables. In Table 2 three categories are suggested; the numerical values of doses chosen have their counterparts in common clinical experience, and the three groups are similar to those chosen by others.[12]

TABLE 2
Dosimetric Overexposure Categories

	I: 25.0—250 rad[a] (0.25—2.5 Gy)	II: 250—750 rad[a] (2.5—7.5 Gy)	III: 750—2000 rad[a] (7.5—20 Gy)
Therapeutic needs	Minimal	Substantial	Major
Patient status	Ambulatory	Hold for observation	Prepare for reverse isolation
Clinical picture	Anxiety	Add:	Add:
	Nausea	Hematologic damage	Diarrhea
	Malaise		Skin erythema
	Vomiting		Disorientation
	Fever		
Lab needs	Standard trauma	Blood counts	Full physiologic monitoring
	Cytogenetics	Marrow biopsies	
	HLA typing	HLA typing	
Prognosis	Excellent	Good	Guarded

[a] Estimated whole-body dose.

1. Category I

Those patients with doses in the range of 25 to 250 rad (0.25 to 2.5 Gy) will need minimal specific treatment. Doses in this range (or the whole-body equivalent) to a limited body field are given commonly to ambulatory radiation therapy patients with few if any symptoms. Even if the estimated dose subsequently may be proven incorrect, securing appropriate blood samples at presentation is to be recommended. Pending evaluation of data accumulated over a period of time, no prognosis should be rendered. Nevertheless, the clinician whose data make him secure about a dose in this range can work knowing that the immediate prognosis will be excellent and can anticipate no long-term disability for the patient.

2. Category II

When an accidental exposure falls within the range from 250 to 750 rad (2.5 to 7.5 Gy), therapeutic needs will be great, and the patient should certainly be held for observation and biological verificiation of the dose. Although serious hematologic damage to the bone marrow is anticipated, we believe that sufficient experience from therapy and from accidents is available to suggest that recovery will occur with good supportive care. The severity of the aplastic anemia will be judged by sequential bone marrow biopsies, and every effort will be made to support the patient, to use blood components judiciously, to treat infection, and to prevent gastrointestional bleeding, anticipating recovery of the bone marrow. Precipitous management decisions are not appropriate.

3. Category III

Whole-body doses over 750 rad (7.5 Gy) are accidents requiring major therapeutic commitment. Because the patient's granulocytes will be lost promptly and his immune competence seriously compromised, the patient must be prepared for reverse isolation with high probability of requiring bone marrow transplantation if a suitable donor is found. Diarrhea, skin erythema, and disorientation may require treatment, and many weeks later radiation pneumonitis may require antibacterial and pulmonary supportive therapy.

Full physiologic monitoring should be instituted at an early point in order that rapid shifts in fluids, pulmonary damage, and renal damage do not begin without detection, allowing treatment at the earliest point. The prognosis is guarded, because of the difficulty anticipating which organ systems may be struck by opportunistic infection and because of the difficulty anticipated in finding a reasonably compatible marrow donor.

For exposures less than about 750 rad (7.5 Gy) and causing unresponsive bone marrow aplasia, it is possible that some immune competence may be retained by patients. Then, prior to bone marrow transplantation, the usual conditioning with cyclophosphamide (or additional radiation) may be necessary to ensure transplant survival.

III. LESSONS FROM CLINICAL EXPERIENCE

A. HALF-BODY RADIATION

Clinical experience suggests that the consequences of severe or extensive half-body radiation therapy may cause symptoms similar to those of whole body exposure. Salazar and associates[13,14] reported their findings with 40 patients given 8 Gy at 30 to 40 cGy/min. The acute radiation syndrome was clearly manifest for those who were irradiated in the upper half of the body. Nausea and vomiting were observed with some tachycardia, pyrexia, and diminished blood pressure. These symptoms began shortly after the initiation of treatment and lasted for 10 h. However, peripheral blood counts were back to normal within 6 to 8 weeks. They estimated that a total of 8 Gy to the upper or lower half-body would lead to a 10 to 20% fatality occurrence.

It is of some interest that the stimuli for bone marrow regeneration can require a substantial volume of a normal hematopoietic system be destroyed before full regeneration may occur. Sacks et al.[15] described 48 patients given radiation but not chemotherapy. Their data suggested that if large sections of the bone marrow are left intact, full regeneration of the portion irradiated may *not* occur with doses less than 3500 rad (35 Gy). This was consistent with the work of others, indicating that recovery appears to occur fully after 4000 rad (40 Gy) delivered to only a part of the bone marrow.

B. TOTAL LYMPHOID IRRADIATION

The rather minimum number of major treatment imperatives involved in large partial-body irradiation exposure is dramatized by two reports of total lymphoid irradiation given for intractable lupus nephritis[16] and for rheumatoid arthritis.[17] Ten and thirteen patients (with each disease, respectively) were exposed to a total of 2000 rad (20 Gy) given at 200 rad (2 Gy) per day for 5 d/week in the mantle area (above the diaphragm) followed by a total dose of 2000 rad (20 Gy) given below the diaphragm at 150 to 200 rad (1.5 to 2 Gy) per day for 4 d/week.

These massive doses were delivered with medical therapy machines, i.e., high-energy linear accelerators, were delivered to limited fields, and were protracted in time. All the patients were said to have one or more of the following radiological side effects: fatigue, nausea, vomiting, loss of appetite, skin irritation, xerostomia, dysphagia, and transient hair loss. None of the symptoms was severe enough to interrupt the treatment course, require hospitalization, or interrupt the patients' normal activities. All *acute* symptoms disappeared within 1 month after the completion of the radiation. Depression of peripheral circulating blood cell components was not severe; only 3 patients had to suspend radiation temporarily to permit restoration of their white cell count to greater than 2000/μl. Herpes zoster occurred in five of the patients.

C. [131]I TREATMENT FOR THYROID CANCER

Yet another medical analog for the body response to radiation and therapeutic demands for treatment is afforded by the experience with ^{131}I treatment for metastatic thyroid cancer. Although this radiopharmaceutical therapy aims to take advantage of the biological concentration of the radioisotope by the thyroid cells, the administered quantity of ^{131}I, today typically 100 to 200 mCi (3.7 to 7.4 GBq), may result in effective whole-body and/or bone marrow doses in the range of 50 to 200 rad (0.5 to 2 Gy) at dose rates of 3 to 10 rad (30 to 100 mGy) per hour. Experience has taught that complications and symptoms requiring treatment are minimal at administered doses of 7.4 GBq or less. However, summaries of the complications of higher doses are instructive.[18] Those that are not unique to thyroid disease include nausea and vomiting, inflammation of the salivary glands, and fatigue and headache occurring in as many as 75% of patients. Bone marrow suppression, as judged by leukopenia, lymphopenia, and thrombocytopenia, occurs but is generally reversible. The subsequent doses — typically two to seven courses — are not given until the circulating blood cells show recovery from any depression. Because these patients have had prior thyroidectomies, retention of the radioiodine by the body is generally brief and most of the serious complications have occurred when there was greater than expected delay in excretion, particularly with retention of over 5.6 GBq in the body at 48 h.

The report of Benua and associates[19] reviewed the radiation complications observed in 59 patients administered doses averaging about 7.4 GBq but ranging up to 594 mCi (22.2 GBq). Nausea was observed after 44 such treatments, usually accompanied by vomiting. Bone marrow depression occurred in two thirds of the patients. Keratitis, unpleasant taste, and dry mouth were also observed. Only a single case of diarrhea was reported. Serious bone marrow depression was observed eight times and radiation pneumoniitis five times, with two fatalities thought to have arisen from each complication.

IV. APLASTIC ANEMIA

The bone marrow is the body organ most sensitive to the effects of uniform whole-body radiation, hence its response plays a major role in determining treatment. Because accident situations are so complex etiologically and dosimetrically, we look again to medical models for guidance. There are two, neither perfect: (1) therapeutic whole-body radiation, generally applied to persons with severe illnesses, and (2) aplastic anemia, occurring with or without known exposure to a toxic agent, an imperfect model by virtue of the lack of prior radiation. Nevertheless, many aspects of conventional medical treatment for aplastic anemia are those which would be put in place in support of severe bone marrow damage due to radiation. In the case of a typical worker, the presumption is that the individual was initially in good health and that the only new conditions are those arising from the circumstances leading to or accompanying the radiation exposure.

Aplastic anemia is defined operationally as a decrease in the numbers of circulating red cells, granulocytes, and platelets, together with a bone marrow biopsy indicating hypocellularity and decrease in the numbers of all hematopoietic cell lines. Simple depression of the numbers of peripheral cells measured by automatic counting machines is inadequate for the diagnosis because lymphocytes, whose origin is not the bone marrow, may remain normal. It should be pointed out that not only high radiation exposures, but also severe trauma (such as burns) may depress the lymphocyte population markedly and give a falsely low white blood cell population unless the specific nature of the blood cells is documented. Other causes of pancytopenia should be ruled out as early as possible even after an accident; these would include, for example, hypersplenism, bone marrow replacement by malignancies or fibrosis, vitamin B-12 or folate deficiency, and paroxysmal nocturnal hemoglobinuria.

In typical aplastic anemia that does not follow radiation, bacterial infection due to granulocytopenia is a much less common presenting problem than are weakness and fatigue attributable to anemia, easy bruising, or hemorrhage from the gastrointestinal or genitourinary tract. Presumably the immune system remains intact.

It is likely that several pathogenetic mechanisms are operating both in spontaneously occurring aplastic anemia and following radiation: (1) defective stem cells (the success of bone marrow transplantation for some cases of aplastic anemia is support for this mechanism), (2) a defective or hostile microenvironment (it is possible that radiation may initiate changes

TABLE 3
Detailed Treatment Summary

Problem	Treatment suggested
Nausea, vomiting	Diphenhydramine 25—50 mg i.v.
	Nembutal 100 mg i.v.
	Lorazepam 1—2 mg i.v.
	Perphenazine 10 mg i.v.
Apprehension	Oxazepam 10—20 mg p.p.
	Lorazepam 1—2 mg i.v.
Fever	Acetaminophen, 650 mg p.o.
GI bleeding	Aluminum hydroxide/simethicon 30 ml q4h
	Sucralfate 1g q4h
Pain, cramps from mucositis, parotitis, GI inflammation	Morphine 5 mg i.v. drip, 1—10 mg/h
Pancytopenia	Blood component therapy (irradiated to 50 Gy)
GI sterilization	Gentamicin/vancomycin/nystatin bowel prep
Mucosal infection	Nystatin suspension
	Betadine/chlorhexadine washes
Opportunistic infections	Reverse isolation
	Sterilization of foods, personal items
	Acyclovir 5 mg/kg/q8h
	Trimethoprim-sulfamethoxazole b.i.d
Bone marrow aplasia	Bone marrow transplantation

in the microenvironment of progenitor cells, thereby leading to failure of cell production), or (3) an autoimmune basis, which might not apply to persons for whom there is a directly identifiable agent such as radiation.

The aim of treatment in aplastic anemia is to provide support with expectation of spontaneous recovery.[21,22] Only after all support fails would there be an effort to consider bone marrow transplantation.

The elements of supportive treatment are shown in Table 3.

A. PREPARATION OF THE PATIENT AND HIS ENVIRONMENT

Depending upon the passage of time, the severity of the pancytopenia, and the onset of complications, efforts are made to prevent infection of the patient from inhaled or ingested materials by means of air filtration, food and material sterilization and scrupulous use of sterile techniques. For prolonged granulocytopenia (granulocytes $<500/\mu l$) following radiation, good practice would employ some sort of laminar air flow room in which all air presented to the patient has been filtered in advance and is directed out of the room. It is to be emphasized that both the bone marrow *and* the body's immunocompetence are damaged by high-dose total-body radiation.

B. BLOOD COMPONENT THERAPY

Blood component therapy should be minimized, i.e., administered only when pressed by severity or obvious complications.[23]

C. PHARMACOLOGIC AGENTS

For extreme aplastic anemia, androgens have not proven as effective as they have for other less severe anemic conditions accompanying other diseases, such as chronic renal failure. If bone marrow biopsies indicate some remaining hematopoietic elements, androgens (as oxymetholone) may be administered on trial.

Some patients with aplastic anemia have responded to clinical steroid treatment or to lithium administration at 900 mg/d. For other patients, antilymphocyte globulin seems to have had some beneficial effect, particularly when there appeared no reasonable anticipation of availability of a bone marrow donor.

Storb and co-workers[24] have suggested recently that flow microfluorometry can identify the presence of a population of peripheral blood mononuclear small cells associated with the erythroid lineage and with clinical recovery from severe aplastic anemia. It would seem appropriate to apply this technique of fluorescence-activated cell sorting (FACS) analysis for prognostic and planning purposes.

Nuclear magnetic resonance imaging of the bone marrow exhibits promise as a noninvasive alternative to biopsy for evaluating bone marrow status and recovery. Healthy marrow and its fatty replacement generate low- and high-intensity signals, respectively, when signals from T1-weighted images are analyzed.[25]

The most convincing indication of the efficacy of bone marrow transplantation for severe aplastic anemia has been the experience reported by Thomas and co-workers.[26] Fifty patients with severe aplastic anemia who had no transfusions of blood products until just before bone marrow transplantation from HLA-identical family members exhibited an actuarial 10-year survival of 82%. Graft vs. host disease (GVHD) was the predominant cause of death among the 8 fatalities. This experience is also consistent with the theory that transfusion-induced sensitization to minor transplantation antigens is a major pathogenic mechanism for marrow graft rejection.

V. BLOOD COMPONENT THERAPY

For the patient whose peripheral blood counts indicate a severe deficiency of red cells, platelets, or granulocytes, blood component therapy may be required.

A. ERYTHROCYTES

Depending upon the rapidity with which the anemia develops, young healthy workers may be able to tolerate a rather low hematocrit, perhaps even in the range 10 to 20%, provided that their activities are circumscribed and appropriate care given to other traumatic injuries and to the gastrointestinal tract. Good practice dictates that packed red cell preparations be used, either washed packed cells or frozen washed cells. For those patients who have had prior transfusions and are having nonspecific, nonhemolytic transfusion reactions, apparently due to sensitization to human leukocyte antigens (HLA), the use of frozen deglycerolyzed washed cells may reduce such reactions. If the requirement for red cells is progressively increasing, it is possible that distruction of red cells in the spleen or by development of anti-erythrocyte antibodies may be occurring; this would be unlikely in an accident victim. Prior to the initial transfusion and at periodic intervals following, complete red cell and HLA typing should be done.

B. PLATELETS[29,30]

Serious bleeding from thrombocytopenia occurs generally at platelet counts less than 20,000/μl, although many patients have sustained lower platelet counts without evidence of bleeding. In the absence of a clinical imperative or associated injuries, and with restriction of activity and care of the gastrointestinal tract, slightly lower platelet counts may be tolerated.

The most common sources of platelet preparations are single units obtained from random donors. However, the technology exists to obtain (-*pherese*) as many as 12 units from a single donor, whether it be a random donor, family member, or a specific HLA type donor.

The platelet increment with each transfusion should be about 10,000/μl, but such a response may be compromised by sepsis, trauma, or sensitization. Platelets do carry HLA antigens, hence sensitization may arise through prior pregnancy or transfusions.[31] This may require testing random donors, family members, or specifically identified compatible individuals.

C. GRANULOCYTES

The occurrence of infection in aplastic anemia is related to the severity of granulocytopenia, its length in time, and predisposing conditions such as infected burns, pneumonitis, or urinary tract infections. Several methods for processing granulocytes of normal donors are available. However, their explicit clinical efficacy in humans is still a matter of some debate. Moreover, granulocyte transfusions do contain HLA antigens, potentially limiting their usefulness. If it is anticipated that bone marrow transplantation will be needed, platelets and granulocytes should not be obtained from family members.

Granulocyte transfusions are used therapeutically, rather than prophylactically. As a rule they are reserved for patients who also have persistent absolute granulocyte counts <500/μl. A common indication is proven Gram negative bacterial infections. The facility should be prepared to continue granulocyte transfusions for 3 to 6 d.

D. IRRADIATION OF BLOOD COMPONENTS

Our practice for immunosuppressed patients, or those for whom transplantation may be required, is to irradiate all components with 50 Gy prior to transfusion.[32] We believe this is associated with diminished immunogenicity and a decreased prevalence of later GVHD. It has been presumed that lymphocytes contaminating transfused units of red cells, granulocytes or platelets may survive and contribute to GVHD for patients whose immune mechanisms are unable to destroy these foreign cells. Because GVHD is such a serious threat to patients receiving bone marrow transplants, any such easily accomplished preventive measure is welcome. Of course, all donors are tested for antibodies to cytomegalovirus (CMV).

VI. BONE MARROW TRANSPLANTATION

A. GENERAL COMMENTS

Because the bone marrow appears to be the most sensitive organ to whole-body irradiation within survivable doses, it is appealing to look to bone marrow transplantation as a principal therapeutic modality. Moreover, hospitals around the world now have experience with several thousand such procedures, and it is reasonable that it be applied when appropriate. Also, planned therapeutic radiation overexposures are an important component of preconditioning therapy for a transplantation, thus linking the medical analog of the accident with definitive therapy.

Marrow transplantation is a developing technology. As indicated in the section on aplastic anemia, every effort should be made to facilitate regrowth of the accident victim's own bone marrow; this principle should not be violated in the rush to apply dramatic, newsworthy experimental technology.

Second, marrow transplantation requires enormous technical and professional support. For this reason, it would seem mandatory that no more than one or two victims from each radiation accident be sent to even the most experienced and capable medical center. Triage using facilities around the world should be done if required, although history suggests that serious overexposures typically involve very small numbers of workers.

Third, it is correct to use methodically every available means for evaluating the patient's marrow. Multiple biopsies and assessment of potential locations of viable marrow by means of ^{111}In imaging, nuclear magnetic resonance imaging, etc., should be engaged.

During this period of evaluation, it should be possible to enlist substantial resources toward fully evaluating the nature of an exposure, including reenactment with measurements where possible. The evaluation period will also permit selection of donors and surveys of donor registries for persons compatible at the HLA surface antigen cell loci.

Depending upon the state of the recipient's immunity after the radiation accident and a full evaluation of the homogeneity and total dose delivered, additional immunosuppression and/or radiation may be required prior to transplantation.

TABLE 4
HLA Relationships

Gene region	Class	Polypeptide product
A, B, C	I	Cell surface antigens (α chain): when transplanted, elicit host antibody response and T-cell proliferation
DR, DQ, DP	II	Other cell surface antigens (α and β chains): stimulate antibodies; activate lymphocytes in GVHD; augment and inhibit immune responses
Bf, C4, C2	III	Complement C4, C2, B, and other factors

The procedural details of obtaining bone marrow are simple.[33] In an operating room under general anesthesia, bone marrow is aspirated from the pelvic bone with an effort to obtain 800 to 900 ml from an adult. The marrow thus harvested is transferred by syringe into a sterile heparinized medium, centrifuged and filtered to remove bone spicules and large tissue fragments, and returned intravenously to the recipient through a standard blood administration filter. Viable bone marrow progenitors somehow pass the lungs and find a comfortable site for growth. In the ensuing period, effort is made to prevent infection of the patient and to treat complications promptly.

Although restoration of granulocyte and platelet counts with the appearance of reticulocytes in the peripheral blood are acceptable clues to a viable bone marrow graft, other observations are important. The direct indications of success are the appearance of donor red cell antigens, HLA cell surface antigens, sex chromosomes, and granulocyte markers in the patient's blood. In a sense, the occurrence of GVHD is itself indirect evidence for viability of the donor graft. A somewhat less clear indicator would be tolerance to donor diseases and appearance of some measurable marker for donor immune function.

What are the results to be expected from the procedure? The three major contributors to success are lack of severe complicating conditions, young age, and the availability of closely matched donors. An approximate anticipation of survival under such favorable circumstances would be 70%. Although less than optimal, when compared to the very poor survival otherwise, the 70% would appear to be acceptable. Moreover, as discussed later, progressive improvements in therapeutic technology may be anticipated to permit access to a wider range of donors and to diminish complications.

B. HLA TYPING

The survival or rejection of any transplanted tissue within a new host depends on many factors, including its immunologic compatibility with the host. A greater genetic similarity permits better survival and functional capacity. As a consequence, many tests have been developed to predict and monitor these factors.

The mammalian immune network is regulated in part by a large number of molecules whose synthesis is directed by genes residing within the major histocompatibility complex (MHC).[34-36] Cell surface molecules that are MHC gene products act as antigens and are the basis by which immunocompetent cells discriminate themselves from foreign cells.

The human MHC is located on the short arm of chromosome 6. It is divided into four regions comprising two classes named for their product antigens by HLA designation (Table 4). The Class I genes (HLA-A, HLA-B, HLA-C) are responsible for production of cell surface antigens that are present on all nucleated cells. Class II genes (HLA-D related genes) encode for differentiation antigens primarily present on B-lymphocytes and macrophages.

Viewed in very simple fashion, these immune response HLA genes act as follows: host T-lymphocytes recognize a foreign antigen when macrophages present the antigen. The products of Class II genes are involved in the initial recognition, and the Class I gene products participate in the later phase of T-lymphocyte responses. Class I molecules are markers of self for the T-lymphocytes with a cytotoxic T-cell phenotype (T-8), and Class II molecules are markers for helper T-cells (T-4).

To characterize the HLA compatibility of donor cells, complement-dependent microcytotoxicity tests are employed, using antigens and antibodies of known class.

An identical twin is rarely available for a bone marrow transplant, and it is customary to survey sibling or family donors for HLA markers that are genotypically identical and of sufficient compatibility to allow engraftment of the allogeneic bone marrow. Only about 25 to 35% of potential candidates for allogeneic bone marrow transplantation will have an HLA-identical sibling donor. For this reason, large files of persons with known HLA characteristics are being developed, in particular by the National Bone Marrow Donor Registry in Minneapolis. Due to this donor pool limitation, much effort has been directed toward achieving marrow transplantation with HLA-nonidentical marrow grafts.

C. RADIATION DETAILS

Total-body irradiation (TBI) has been a major component of preparative conditioning therapy prior to syngeneic (identical twin) or allogeneic (non-genetically identical human) bone marrow infusion. Generally, chemotherapy, with agents such as cyclophosphamide, also has been included. More recently, when autologous (to self) transplants have been used for solid tumors of restricted distribution, chemotherapy in high doses alone has been employed.

The major aim of this conditioning therapy is twofold: (1) in those patients with a malignant disease, to destroy all malignant cells and their precursors and (2) to impair the function of the body's cellular immune system so as to permit acceptance of the transplant.

In light of these goals, it is necessary to deliver a very large dose of radiation rather uniformly to all areas of the body. Two general modes of delivery of 1000 to 1400 rad (10 to 14 Gy) radiation doses have been employed, opposing ^{60}Co sources and modified medical linear accelerators. The dose rates have varied widely from 3 to 30 rad (30 to 300 mGy) per minute, but 5 to 10 rad (50 to 100 mGy) per minute is the dose rate typically used today.

At our institution, two Clinac 4 MeV linear accelerators have been modified to deliver parallel opposed fields for a wide variety of very large field sizes, dose rates, and source-to-subject distances. One unit is installed in the ceiling and the second in a floor pit. Each device can travel vertically along the common axis so the source distance can be varied to encompass large whole-body field sizes. Modified fixed and independently movable collimators permit well-defined fields from as small as 5 × 5 up to 75 × 210 cm. To provide a uniform dose rate along the coronal plane section of the body, special beam-flattening filters were made.

Patients can be treated on a conventional type couch or stretcher, but we have found it useful to employ a modified support of sail cloth, thereby minimizing scatter from and attenuation by the support structure. At a dose rate of 10 mGy per minute, treatments are typically 2-Gy doses twice a day on 3 or 4 consecutive days.

These doses are rather well tolerated by patients who generally have undergone high-dose chemotherapy as well. Mild nausea, malaise, and fever have been the typical symptoms, despite the nearly simultaneous delivery of very high doses of cyclophosphamide.

Whatever the technique used, great care is needed to assure uniformity of the dose rate delivered to all parts of the body. Lead shields are generally used for the central portions of the lungs to diminish or eliminate the occurrence of radiation pneumonitis.

D. NURSING PROCEDURES
1. Preparation and Care of the Isolation Room

Periodic maintenance, regular surveillance cultures, washdowns, and upgrading of laminar air flow rooms are important components of providing a protective environment that minimizes infection yet permits efficient patient care. These should be the most nearly sterile rooms in the hospital.

2. Personal Assessments

Prior to undertaking the transplant (and continually thereafter), a detailed assessment must be made of the capacity of the patient and his family for adaptation to the prolonged and delibitating treatment sequence. This involves largely the primary nurse, assisted by numerous other professionals. Evaluations should include interpreting the meaning of the illness for the patient and his family, explaining their role assignments, consideration of their ethical and cultural norms, family communication patterns, their present and future financial situation, and ways for developing the patient's relationship to the care team. For the accident victim, many aspects of this adaptation assessment will differ markedly from those of the patient with leukemia. The patient's expectations must be adjusted to accept the reality of long and often painful confinement.

3. Intravenous Access Lines

Much of the varied therapeutic menu is administered intravenously. Insertion of Hickman lines for large vein access must be done at an early time and maintained with scrupulous care for as long as needed.

4. Body and Materials Sterilization

All foods, personal items, toys, radios, communion wafers, etc., which will be touched or ingested by the patient must be sterilized. Even stuffed animals and articles of clothing must be sterilized on a routine basis to minimize bacterial contamination. Procedures are established prior to transplantation for careful skin care, vigorous oral hygiene, and cleansing of mucous membranes and body orifices (and for corrective procedures when needed). To maintain sterility the patient may not leave the room — for months if necessary — except under exceptional medical circumstances.

5. Transportation and Transfer

Should patients require transportation, as for emergency radiographic studies, the wheelchair or stretcher must be carefully cleaned, the patient must be fully clothed in sterile gowns, and all attending personnel must wear masks, gowns, and gloves. Security will clear a direct route via elevators and halls.

Once the patient is ready to go on to a regular private room, reverse isolation must be continued, sterile water and ice provided, a low bacteria diet maintained, and a private bath made available. All administered blood products continue to be irradiated in advance of administration.

6. Recontamination

When it is clear the patient has improved to the point at which he may reenter the normal hospital environment, distinct stages for skin and gastrointestinal recontamination are initiated. These vary from institution to institution, but the aim is the same: to permit slow regrowth of normal body bacteria.

Discharge home requires the following: (1) successful, durable engraftment of the donated bone marrow, (2) an absolute granulocyte count over $500/\mu l$, (3) absence of severe acute GVHD, and (4) stable cardiovascular, pulmonary, hepatic, and renal function.

7. Nutritional Assessment

The hospitalized patient has access to a wide variety of modern nutritional regimens.

On occasion, total parenteral nutrition may have to be continued at home to maintain adequate caloric intake.

E. COMPLICATIONS OF BONE MARROW TRANSPLANTATION

Despite the dramatic and unique contribution of marrow transplantation, complications arise after the procedure. These pose major threats to the survival of each patient and consume enormous staff efforts.

1. Engraftment Failure

Failure of the transplanted marrow to engraft typically occurs within 1 month after transplantation. It is attributed to antibody- or cell-mediated sensitization to non-HLA transplantation antigens, and very likely arises from a combination of inadequate immunosuppression and sensitization by prior transfusion. Whereas improving therapeutic measures may reduce these sources of trouble, efforts to extend transplantation to less specifically identical donors will tend to increase the problem. Lack of adequate marrow progenitors in the graft, serious systemic infection, and pharmacotherapeutic agents may also contribute to failure. Inadequate hematopoietic stem cell ablation in the recipient may allow recovery of recipient cells and subsequent predominance over the transplanted marrow cells, as occurred in Yugoslavia and Russia.

2. GVHD

The untoward reaction requiring the greatest supportive efforts is GVHD. This complex and heterogeneous reaction is thought to be related to the degree of genetic disparity, to actions of mature donor T-lymphocytes contaminating a marrow infusion, and possibly to other immunoregulatory "imbalances".

The acute form of GVHD occurs within two months of transplantation in 40 to 90% of adult recipients of histocompatible transplants. The characteristic features are an erythematous rash varying widely in severity, evidence of hepatocellular inflammation, fever, and nonspecific gastrointestinal dysfunction. A variety of therapeutic modalities, including steroids, antilymphocyte globulin, cyclosporine, and selected monoclonal antibodies have been employed in efforts to modify GVHD.[37,38] Prednisone and azathioprine are standard pharmacologic therapy.

Chronic GVHD occurs later than two months after transplantation and is manifest by cholestatic serum chemistries, dermatologic changes similar to scleroderma or dermatomyositis, a dry stomatitis, and keratoconjunctivitis. In severe cases, a variety of other organ-specific inflammatory processes may occur. Continued infections via the lung and gastrointestinal tract may require appropriate treatment. Careful and prompt attention should be given to the earliest and most minimal indications of infection.

3. Opportunistic Infections

Opportunistic infections rank second to GVHD as a cause of morbidity and mortality after bone marrow transplantation. These infections are similar to those associated with immunocompromised patients in general, the focus of considerable diagnostic and therapeutic effort today.

The risk of specific infections seems related to the time after the transplant procedure. During the period of severe granulocytopenia and loss of cutaneous or mucous membrane layers, the Gram-negative bacilli are preeminent. Sterilizing the room environment and gastrointestinal tract of the patients plus prophylactic or specific antibiotics have been used to manage these infections (Table 3).

A successful transplant may have return of granulocytes, but with GVHD and continued compromise of the immune system, the bacterial complications may yield to fungal and viral infections. After the first 6 weeks, the variety of interstitial pneumonias (not those related to radiation), are the major risk from infection: *Pneumocystis carinii*, CMV, and herpes simplex infections have been problematic.[39-41] Acyclovir has been useful for some of these complications. However, there is no effective therapy for CMV infection and CMV-negative donors are preferred for any required component transfusions.

Months after transplant, a number of opportunistic infections may involve the liver: CMV, hepatitis B or A virus, and Epstein-Barr virus have been reported. Infections occurring even later are generally secondary to GVHD. Because each patient's cellular memory for prior donor infections and immunization is absent, revaccination should be considered after the first year, avoiding the use of live attenuated viruses.

4. Other Complications

Hepatic veno-occlusive disease has been noted in some patients, occasionally as many as 20% shortly following marrow transplantation.[42] Whether this is purely due to the high-dose cyclophosphamide treatment and/or irradiation has not been fully elucidated. Treatment is purely supportive, yet the nature of the liver disease has to be elucidated to exclude other important forms, especially that due to GVHD.

Late onset of restrictive and obstructive pulmonary disease has been noted and is postulated to be due to chemotherapy, in the absence of evidence for radiation pneumonitis. There have been rare reports of secondary tumors following marrow transplantation,[43] including the occurrence of B cell proliferation in cells of both donor and recipient origin.[44]

Radiation pneumonitis is a sufficiently common complication in that it has been the major impetus for dose fractionation and for use of midlung shields for patients receiving ablative irradiation.[45] Also, the occurrence and severity of the pneumonitis appears dose related, being relatively uncommon with dose rates less than 5 rad (50 mGy) per minute or <800 rad (8 Gy) total.

Cataracts are observed in as many as 50% of patients treated by a single dose of 900 to 1000 rad (9 to 10 Gy).[46] Dose fractionation appears to diminish this distressing complication.

A variety of nonspecific gastrointestinal manifestations — persistent nausea, vomiting, and diarrhea — also may be observed. These perhaps represent one end of the spectrum of sequelae which, at the extreme, are represented by obstructing strictures, fistulas, perforation, and bleeding that are seen in 2 to 11% of instances of therapeutic abdominal or pelvic irradiation (usually over 2000 rad [20 Gy] locally). Severe lower intestinal complications require careful judgment and repeated selective surgical operations. More recently, endoscopic laser therapy has been described as a successful means for terminating severe chronic bleeding from rectal radiation injury.[47] A simple colostomy may not suffice to stop bleeding. It would be appropriate to follow the patient by periodic endoscopic exams.

5. Therapy Toxicity

The pharmacotherapeutic menu for bone marrow transplantation is a long one, including conventional drugs with well known hazards and investigational pharmaceuticals of less well defined danger. Aminoglycosides, cyclosporine, immunosuppressives, and chemotherapeutic agents require careful judgment and frequent observation.

VII. ASSOCIATED BURNS AND RESPIRATORY INJURIES

No discussion of radiation accidents is complete without reference to associated traumatic injuries. In particular, because a number of radiation accidents have involved burns, it is appropriate to comment on the critical nature of initial treatment of these injuries. It is now appreciated that as many as 50% of burn deaths are attributable to inhalation injury.[48,49]

Moreover, the early symptoms of carbon monoxide intoxication, such as might occur from exposure to burning organic matter, include headache, confusion, malaise, fatigue, and nausea, symptoms familiar by now as manifestations of serious acute radiation exposure.[49]

A. BURNS

When burns or explosions complicate a radiation accident, high-flow oxygen should be administered to the patient until carbon monoxide toxicity is ruled out. As early as possible, it should be determined whether there is either thermal or chemical inhalation injury. Endotracheal intubation is indicated for substantial facial burns, smoke inhalation with endoscopic evidence of airway edema, and severe circumferential chest burns where ventilatory assistance is needed. Bronchodilators and liberal use of positive pressure ventilation to maintain lung volumes are indicated. Central venous pressure and blood gases should be frequently measured, and a nasogastric tube put in place for suction to avoid aspiration and gastric distension.

Whereas for a serious radiation injury the major support problems occur much later in time, the initial fluid replacement requirements for serious burns are urgent.[51,52] Venous catheters are placed in nonburned extremities for administration of primary (crystalloid) and secondary (colloid) fluids to improve perfusion and help minimize edema. By whatever route fluid volume is administered, the urine output should be kept above 0.5 ml/kg/h and the pulse rate less than 120/min. Intravenous dopamine or dobutamine may be required as needed for circulatory support. Body temperature should be maintained and mixed venous pO_2 kept above 35 mmHg.

Hospital personnel rarely are with the patient during the first 10 to 20 min after a severe burn, during which cooling is indicated. Later, hypothermia is a greater threat and should not be enhanced by efforts to cool the body. Decontamination and evaluation of contamination in the wound can proceed at the same time that the usual cleansing and debridement are performed. Once washed down, burn wounds are covered with topical antibiotics or temporary skin substitutes followed by dry dressings. Final open wound treatment is begun only after the patient is physiologically stable and in a warm surgical environment.

Because large burns require major medical support, the simultaneous occurrence of several such injuries is an absolute requirement for triage to several trauma center hospitals.

B. INHALATION INJURY

Inhalation injury may present as one or all of a sequence of three stages.[53] First, in the case of carbon monoxide, carbon dioxide, or cyanide exposures, the onset of noncyanotic lethargy, disorientation, and nausea with a normal chest examination may be immediate. After 12 to 24 h, internal thermal injury may become manifest as dyspnea, tachypnea, stridor, and possible cyanosis — despite a normal chest radiograph. Finally, the delayed chemical effects may cause similar symptoms together with wheezing, rhonchi, and progressive development of atelectasis, alveolar edema, or bronchopneumonia.

In cases of major trauma, endotracheal intubation may be indicated if there is even moderate airway concern. A high fraction of inhaled oxygen, at positive pressure if needed, should be maintained to diminish the disorientation and confusion and to reduce carbomonoxyhemoglobin to <10%. Frequent suctioning and bronchodilators, together with the earlier measures, may be required for as long as a week, until edema resolves and gas exchange is normalized.

Due to the paucity of adequate clinical data for evaluating the consequences of severe traumatic injury, i.e., burns, complicated by a severe radiation overexposure, little in the way of explicit guidance can be given. Experimentally, there is evidence to suggest that sepsis superimposed on radiation injury in mice engenders higher mortality, as might be expected.[53] Clinical experience with cancer treatment indicates that adequate wound healing may be obtained even after substantial local radiation, probably after much higher doses than would be survivable if delivered as a whole-body dose. Meticulous hemostasis should be the rule in management of burns and traumatic injuries at any time.

Concomitant antibiotics administered to dogs and to pigs with experimental combined burn and irradiation injuries appear effective in reducing mortality.[55,56] However, both these species are far more susceptible to infection than humans and would normally not get the same routine diagnostic testing and sterile environment available to human subjects. Many of the supportive and protective measures afforded the victim of serious radiation overexposure would also serve to diminish nosocomial infection.

VIII. CASE REPORT

An instructive example of the many therapeutic demands afforded by a single serious radiation accident is the report that appeared in the *New England Journal of Medicine* on April 5, 1965.[57] From a physician's point of view, this is a model of excellence for a useful and readily accessible medical case report. The physical details of the event, the medical findings and course, dosimetry, and laboratory and pathologic findings are summarized with consummate clarity.

An employee of a private sector recovery plant was pouring a mixture containing ^{235}U from a large graduated cylinder into a tank containing sodium carbonate. A fission explosion occurred, and the man recalled sensing a flash of light and being hurled backwards. He ran immediately from the building discarding his clothing as he ran. At an emergency shack 200 yards away, he complained of abdominal cramps and headache, and was observed to vomit and pass a bloody diarrheal stool.

He arrived at a major hospital 1 h and 43 min after the accident. It was later estimated that the patient received a neutron dose of 2200 rad (22 Gy) and a gamma-ray dose of 6600 rad (66 Gy), from 10 to 20 times what was thought to be a lethal dose.

The blood pressure was 160/80, pulse 100 and regular, respiratory rate 20, and the temperature 100.4°F on admission. His skin color and turgor were normal, and he complained of abdominal cramps, headache, thirst, and chilliness, despite perspiring profusely. A slight nonbloody diarrhea was noted, and he had transient difficulty pronouncing some words. His abdomen was rigid, but the remainder of the physical exam was fully normal.

The exposure rate 2 ft from his face and upper chest was 40 mR/h, decreasing to 18 mR/h above the abdomen. These exposures appeared primarily due to contamination with ^{24}Na and ^{32}P.

By 40 h after the exposure, the patient's peripheral white blood cell count had increased to 45,000/ml, but lymphocytes were absent both from peripheral blood and from the bone marrow. The peripheral blood platelets had remained approximately stable, at 170,000/ml, and the hematocrit had increased to 51.5%. In the first 18 h, the patient's total fluid intake was 4575 ml and his output was 3400 ml, 2000 of that being gastric aspirate and vomitus. During the next 12-h period, he received 2500 ml of fluid and excreted only 65 ml in the urine.

Both parenteral and nonabsorable antibiotics were given, but his clinicians felt that diphenhydramine, morphine, methylprednisolone, dimehydrinate, and levarterenol were the only helpful pharmacologic agents. These were required to maintain vital signs at 4 h after the accident, but even as late as 10 h afterward the patient reported that he felt well, despite a temperature rise to 102°F. His left hand and forearm then became edematous and red. Conjunctivitis and periorbital edema appeared on the left side, although his visual acuity for newsprint appeared normal. At 16 h after the accident, a chest radiograph showed some hilar congestion, and the hand and arm were more painful.

On the second day support of the circulation continued to be a problem and the patient was restless, apprehensive, and dyspneic. The left-sided swelling and redness was severe, and he could not read letters 1 in. high. Urine output ceased, and he expired 49 h after the accident.

His blood chemistries were characteristic only of progressive acute renal failure. The electrocardiographic changes late in the 2nd day seemed to indicate progressive right heart strain associated with the clinical appearance of pulmonary congestion.

A postmortem examination showed severe edema of the left side and extremities, acute inflammation of the trachea and esophagus, bilateral pleural effusions, pulmonary interstitial edema, and subserosal and submucosal edema in the gastrointestinal tract. Acute pericarditis involved the anterior right atrium and right ventricle. The liver showed passive congestion and minimal focal fatty metamorphosis; acute pancreatitis was noted. The bone marrow was aplastic and lymphocytes were depleted from their normal sites. Minimal changes in the brain and testes were observed.

Despite normal or elevated peripheral blood counts (except for depletion of lymphocytes), it would appear this patient's bone marrow was destroyed. The major cause of death was circulatory, complicated by renal failure with minimal morphologic changes in the kidneys. Many evaluative and therapeutic modalities routinely available today were not available to this patient in 1964, and it is tempting to think that these cardiorenal problems might be surmounted. Moreover, in light of the postmortem findings, it is interesting that the possibility of respiratory tract thermal injury and/or damage by inhaled chemicals or isotopes appeared not to be considered by his physicians. The rapid depletion of peripheral lymphocytes suggests that adequate blood samples for HLA typing must be obtained as early as possible after such an extreme overexposure.

This accident raised many issues in hospital radiation safety and administrative control during such an incident. However, these would appear to be well known today and should present no insurmountable problems at accredited institutions.

IX. PROSPECTS FOR THE FUTURE

Extreme doses of radiation or chemotherapy separately are highly effective in eliminating cancer cells wherever they may be in the human body. For this reason they offer great promise in cancer treatment, and enormous investigative and clinical work aims to exploit this promise during the next decade. Unfortunately, the price sometimes paid is destruction of the bone marrow, hence equally intense efforts are being made to find ways to salvage bone marrow or to improve the efficacy and general applicability of bone marrow transplantation. Capability for treating the hematologic and other effects of whole-body irradiation will be an important secondary gain from this vigorous area of worldwide medical research. One major contribution now developing is the establishment of large bone marrow donor registries to increase the pool of transplant sources.

Various treatments of donor bone marrow specimens prior to infusion are being tested. Purging of T cells contaminating donor marrow by admixture with specific single and mixed monoclonal antibodies with and without complement is being studied,[37,58] and antibodies to interleukin-1 have contributed to some experimental success.[59] It also appears that freezing in itself may decrease the numbers of active T-cells in a marrow preparation.

Many bone marrow cells can be propagated in cell culture. By using joint application of a variety of media ingredients and intrinsically different growth cycles, it would seem likely that selective marrow cultures might develop so as to maximize engraftment and minimize GVHD.

Next to failure of engraftment, GVHD is the major threat to successful transplantation. Cyclosporine A appears useful for improving graft survival by as yet unidentified effects on the consequences of GVHD even when the GVDH itself appears no less severe.[38,60] Other pharmaceuticals are under development and will undoubtedly prove even more effective.

Stimulatory molecules may play a therapeutic role in enhancing the viability of transplanted marrow. Recombinant erythropoietin[61] would appear to be a useful means for maximally stimulating red cell precursors remaining after a radiation accident or for stimulating transfused donor marrow cells after very high dose whole-body irradiation. Several agents, called colony stimulating factors (CSF) have been described as stimulants of myelopoiesis.[62] These include granulocyte-monocyte CSF (GM-CSF), granulocyte-CSF, and macrophage-CSF.

Evaluation of bone marrow through ^{111}In chloride imaging[63] and magnetic resonance imaging,[25] previously cited, has not been widely utilized. They or analogous diagnostic procedures will surely be used in conjunction with other means for judging the need for and evaluating the success of marrow transplantation.

One fundamental therapeutic need for accidental whole-body irradiation is as yet unmet and the subject of little investigation: pharmacologic agents that directly protect against the effects of radiation would be a welcome adjunct. Radiobiologists and radiochemists have long employed a variety of alcohols, thiols, and amines as radical scavengers, effectively diminishing experimentally the biological effects of radiation. No one has yet suggested that radiation workers should be kept permanently intoxicated to minimize the effects of whole-body radiation, yet the principle of having available a simple, harmless, and acceptable pharmaceutical for this purpose is attractive.

Likewise, no effective means for enhancing the ability of the body to repair the sequence of events initiated by whole body irradiation has yet become available. However, with the wide availability of many means for characterizing the functional activities of DNA molecules and with advent of direct gene repair, it may be anticipated that many of the techniques of genetic engineering may become just as effective in repairing some acute effects of radiation as they are anticipated to be for detecting and correcting static, inherited genetic anomalies.

REFERENCES

1. **Mettler, F. A. and Ricks, R. C.,** History of radiation accidents, in *Medical Management of Radiation Accidents*, Mettler, F. A., Kelsey, C. A., and Ricks, R. C., Eds., CRC Press, Boca Raton, 1989.
2. **Thomas, E. D., Storb, R., Clift, R. A., et al.,** Bone-marrow transplantation, *N. Engl. J. Med.*, 292, 832, 1975.
3. **Blume, K. G., Beutler, E., Bross, K. J., et al.,** Bone-marrow ablation and allogeneic marrow transplantation in acute leukemia, *N. Engl. J. Med.*, 302, 1041, 1980.
4. **Thomas, E. D.,** Bone marrow transplantation. A lifesaving applied art, *JAMA*, 249, 2528, 1983.
5. **Arthur, C. K.,** Bone marrow transplantation for leukemia, *Bone Marrow Transplant.*, 1, 329, 1987.
6. **Bloomer, W. D. and Hellman, S.,** Normal tissue responses to radiation therapy, *N. Engl. J. Med.*, 293, 80, 1975.
7. **Little, J. B.,** Cellular effects of ionizing radiation, *N. Engl. J. Med.*, 278, 308, 1968.
8. **Finch, S. C.,** Acute radiation syndrome, *JAMA*, 258, 664, 1987.
9. A Guide to the Hospital Management of Injuries Arising from Exposure to or Involving Ionizing Radiation, American Medical Association, Chicago, 1984.
10. International Commission on Radiological Protection, The principles and general procedures for handling emergency and accidental exposures of workers, ICRP Publ. 28, Pergamon, New York, 1978.
11. National Council on Radiation Protection and Measurements, Management of Persons Accidentally Contaminated with Radionuclides, NCRP Rep. 65, Washington, D.C., 1980.
12. **Mettler, F. A.,** Effects of Whole Body Irradiation, in *Medical Management of Radiation Accidents*, Mettler, F. A., Kelsey, C. A., and Ricks, R. C., Eds., CRC Press, Boca Raton, 1989.
13. **Salazar, O. M., Rubin, P., Keller, B., et al.,** Systemic (half-body) radiation therapy: response and toxicity, *Int. J. Radiat. Oncol. Biol. Phys.*, 4, 937, 1978.
14. **Salazar, O. M. and Poussin-Rosillo, H.,** Systemic half-body irradiation: a new dimension in oncology, *Appl. Radiol.*, 16, 67, 1987.

15. **Sacks, E. L., Goris, M. L., Glatstein, E., et al.,** Bone marrow regeneration following large field radiation. Influence of volume, age, dose, and time, *Cancer,* 42, 1057, 1978.

16. **Strober, S., Field, E., Hoppe, R. T., et al.,** Treatment of intractable lupus nephritis with total lymphoid irradiation, *Ann. Intern. Med.,* 102, 450, 1985.

17. **Strober, S., Tanay, A., Field, E., et al.,** Efficacy of total lymphoid irradiation in intractable rheumatoid arthritis. A double-blind, randomized trial, *Ann. Intern. Med.,* 102, 441, 1985.

18. **Freitas, J. E., Gross, M. D., Ripley, S., et al.,** Radionuclide diagnosis and therapy of thyroid cancer: current status report, *Semin. Nucl. Med.,* 15, 106, 1985.

19. **Benua, R. S., Cicale, N. R., Sonenberg, M., et al.,** The relation of radioiodine dosimetry to results and complications in the treatment of metastatic thyroid cancer, *Am. J. Roentgenol.,* 87, 71, 1962.

20. **Casale, T. B.,** Aplastic anemia. The disease and its management, *Postgrad. Med.,* 71, 59, 1982.

21. **Gale, R. P., Champlin, R. E., Feig, S. A., et al.,** Aplastic anemia: biology and treatment, *Ann. Intern. Med.,* 95, 477, 1981.

22. **Camitta, B. M., Storb, R., and Thomas, E. D.,** Aplastic anemia. Pathogenesis, diagnosis, treatment and prognosis, *N. Engl. J. Med.,* 306, 645, 1982.

23. **Storb, R., Thomas, E. D., Buckner, C. D., et al.,** Marrow transplantation in thirty "untransfused" patients with severe aplastic anemia, *Ann. Intern. Med.,* 92, 30, 1980.

24. **Storb, B., Doney, K., Sale, G., et al.,** Subsets of patients with aplastic anemia identified by flow microfluorometry, *N. Engl. J. Med.,* 312, 1015, 1985.

25. **Kaplan, P. A., Asleson, R. J., Klassen, L. W., et al.,** Bone marrow patterns in aplastic anemia: observations with 1.5-T MR imaging, *Radiology,* 164, 441, 1987.

26. **Thomas, E. D., Anasetti, C., Doney, K. C., Storb, R., et al.,** Marrow transplantation for severe aplastic anemia, *Ann. Intern. Med.,* 104, 461, 1986.

27. **Horwitz, C. A.,** Blood transfusion therapy, *Postgrad. Med.,* 69, 155, 1981.

28. **Blumberg, N., Borucki, D. T., Lichtiger, B., et al.,** *Blood Transfusion Therapy. A Physician's Handbook,* Snyder, E. L., Ed., American Association of Blood Banks, Arlington, 1983.

29. Platelet transfusion therapy. Consensus conference, *JAMA,* 257, 1777, 1987.

30. **Pineda, A. A.,** Blood component therapy: granulocyte and platelet transfusion, *Mayo Clin. Proc.,* 56, 645, 1981.

31. **Kickler, T. S.,** Platelet-compatibility testing: an update, *Lab. Manage.,* 25, 33, 1987.

32. **Button, L. N., DeWolf, W. C., Newburger, P. E., et al.,** The effects of irradiation on blood components, *Transfusion,* 21, 419, 1981.

33. **Thomas, E. D. and Storb, R.,** Technique for human marrow grafting, *Blood,* 36, 507, 1970.

34. **Dausset, J.,** The major histocompatibility complex in man, *Science,* 213, 1469, 1981.

35. **Goldman, J. N. and Goldman, M. B.,** What the clinician should know about the major histocompatibility complex, *JAMA,* 246, 873, 1981.

36. **Bach, F. H. and Sachs, D. H.,** Transplantation immunology, *N. Engl. J. Med.,* 317, 489, 1987.

37. **Mitsuyasu, R. T., Champlin, R. E., Gale, R. P., et al.,** Treatment of donor bone marrow with monoclonal anti-T-cell antibody and complement for the prevention of graft-versus-host disease, *Ann. Intern. Med.,* 105, 20, 1986.

38. **Storb, R., Deeg, H. J., Whitehead, J., et al.,** Methotrexate and cyclosporine compared with cyclosporine alone for prophylaxis of acute graft versus host disease after marrow transplantation for leukemia, *N. Engl. J. Med.,* 314, 729, 1986.

39. **Weiner, R. S., Bortin, M. M., Gale, R. P., et al.,** Interstitial pneumonitis after bone marrow transplantation, *Ann. Intern. Med.,* 104, 168, 1986.

40. **Masur, H., Shelhamer, J., and Parrillo, J. E.,** The management of pneumonias in immunocompromised patients, *JAMA,* 253, 1769, 1985.

41. **Rosenow, E. C., Wilson, W. R., and Cockerill, F. R.,** Pulmonary disease in the immunocompromised host, *Mayo Clin. Proc.,* 60, 473, 1985.

42. **Woods, W. G., Dehner, L. P., Nesbit, M. E., et al.,** Fatal veno-occlusive disease of the liver following high dose chemotherapy, irradiation and bone marrow transplantation, *Am. J. Med.,* 68, 285, 1980.

43. **Deeg, H. J., Saunders, J., et al.,** Secondary malignancies after marrow transplantation, *Exp. Hematol.,* 12, 660, 1984.

44. **Schubach, W. H., Miller, G., et al.,** Epstein-Barr virus genomes are restricted to secondary neoplastic cells following bone marrow transplantation, *Blood,* 65, 535, 1985.

45. **Fryer, C. J. H., Fitzpatrick, P. J., Rider, W. D., et al.,** Radiation pneumonitis: experience following a large single dose of radiation, *Int. J. Radiat. Oncol. Biol. Phys.,* 4, 931, 1978.

46. **Deeg, H. J., Storb, R., and Thomas, E. D.,** Bone marrow transplantation: a review of delayed complications, *Br. J. Hematol.,* 57, 185, 1984.

47. **Ahlquist, D. A., Gostout, C. J., and Viggiano, T. R.,** Laser therapy for severe radiation-induced rectal bleeding, *Mayo Clin. Proc.,* 61, 927, 1986.

48. **Zawecki, B. E., Jung, R. C., Joyce, J., et al.,** Smoke, burns, and the natural history of inhalation injury in fire victims: a correlation of experimental and clinical data, *Ann. Surg.,* 185, 100, 1977.

49. **Trunkey, D. D.,** Inhalation injury, *Surg. Clin. N. Am.,* 58, 1133, 1978.

50. **Cahalane, M. and Demling, R. H.,** Early respiratory abnormalities from smoke inhalation, *JAMA,* 251, 771, 1984.

51. **Demling, R. H.,** Fluid resuscitation after major burns, *JAMA,* 250, 1438, 1983.

52. **Demling, R. H.,** Burns, *N. Engl. J. Med.,* 313, 1389, 1985.

53. **Demling, R. H.,** Smoke inhalation injury, *Postgrad. Med.,* 82, 63, 1987.

54. **Miller, C. P., Hammond, C. W., and Thompkins, M.,** The incidence of bacteremia in mice subjected to whole body X-radiation, *Science,* 3, 540, 1950.

55. **Brooks, J. W., Evans, E. I., Ham, W. T., et al.,** The influence of external body radiation on mortality from thermal burns, *Ann. Surg.,* 136, 533, 1952.

56. **Baxter, H., Drummond, J. A., Stephens-Newsham, L. G., et al.,** Reduction of mortality in swine from combined total body radiation and thermal burns by streptomycin, *Ann. Surg.,* 137, 450, 1953.

57. **Karas, J. S. and Stanbury, J. B.,** Fatal radiation syndrome from an accidental nuclear excursion, *N. Engl. J. Med.,* 272, 755, 1965.

58. **Reinherz, E. L., Geha, R., et al.,** Reconstitution after transplantation with T-lymphocyte-depleted HLA haplotype-mismatched bone marrow for severe combined immunodeficiency, *Proc. Natl. Acad. Sci. U.S.A.,* 79, 6047, 1982.

59. **Smith, B. R., Rappeport, J. M., et al.,** Marrow T cell depletion with anti-leu-1 monoclonal antibody and complement in matched and mismatched transplantation, *Blood,* 64(Suppl.), 221A, 1984.

60. **Atkinson, K.,** Cyclosporin in bone marrow transplantation, *Bone Marrow Transplant.,* 1, 265, 1987.

61. **Eschbach, J. W., Egrie, J. C., Downing, M. R., et al.,** Correction of the anemia of end-stage renal disease with recombinant human erythropoietin, *N. Engl. J. Med.,* 316, 73, 1987.

62. **Nathan, D. G.,** Hope for hematopoietic hormones, *N. Engl. J. Med.,* 317, 626, 1987.

63. **McNeil, B. J., Rappeport, J. M., and Nathan, D. G.,** Indium chloride scintigraphy: an index of severity in patients with aplastic anemia, *Br. J. Hematol.,* 34, 599, 1976.

Chapter 8

CYTOGENETIC TECHNIQUES IN BIOLOGICAL DOSIMETRY: OVERVIEW AND EXAMPLE OF DOSE ESTIMATION IN TEN PERSONS EXPOSED TO GAMMA RADIATION IN THE 1984 MEXICAN ^{60}Co ACCIDENT

L. G. Littlefield, E. E. Joiner, and K. F. Hubner

TABLE OF CONTENTS

I. INTRODUCTION

Although there are many excellent physical means for measuring radiation dose, situations often arise when there is reason to suspect that exposures registered on personal monitors, such as film badges or thermoluminescent dosimeters (TLDs), do not reflect dose received by the wearer, or when persons having suspected overexposures were not wearing any type of physical dosimeter. In such instances, biological indicators may provide the only means for determining whether or not a suspected overexposure actually occurred. At present, the analysis of radiation-induced chromosome aberrations in cultured lymphocytes is the most sensitive biological technique for quantifying dose in persons having whole-body exposures to penetrating radiation.

The applicability of the cytogenetic dosimetry system is based on over four decades of scientific research in radiation biology. It was established in work conducted in the 30s and 40s that ionizing radiation induces structural aberrations in the chromosomes of exposed cells, and that the incidence of induced aberrations shows a strict dependency on radiation dose. Elegant early studies in plant cells[1-4] defined not only the complex array of aberration types induced when exposures were delivered at differing stages of the cell cycle, but also determined the dose dependency for radiations of differing qualities, delivered at high or low dose rates, and under differing conditions of oxygen tension. In 1960 a technique was introduced for culturing human lymphocytes which reliably produced high-quality preparations of metaphase chromosomes.[5] Shortly thereafter, it was determined that radiation-induced chromosome aberrations could be quantified in cultured lymphocytes from X-irradiated patients,[6] and in 1964, Bender[7] first proposed that the evaluation of induced aberrations could provide a biological method for estimating radiation dose. Since then, hundreds of studies have been conducted in mammalian and human lymphocytes exposed to various qualities of radiation delivered under a variety of experimental conditions. These have firmly established the utility of cytogenetic methods as a dosimetric tool, and have defined numerous physical and biological factors that must be considered in interpreting data from exposed persons.

During the last 20 years, cytogenetic dosimetry studies have been conducted in a number of radiation accidents,[8-13] including very recent evaluations in persons exposed at Chernobyl in 1986.[14] Presently, cytogenetic dosimetry techniques are routinely applied by several laboratories (most notably the National Radiological Protection Board [NRPB] in Great Britain[15] and the Radiation Emergency Assistance Center/Training Site [REAC/TS] Laboratory in Oak Ridge[16]) for estimating dose in persons having real or suspected radiation overexposures.

Several excellent discussions of radiation cytogenetics and of the application of cytogenetic techniques in dosimetry are available,[17-25] and an International Atomic Energy Agency (IAEA) technical report describing detailed methodological approaches for the use of chromosome aberration analysis for dose assessment has recently been published.[26] The purposes of the present chapter are to provide an overview of biological dosimetry applications, and, as an example of the use of the technique in estimating radiation dose, to describe data our laboratory obtained in studies of ten persons exposed in the 1984 Mexican ^{60}Co accident.

II. GENERAL CONSIDERATIONS

A. THE LYMPHOCYTE CULTURE SYSTEM

Although metaphase preparations of human chromosomes may be obtained from mitotic cells derived from other tissues (i.e., marrow or cultured fibroblasts), the lymphocyte culture system forms the basis for the cytogenetic dosimetry technique. Numerous modifications of the original lymphocyte culture method[5] are in use by various laboratories. For initiation of cultures from persons having suspected radiation exposures, aliquots of whole blood, leukocyte-rich plasma, or purified lymphocytes are sterilely introduced into formulated tissue culture medium (such as TC 199, RPMI 1640, Hams F-10, etc.) which is generally supplemented with 10 to 20% human or bovine serum and antibiotics. Immunocompetent T lymphocytes are stimulated to undergo blast transformation and to enter mitotic cell division by the addition of an appropriate mitogen (most commonly phytohemagglutinin [PHA]) to the culture medium. Many radiation cytogenetics laboratories have adopted the protocol of adding the pyrimidine base analog 5-bromodeoxyuridine (BrdU) to the medium at the time of culture initiation.[21,23-25] The use of BrdU substitution into the chromosomes of dividing lymphocytes,[27] when combined with appropriate specialized staining techniques,[28] makes it possible to select for analysis those metaphases that have divided only once during the period of *in vitro* culture.[29] This procedure avoids problems inherent in analyzing metaphases of lymphocytes that may have divided two or more times *in vitro,* and consequently which may have lost a proportion of radiation-induced aberrations as a result of reproductive death.[30-35]

Cultures are incubated at 37°C for sufficient time to allow a large proportion of the lymphocytes to complete one round of DNA synthesis (about 44 to 48 h), and a mitotic inhibitor such as colchicine is added to arrest cells at the metaphase stage of cell division. One to several hours later, cells are harvested by exposure to a hypotonic solution, and fixed to preserve morphology of the chromosomes. Cells are then resuspended in fixative and dropped onto the surface of a microscope slide. After staining, slides are scanned under the microscope to locate well-spread first division metaphases and these are counted and evaluated for radiation-induced chromosome aberrations at a magnification of about $1,000 \times$. Depending on the level of exposure and degree of statistical certainty desired, it may be necessary to score several hundred metaphases to obtain valid estimates of the proportions of cells bearing aberrations.

The lymphocyte culture method has several advantages in biological dosimetry studies. Among these are the facts that PHA-responsive lymphocytes have uniform radiation sensitivity,[29] that the technique requires only a small amount of venous whole blood, and that lymphocytes can be cultured from transported blood as long as samples are properly packaged and received within about 24 to 48 h after the blood sample is drawn.[16] Lastly, because human T lymphocytes have a relatively long lifespan in the body,[36] reliable estimates of the initial amount of radiation-induced chromosome damage can be made for up to about 5 weeks after an acute exposure.[9]

B. RADIATION-INDUCED CHROMOSOME ABERRATIONS

A complex variety of chromosome and chromatid breaks and rearrangements may be observed following exposures to ionizing radiation. The types of aberrations that are induced *directly* or *derived* in the second post-radiation mitosis depend upon the stage of the cell cycle during which the exposure occurred (for detailed descriptions of all classes of radiation-induced chromosome aberrations see Reference numbers 37-38). Because peripheral blood lymphocytes comprise a virtually homogeneous population of cells in a resting, premitotic stage of the cell cycle, only chromosome-type aberrations are induced following *in vivo* exposure. Seven types may be observed in conventionally stained metaphase preparations from exposed persons. These aberrations are shown diagrammatically in Figures 1 and 2, and are described briefly below.

1. Asymmetrical Chromosome-Type Aberrations
a. Acentrics

Three types of acentric aberrations may be observed at metaphase following exposure of human G_o lymphocytes to ionizing radiation. These result from single or double scissions

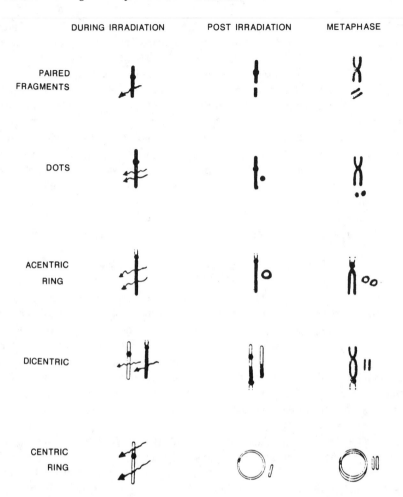

FIGURE 1.   Schematic representation of the formation of asymmetrical chromosome-type aberrations in lymphocytes exposed to ionizing radiation. The solid circle depicts the location of the centromere. See text for discussion.

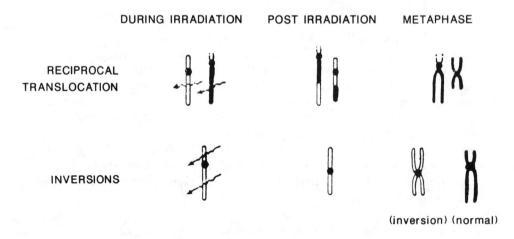

FIGURE 2.   Schematic depiction of the formation of symmetrical chromosome-type aberrations in lymphocytes exposed to ionizing radiation. See text for discussion.

in the DNA-backbone of a single chromosome, resulting in a deletion of a terminal or interstitial segment. At metaphase these deletions appear as paired fragments, ''dots'', or various sizes of acentric rings. Because it is often not possible to distinguish between small terminal and interstitial deletions, these classes of aberrations are generally pooled and classified as *excess acentrics*.

b. Dicentric (or Polycentric) Chromosomes (Asymmetrical Interchanges)
During radiation exposure, one or more radiation tracks may induce breaks in two chromosomes within the same cell nucleus. If the ''broken ends'' are within close spatial proximity, and if the breaks occur within a finite time interval, the broken ends may rejoin in an abnormal configuration, giving rise to a dicentric chromosome with an accompanying fragment. More rarely, three or more chromosomes may be involved in asymmetrical interchange formation, in which case the number of accompanying fragments will be equal to the number of centromeres minus one. Dicentric chromosomes are easily identified, occur with a low background frequency of about 1 or 2/1000 metaphases,[39,40] and are only rarely observed following exposure to chemical clastogens. For these reasons the dicentric is considered to be the most sensitive and reliable indicator of dose in persons having recent radiation exposures.

c. Centric Rings (Asymmetrical Intrachanges)
Asymmetrical intrachanges are formed when broken ends of the same chromosome are rejoined to give rise to a ring structure with its accompanying fragment. The ratio of induction of rings to dicentrics is approximately 1:8 to 1:10. Thus, although centric rings are highly typical of radiation exposure of nondividing cells, this aberration type is not as sensitive an indicator as the dicentric. An example of a metaphase exhibiting multiple asymmetrical chromosome type aberrations is shown in Figure 3. This metaphase was observed in cultured lymphocytes of a radiation accident victim contaminated with [241]Am.

2. Symmetrical Chromosome-Type Aberrations
a. Reciprocal Translocations (Symmetrical Interchanges)
Translocations are the symmetrical counterparts of dicentrics, resulting from breakage and reciprocal interchange of the telomeric segments of two chromosomes. While dicentrics and reciprocal translocations are induced with equal frequencies, microscopic ascertainment is greatly reduced in the scoring of translocations. This results from the fact that reciprocal exchanges involving equal-sized or small pieces of chromatin material can only be detected in banded metaphase preparations. On the other hand, if the exchange involves large and unequal chromatin segments, the reciprocal translocation can be readily identified via detailed microscopic analyses of unbanded metaphase preparations.

b. Inversions (Symmetrical Intrachanges)
Pericentric inversions are formed as a result of breakage and intrachange of both telomeres of a single chromosome and are, therefore, the symmetric equivalent of the centric ring. As is the case for reciprocal translocations, only those pericentric inversions which result in altered centromere ratios are detectable in nonbanded preparations. Similarly, paracentric inversions (intra-arm inversions) cannot be observed in conventionally stained metaphase preparations.

C. DOSE RESPONSE RELATIONSHIPS
To provide various ''calibration standards'' for use in dose estimation, human whole blood is exposed *in vitro* to various qualities of ionizing radiation to establish the dose dependency for aberration induction by radiations of differing linear energy transfer, or LET.

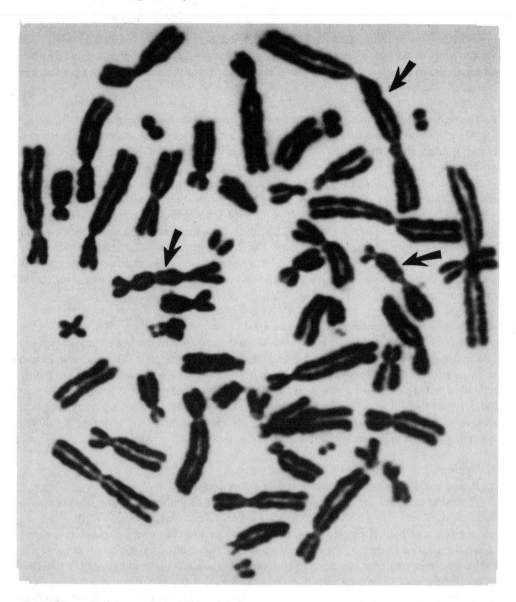

FIGURE 3.   Metaphase from lymphocyte preparations from an accident victim internally contaminated with [241]Am. Arrows identify multicentric chromsomes, also note numerous acentric fragments. Metaphases with such extensive chromosome damage are typically observed following *in vivo* or *in vitro* exposures to high-LET α particles.

Since aberration induction in lymphocytes may be influenced by a number of experimental variables (i.e., temperature[41,42] and oxygen tension,[43,44]) for such exposures, it is necessary to mimic as closely as possible the *in vivo* exposure condition. Promptly after irradiation, lymphocyte cultures are initiated and the frequencies of aberrations are quantified by scoring a representative sample of first division metaphases from each applied radiation dose.

During the past few years our laboratory at REAC/TS has derived *in vitro* dose response curves for several radiation qualities, including gamma radiation from ^{60}Co and ^{192}Ir, shielded and unshielded 220 keV X-rays, and 1.2 MeV fission spectrum neutrons. A portion of these data is described as an illustration of methods used in generating calibration curves.

For exposures to ^{60}Co and X-radiation, venous whole blood from normal adult donors was aerated for approximately 45 min, transported to a radiation facility in prewarmed

TABLE 1

Dose Dependency for Asymmetrical Aberrations in Human Lymphocytes Exposed to
⁶⁰Co Gamma or 220 kev X-Radiation

⁶⁰Co[a] dose (rad)	Cells scored	Cells with aberrations	Aberrations[b]		
			Dicentrics	Excess acentrics	Total
0	1100	2	2	1	3
25	1721	40	17	22	41
50	2230	102	51	46	107
100	689	86	54	35	96
198	500	165	122	69	207
299	500	306	289	146	472
399	650	513	626	370	1081

X-ray[c] dose (rad)	Cells scored	Cells with aberrations	Aberrations		
			Dicentrics	Excess acentrics	Total[b]
0	500	1	0	1	1
25	1500	59	26	28	63
49	1500	85	46	37	89
94	500	81	52	32	88
188	500	199	169	85	277
281	500	325	323	185	552
376	500	412	533	299	895

[a] Barnes ⁶⁰Co teletherapy unit, exposure rates measured using 621 R-chamber, roentgen-to-rad conversion factor 0.98.

[b] Aberrations scored in selected first division metaphases from BrdU substituted lymphocyte cultures. Acentrics in excess of those associated with exchanges. Total aberrations include dicentrics, acentrics, and rings.

[c] Westinghouse 250 kVp X-ray teletherapy unit operated at 220 kV and 15mA, filtration 1.0 mm Al, 1.0 mm Cu, exposure rates measured with Victoreen R-chamber, roentgen-to-rad conversion factor 0.93.

styrofoam containers (37°C), and exposed to varying radiation doses ranging from 25 to about 500 rad (0.25 to 5 Gy). Afterwards, lymphocyte cultures were established and harvested at 48 h. The frequencies of radiation-induced chromosome aberrations of the asymmetrical type were quantified by scoring first division metaphases having a complete chromosome complement (Table 1). Poisson regression analyses[45] were used to estimate the dose response parameters for various models for the dicentric/cell data for lymphocytes exposed to X- or gamma radiation. For both sets of data the dose dependency for yield of dicentrics was adequately described by the linear-quadratic model $Y = \alpha D + \beta D^2$, where Y = dicentric yield (dicentrics/cell), D = radiation dose in rad, and α and β = the slope coefficients derived from the curve fittings. In Table 2 the values for the coefficients derived from ⁶⁰Co gamma and 220 kV X-ray are compared with our earlier data obtained from *in vitro* exposures of human lymphocytes to ¹⁹²Ir gamma radiation,[24] or to 1.2 MeV, fission-spectrum neutrons.[25]

As is demonstrated by comparisons of these coefficients, dicentric yield in exposed human lymphocytes varies as a function of radiation LET with neutrons being considerably more efficient than the various low-LET radiation qualities. Similarly, these data demonstrate that, as expected, the yields of dicentrics vary as a linear function of dose following *in vitro* exposure to fission neutrons. Fitted dose response curves for these various radiation qualities are shown in Figures 4 and 5. The observed dose response relationships and coefficients from these studies are in good agreement with published data from several laboratories. For an excellent review, compilation, and discussion of published *in vitro* dose response data for human lymphocytes exposed to radiations of a wide range of LET, the reader is referred

TABLE 2
Coefficients Derived from Maximum Likelihood Fits of Dicentric Cell^{-1} Data to
Dose Response Model Y = αD + βD²

Radiation quality	Mean energy (e)	Dose rate	α(±SE) × 10⁻⁴	β(±SE) × 10⁻⁶
⁶⁰Co gamma	1.2 MeV	~50 R/min	1.57 ± 0.66	5.70 ± 0.29
¹⁹²Ir gamma	0.3 MeV	12.8 R/min	3.18 ± 1.80	6.09 ± 0.72
X-ray	220 keV	~50 R/min	4.34 ± 0.81	6.55 ± 0.39
Neutron	1.28 MeV	2 to 8 R/min	79.7 ± 1.5	—

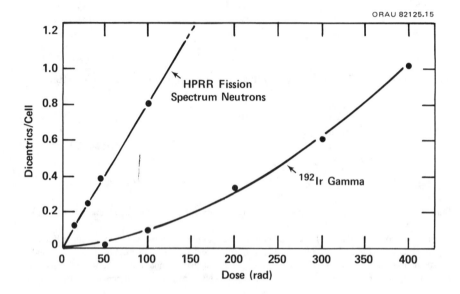

FIGURE 4.   Dose response curves for dicentric chromosomes in human lymphocytes exposed to gamma or neutron radiation. Note that the dose response relationship is linear for neutrons and curvilinear for gamma rays. Note also the increased efficiency of the neutron relative to gamma rays in the induction of chromosome aberrations.

to the report of Lloyd and Edwards.[21] The justification for use of such *in vitro* calibration curves as reference standards for estimating absorbed dose in exposed persons is based on observations in experimental animals and man that the yields of aberrations induced in lymphocytes after *in vitro* exposures are both qualitatively and quantitatively identical to those observed after *in vivo* exposures.[46-50]

Following acute whole-body exposures to penetrating radiations of a single quality, cytogenetic dosimetry studies can provide reasonably accurate estimates of radiation doses ≥ about 20 rem (0.2 Sv) when 300 to 500 metaphases are scored from the patient's cultured lymphocytes. To derive estimates of dose, the yield of aberrations/cell (usually dicentrics) observed in cultured lymphocytes from the patient is substituted for Y in the appropriate *in vitro* calibration equation which is solved for D to obtain a point estimate of dose. The statistical accuracy of the dose estimate will depend on the Poisson error associated with the estimate of aberration frequency in cells from the patient, as well as the attendant errors in the estimates of α and β coefficients derived from the dose response curves. Detailed discussions of methods for estimating confidence intervals are discussed in reference numbers 24, 26, and 45. While such calculations are straightforward in most instances of accidental exposure, attention must be given to a number of physical and biological variables that may influence the frequency of radiation-induced aberrations and thus affect the accuracy of dose estimates.

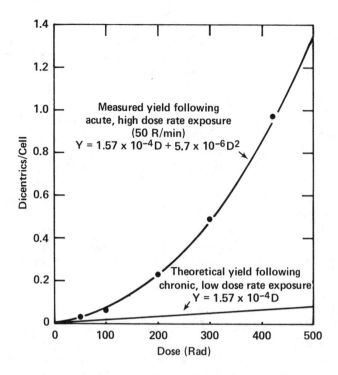

FIGURE 5.   Dose response curve for dicentrics induced in human lymphocytes exposed *in vitro* to ^{60}Co gamma radiation, compared with predicted response at very low dose rates.

D. PHYSICAL AND BIOLOGICAL FACTORS TO BE CONSIDERED IN DERIVING DOSE ESTIMATES

1. Radiation Quality

As demonstrated in the preceding paragraphs, induced aberrations in human lymphocytes vary as a function not only of radiation dose magnitude, but also of LET. Because radiation qualities having differing LET vary considerably in their relative efficiencies in inducing aberrations, the relative "sensitivity" of the lymphocyte dosimetry system will also vary, depending upon whether exposures were to penetrating high- or low-LET radiations.

Radiation LET is also important when considering the distribution of chromosome aberrations observed in lymphocytes from exposed persons. For example, when persons receive uniform whole-body exposures to penetrating low-LET radiations, all of their lymphocytes are at equal and random risk for being traversed by one (or many) sparsely ionizing radiation tracks. Thus, the relative proportion of their lymphocyte metaphases that have 0, 1, 2, or more aberrations will depend on their average whole-body dose, and the dispersion of aberrations among their cells will conform to a random "count" or Poisson distribution.[51-54] In contrast, following *in vivo* exposures to similar total doses of some types of high-LET radiations, for example, α particles emitted by various isotopes such as radium, plutonium, or americium, fewer lymphocytes will be traversed by densely ionizing tracks, and those that are traversed will probably receive larger and more variable depositions of energy. Thus the dose distribution among individual cells that are "hit" by the α particles will be quite uneven. This will result in an "overdispersion" of aberrations in cultured lymphocytes, i.e., an excess number of metaphases having multiple chromosome aberrations, as well as an excess number having no damage at all.[55-59] A further complication in applying cytogenetic dosimetry in persons having internal depositions of α particle-emitter radionuclides is that only those lymphocytes that pass within approximately 45 μm of the site(s) of deposition will be at risk for radiation exposure which results in further "nonrandomness" in the dose received by circulating lymphocytes. Because of the localized nature of the dose deposition in the body, and the unevenness of dose distribution in traversed cells, evaluations of radiation-induced aberrations in their lymphocytes will provide little information regarding whole-body dose.

2. Temporal Distribution of Dose (Dose Rate, Fractionation Effects)

In persons having potential overexposures to moderate to high doses of low-LET radiation, the distribution of dose in time becomes another important physical factor that may influence aberration yield. As a general rule, more inter- and intrachange-type aberrations are observed in lymphocytes after single, acute exposures to X- or gamma radiation delivered at high dose rates than when exposures are received in fractions, or as a single dose delivered at low dose rates (see reference numbers 61-65 for recent studies in human lymphocytes). Thus, when applying cytogenetic data for dose estimation, it is important to take into account whether the radiation dose was received acutely, in fractions, or from chronic exposures at low dose rates. Methods for estimating doses in such situations are discussed in later paragraphs.

3. Uniformity of Exposure

Many biological factors can also impact on the number of aberrations that may be observed in lymphocytes from exposed persons. Among these, degree of homogeneity (or inhomogeneity) of exposure is of major importance. In many accidental overexposures to penetrating low-LET radiations, a victim will receive a radiation dose to only a portion of the body. In these situations, only those circulating lymphocytes that pass through the radiation field will be exposed. Afterwards, the populations of exposed and nonexposed lymphocytes will be mixed as the blood circulates. The mixing will result in a "contamination" of the irradiated lymphocyte population with undamaged cells from the nonirradiated lymphocyte compartment, which will also create an "overdispersion" of aberrations similar to that observed for α particles. In exposure situations involving only a small portion of the body, such as the fingers or part of an extremity, the number of exposed lymphocytes may be so few as to preclude their detection by cytogenetic methods. However, when partial-body exposures involve one third to one half the body or more, it is possible to use degree of deviation from the Poisson distribution as a basis for estimating dose to the fraction of exposed lymphocytes.[18] A second method for estimating dose in persons having partial-body exposures employs calculations based on the relative number of aberrations/metaphase with aberrations (i.e., Qdr method[66]). An excellent discussion of these mathematical models and of their application in estimating dose to exposed fraction of lymphocytes is presented in an IAEA report.[26]

4. Time of Sampling

With increasing time after an *in vivo* radiation exposure, varying numbers of irradiated mature lymphocytes will live out their normal lifespan and be eliminated from the circulating blood. As a result of this normal lymphocyte turnover, a time-course-dependent diminution in the proportion of mitogen-responsive lymphocytes bearing unstable aberrations is observed in preparations from persons having radiation exposures. Longitudinal cytogenetic evaluations in a radiation accident victim who received an acute whole-body dose of appoximately 150 rad (1.5 Gy) gamma radiation demonstrated a significant reduction in unstable aberrations beginning at 5 to 6 weeks after exposure,[9] and long term followup evaluations in patients irradiated for ankylosing spondylitis have demonstrated a 40% decrease in the proportion of lymphocytes bearing unstable aberrations per year during the first 4 years after exposure.[36] Thus, accurate *direct* estimates of the proportion of unstable aberrations induced in circulating lymphocytes can be made only when blood samples are obtained for cytogenetic evaluation within the first several weeks after exposure. With later sampling times, one must apply corrections for the loss of aberrations as a function of elapsed time since exposure.[38] Because the rate of lymphocyte turnover may vary considerably between individuals, any corrections based on estimates of lymphocyte lifespan will carry large errors of uncertainty.

III. EXAMPLE OF DOSE ESTIMATION USING *IN VITRO* CALIBRATION CURVES: STUDIES IN TEN PERSONS EXPOSED TO ⁶⁰Co GAMMA RADIATION IN THE 1984 MEXICAN ACCIDENT

As previously noted, cytogenetic dosimetry estimates accurately reflect dose in instances of acute whole-body exposures to penetrating radiations of a single radiation quality. However, cytogenetic dose estimation becomes more complicated in situations involving intermittent or protracted exposures to sparsely ionizing radiation. To illustrate factors that must be taken into account in the use of calibration curves for estimating dose in such instances, we will describe our cytogenetic evaluations in ten persons exposed to ⁶⁰Co gamma radiation in the 1984 Mexican accident.

A. DESCRIPTION OF ACCIDENT

The circumstances surrounding the Mexican ⁶⁰Co radiation accident have been described in detail in a technical report prepared by The Mexican *Direccion General de Communicacion Social*[67] and will be described only briefly here. The radioactive source involved was a Picker® C-3000 teletherapy unit that contained about 6010 pellets of ⁶⁰Co. Each pellet was approximately 1 mm² in size, and had an estimated activity of 0.07 Ci. In late November, 1983, the source head was removed from a warehouse, and on or about December 6, 1983, the ruptured source capsule and various other pieces of scrap metal were sold to the Yonke Fenix scrap yard in Juarez. Several hundred ⁶⁰Co pellets had been scattered in the rear of the pickup truck used for delivery, while the remainder became mixed with other scrap metal during processing in the junkyard. The junkyard grounds were found to have varying amounts of radioactivity including hot spots emitting surface exposures of up to 600 R/h in an area near the scales that were used to weigh scrap metal. The contaminated truck was parked on a residential street for appoximately 5 to 6 weeks. When the truck was discovered on January 26, 1984, exposure rates measured at a distance of 1 m from the truck ranged from 8 R/h on the righthand side to 50 R/h on the lefthand side.

B. EXPOSURE HISTORIES OF TEN PERSONS ON WHOM CYTOGENETIC EVALUATIONS WERE CONDUCTED

Blood samples were collected on February 18, 1984, from four persons having suspected overexposures, and on March 24, 1984, from six additional persons. Immediately afterwards the vacutainer tubes were packaged in ice in insulated containers and hand carried to Oak Ridge. Within 24 h, lymphocyte cultures were initiated for evaluation of radiation-induced aberrations. The ten persons evaluated included five male employees who had worked at the Yonke Fenix junkyard for approximately 1 to 2 h/d for an estimated interval of 10 to 15 working days before the ⁶⁰Co contamination was discovered (Table 3). Four of these men were subsequently found to have a depression of lymphocyte counts, and two (MEX 1 and MEX 2) were found to be azospermic. Cytogenetic evaluations were also undertaken on the 14-year-old son of MEX 3, who was a frequent visitor to the junkyard; the 31-year-old driver of the contaminated truck; his 5-year-old son, who had played on the truck; his 28-year-old wife, who had been at risk for exposure during the one-week time period that the truck (8 R/h side) was parked in front of her residential dwelling; and a 64-year-old neigh-

TABLE 3
Exposure Histories of Persons for Whom Cytogenetic Analyses were Done

Code	Age	Sex	Identification
MEX 1	16	M	Junkyard worker
MEX 2	28	M	Junkyard worker
MEX 3	39	M	Junkyard worker
MEX 4	24	M	Junkyard worker
MEX 5	14	M	Son of MEX 3, visitor to junkyard
MEX 6	44	M	Junkyard worker
MEX 7	31	M	Driver of contaminated truck
MEX 8	5	M	Son of MEX 7, played on contaminated truck
MEX 9	28	F	Wife of MEX 7, truck parked across street from dwelling ~1 week
MEX 10	64	F	Neighborhood resident, truck parked in front of dwelling ~5 to 6 weeks

TABLE 4
Frequencies of Radiation-Induced Aberrations in First Division Lymphocyte Metaphases

Subject	No. metaphases	Metaphases with damage	No. dicentrics	No. centric rings	No. acentrics[a]
		February 18, 1984			
MEX 1	500	104	69	9	37
MEX 2	500	145	119	11	37
MEX 3	500	7	4	1	2
MEX 4	500	4	2	0	2
		March 24, 1984			
MEX 5	500	28	16	4	9
MEX 6	500	16	10	1	4
MEX 7	500	69	48	4	20
MEX 8	500	28	13	4	13
MEX 9	500	6	1	0	5
MEX 10	500	114	59	9	53

[a] Acentric rings, + terminal deletions, + interstitial deletions.

borhood resident, who was at risk for exposure for a period of 5 to 6 weeks during which the contaminated truck (50 R/h side) was parked within 20 ft of the front of her dwelling.

C. RESULTS

A total of 500 diploid first division metaphases was scored from cultures from each patient (Table 4). The observed numbers of metaphases with chromosome-type aberrations ranged from 4 to 145 in the 500 cell samples from individual subjects, while the frequencies of dicentrics ranged from 1 to 119. The greatest amount of cytogenetic damage was observed in lymphocytes from two of the junkyard workers (MEX 1 and 2), the truck driver (MEX 7) and the 64-year-old woman whose residence was across the street from the contaminated truck (MEX 10). When the frequencies of metaphases with 0, 1, 2, etc. rings and dicentrics were compared to the expected values from the Poisson distribution, the test statistics demonstrated a highly significant overdispersion in preparations from MEX 2 and MEX 8 (Table 5). In contrast, only a single metaphase having two aberrations was observed in cultures from MEX 10, while four were expected.

TABLE 5
Distribution of Rings and Dicentrics in Damaged Metaphases

Subject	No. metaphases	No. R + D	$\bar{X}$		Number of metaphases with 0, 1, 2, etc.			
					0	1	2	3
MEX 1	500	78	0.156	Obs.[a]	430	62	8	0
				Exp.[a]	427	68	5	0
MEX 2[b]	500	130	0.26	Obs.	392	90	14	4
				Exp.	385	101	13	1
MEX 3	500	5	0.01	Obs.	495	5	0	0
				Exp.	495	5	0	0
MEX 4	500	2	0.004	Obs.	498	2	0	0
				Exp.	498	2	0	0
MEX 5	500	20	0.04	Obs.	480	20	0	0
				Exp.	480	20	0	0
MEX 6	500	11	0.022	Obs.	489	11	0	0
				Exp.	489	11	0	0
MEX 7	500	52	0.104	Obs.	452	45	2	1
				Exp.	450	48	2	0
MEX 8[b]	500	17	0.034	Obs.	485	13	2	0
				Exp.	483	17	0	0
MEX 9	500	1	0.002	Obs.	499	1	0	0
				Exp.	499	1	0	0
MEX 10	500	68	0.136	Obs.	433	66	1	0
				Exp.	436	60	4	0

[a] *Observed* number of metaphases with 0, 1, 2, etc. Ring or dicentric chromosomes compared with *expected* frequencies based on Poisson distribution.
[b] Significantly overdispersed relative to expected distribution.

D. CYTOGENETIC DOSE ESTIMATES: THEORETICAL CONSIDERATIONS

In the present accident it is virtually certain that none of these persons received their dose as a single acute exposure. Because of the uncertainties regarding their respective exposure scenarios, we have used the cytogenetic data to derive point estimates of the upper and lower limits of dose that each person may have received during the several weeks they were at risk for exposure.

Our calculations of minimum and maximum doses are based on the following theoretical considerations. As previously discussed, the dose-response curve for dicentric induction in lymphocytes acutely exposed to high doses of low-LET radiation is accurately described by the linear quadratic model $Y = \alpha D + \beta D^2$ (where Y = the yield of dicentrics and D = radiation dose). When interpreted in terms of the "breakage first theory"[1] the alpha coefficient describes the dose dependency for dicentrics induced by single radiation tracks and is, thus, dose-rate independent. The beta term describes the dose dependency for dicentrics induced by two or more tracks and predominates at high radiation doses. Because the molecular lesions that lead to dicentric formation are available for interaction for a finite period of time (estimated to be approximately 2 h in lymphocytes[62,63]) it follows that the frequency of dicentrics induced by two separate ionizing tracks will be highly dependent on dose rate. If, as a result of the lowering of the dose rate or of increasing the number of fractions, the temporal density of the ionizing tracks is reduced to the point that all dicentrics result from single track events, then the theoretical yield of aberrations would be described by the equation $Y = \alpha D$. For intermediate dose rates delivered within specific lengths of time, it is possible to modify the beta term by applying a time-dependent or "repair" term[62] such as the G function described by Lea and Catcheside.[68] In the present accident situation the dose-rate for any person at any given time was not known, and it was thus not possible to estimate a specific repair term.

TABLE 6

"Limiting" Whole-Body[a] Dose Estimates for Ten Persons Accidentally Exposed to
⁶⁰Co Gamma Radiation

Patient	No. metaphases	No. dicentrics	Dicentric/cell	Dose estimates[a]	
				Acute exposure	Continuous protracted exposure
MEX 1	500	69	0.138	142	~879
MEX 2	500	119	0.238	191	~1,516
MEX 3	500	4	0.008	26	~51
MEX 4	500	2	0.004	16	~25
MEX 5	500	16	0.032	62	~204
MEX 6	500	10	0.02	47	~127
MEX 7	500	48	0.096	117	~611
MEX 8	500	13	0.026	55	~166
MEX 9	500	1	0.002	9	~13
MEX 10	500	59	0.118	131	~752

a   Our preliminary dose estimates for these ten subjects (which were included in tabular form in Reference 67) were calculated using published coefficients of ⁶⁰Co gamma radiation.[34] For these definitive estimates we employed coefficients we derived from subsequent *in vitro* radiations performed in our laboratory. The two sets of coefficients produce remarkably similar point estimates of doses.

E. ESTIMATES OF MINIMUM AND MAXIMUM WHOLE-BODY DOSES

To obtain estimates of the minimum and maximum equivalent whole-body doses that these ten persons may have received, we employed our coefficients for dicentric induction in human lymphocytes exposed *in vitro* to ⁶⁰Co gamma radiation delivered at a dose-rate of 50 R/min (Figure 5).

For these calculations, our "acute exposure" provides the point estimate of the minimum dose of ⁶⁰Co radiation that could have yielded the observed dicentric frequency in human lymphocytes. The dose calculations assume that the persons received a single acute dose delivered at high-dose rates, calculated by the formula:

$$Y = 1.57 \times 10^{-4} D + 5.7 \times 10^{-6} D^2 \tag{1}$$

The "continuous protracted exposure" provides the point estimate of the *maximum* dose of ⁶⁰Co radiation that could have yielded the observed dicentric frequency. This dose calculation assumes that the persons received a continuous, protracted dose, delivered at very low dose rates, calculated by formula:

$$Y = 1.57 \times 10^{-4} D \tag{2}$$

These maximum and minimum estimates produced from the above calculations (Table 6) are useful in describing the upper and lower "limits" of doses that these persons could have received. However, in reality, neither the single acute nor the chronic low dose rate exposure describes the actual exposure conditions for the ten persons, and thus, their true doses should lie somewhere in between these upper and lower estimates. Considerations of distribution of dicentrics in damaged cells and the ratios of dicentrics to acentrics in cultures from several of these persons provide additional information on the nature of their exposures.

For example, statistical comparisons of the distribution of rings and dicentrics in damaged metaphases demonstrated an excess of metaphases with multiple aberrations in preparations from one of the junkyard workers (MEX 2) and from the 5-year-old son of the truck driver (MEX 8). As discussed earlier, such overdispersion of aberrations in lymphocyte cultures is typically observed following nonhomogeneous exposures to low-LET radiation where a portion of the body receives a higher dose than the remainder. Since there were known hot spots in the junkyard, and since the radioactive pellets were scattered nonuniformly in the rear of the truck, it is likely that both the junkyard worker and the 5-year-old child could have received acute high doses to some portions of the body for at least a portion of their total exposure. Similarly, one would not expect to see a high percentage of metaphases with multiple aberrations after chronic exposures to very low dose-rate radiations, since it is highly unlikely that a single low-LET radiation track could induce molecular lesions in several chromosomes that would be required for the expression of multiple dicentrics. Thus the distribution data suggest that MEX 1, 2, 7, and 8 received at least a portion of their dose at very high dose rate and provide evidence that their true doses are probably closer to the minimum than to the maximum estimates.

In contrast, in MEX 10 only a single metaphase with two dicentrics was observed out of a total of 67 cells bearing dicentrics. Based on Poisson expectations, four cells with two dicentrics would have been expected in preparations from this individual. Such a situation could evolve if, as a result of exposures to very low dose-rate radiation, the number of ionizing events per nucleus was so sparse that virtually all exchange aberrations in her lymphocytes resulted from single tracks. That the 64-year-old woman may have received a majority of her exposure as a chronic low dose rate is also suggested by our observations of approximately equal numbers of dicentrics and acentrics in her preparations. It is well known from *in vitro* dose response systems that the induced frequency of dicentrics and excess acentrics are about equal after low-dose magnitude exposures (i.e., when single track aberrations predominate). At high doses of radiation delivered at high dose rates (i.e., when two-track aberrations predominate), higher numbers of exchange aberrations are induced relative to acentrics. In preparations from MEX 1, 2, and 7, the ratio of dicentrics to acentrics was about 2:1, whereas in MEX 10 the ratio was 1:1. This observation also suggests that she received a significant portion of her dose as a chronic low-level exposure. In this particular individual it thus appears that the upper limit of dose may more closely approximate her exposure condition.

IV. SUMMARY

In radiation accidents in which persons are at risk for either intermittent or protracted exposures for periods of several days to several weeks, it is not possible to accurately reconstruct their exposure scenarios, and for this reason physical estimates of dose become quite tenuous. In such instances, biological indicators provide the only realistic measures of dose absorbed by various persons. Our cytogenetic evaluations in ten persons having potential exposures to ^{60}Co gamma radiation in the recent Mexican accident provided evidence that each had received radiation overexposures. To derive limiting estimates of doses for each person from the cytogenetic findings, we used *in vitro* dose-response models for dicentric induction in human lymphocytes. Dose estimates were made assuming that the exposures occurred either as a single acute event or protracted at a continuous low rate. These theoretical calculations provided estimates of the minimum and maximum doses of ^{60}Co radiation that could have yielded the observed dicentric frequency. Statistical analyses of the individual distributions of aberrations in damaged metaphases and comparisons of the ratios of the dicentrics to acentrics also provided information of assistance in interpreting the cytogenetic data to determine biological dose in these exposed individuals.

ACKNOWLEDGMENTS

The authors acknowledge the expert assistance of Dr. E. L. Frome in performing Poisson regression curve fittings and other statistical analyses; and Drs. Cristina de Nava, Patricia Ostrosky, and Osvaldo Mutchinick, Ciudad Universitaria, Mexico City, for all their assistance and helpful discussion of the cytogenetic data. We especially acknowledge Dr. Herbert Ortega, PAHO Field Office in El Paso, who worked closely with REAC/TS staff in these and other studies.

REFERENCES

1. **Sax, K.,** Chromosome aberrations induced by X-rays, *Genetics*, 23, 494, 1938.
2. **Catcheside, D. G., Lea, D. E., and Thoday, J. M.,** The production of chromosome structural changes in *Tradescantia* microspores in relation to dosage, intensity and temperature, *J. Genet.*, 47, 137, 1946.
3. **Giles, N.,** Radiation-induced chromosome aberrations in *Tradescantia*, *Rad. Biol.*, I, 713, 1954.
4. **Lea, D.,** *Actions of Radiations on Living Cells*, The Cambridge University Press, Cambridge, 1955.
5. **Moorhead, P., Nowell, P., Mellman, W., Battips, D., and Hungerford, D.,** Chromosome preparations of leukocytes cultured from human peripheral blood, *Exp. Cell Res.*, 20, 613, 1960.
6. **Tough, I., Buckton, K., Baikie, A., and Court-Brown, W.,** X-ray-induced chromosome damage in man, *Lancet*, 2, 849, 1960.
7. **Bender, M.,** Chromosome aberrations in irradiated human subjects, *Ann. N.Y. Acad. Sci.*, 114, 249, 1964.
8. **Bender, M. and Gooch, P.,** Somatic chromosome aberrations induced by human whole body irradiation: the "Recuplex" criticality accident, *Rad. Res.*, 29, 568, 1966.
9. **Brewen, J., Preston, R., and Littlefield, L.,** Radiation-induced human chromosome aberration yields following an accidental whole-body exposure to ^{60}Co gamma rays, *Radiat. Res.*, 48, 647, 1972.
10. **Jammet, H., Gongora, R., LeGo, R., and Doloy, M. T.,** Clinical and biological comparison of two acute accidental irradiations: Mol (1965) and Brescia (1975), in *The Medical Basis for Radiation Accident Preparedness*, Hubner, K. F. and Fry, S. A., Eds., Elsevier/North Holland, New York, 1980, 91.
11. **Stavem, P., Brogger, A., Devik, F., Flatby, J., van der Hagen, C., Henriksen, T., Hoel, P., Host, H., Kett, K., and Petersen, B.,** Lethal acute gamma radiation accident at Kjeller, Norway: report of a case, *Acta Radiol. Oncol.*, 24, 61, 1985.
12. **Lloyd, D. C., Edwards, A. A., and Prosser, J. S.,** Accidental intake of tritiated water: a report of two cases, *Radiat. Prot. Dosim.*, 15, 191, 1986.
13. **Hirashima, K., Sugiyama, H., Ishihara, T., Kurisu, A., Hashizume, T., and Kumatori, T.,** The 1971 Chiba, Japan, Accident: exposure to Iridium 192, in *The Medical Basis of Radiation Accident Preparedness*, Hubner, K. F. and Fry, S. A., Eds., Elsevier/North Holland, New York, 1980, 179.
14. Summary Report on the Post-Accident Review Meeting on the Chernobyl Accident, Saf. Ser. 75-INSAG-1, International Atomic Energy Agency, Vienna, 1986.
15. **Lloyd, D. C., Edwards, A. A., Prosser, J. S., Moquet, J. E., and Finnon, P.,** Doses in radiation accidents investigated by chromosome aberration analysis. XVII. A review of cases investigated, 1986, National Radiological Protection Board-R207, Chilton, Didcot, Oxon, 1987.
16. **Littlefield, L. G., Joiner, E. E., DuFrain, R. J., Hubner, K. F., and Beck, W. L.,** Cytogenetic dose estimates from *in vivo* samples from persons involved in real or suspected radiation exposures, in *The Medical Basis of Radiation Accident Preparedness*, Hubner, K. F. and Fry, S. A., Eds., Elsevier/North Holland, New York, 1980, 375.
17. **Bender, M.,** Human radiation cytogenetics, *Adv. Radiat. Biol.*, 3, 215, 1969.
18. **Dolphin, G. W.,** Biological dosimetry with particular reference to chromosome aberration analysis, in *Handling of Radiation Accidents*, International Atomic Energy Agency, Vienna, 1969, 215.
19. **Dolphin, G. and Lloyd, D.,** The significance of radiation-induced chromosome abnormalities in radiological protection, *J. Med. Genet.*, 11, 181, 1974.
20. **Lloyd, D. and Purrott, R.,** Chromosome aberration analysis in radiological protection dosimetry, *Radiat. Prot. Dosim.*, 1, 19, 1981.
21. **Lloyd, D. C. and Edwards, A. A.,** Chromosome aberrations in human lymphocytes: effect of radiation quality, dose, and dose rate, in *Radiation-Induced Chromosome Damage in Man*, Ishihara, T. and Sasaki, M. S., Eds., Alan R. Liss, New York, 1983, 23.
22. **Lloyd, D. C.,** An overview of radiation dosimetry by conventional cytogenetic methods, in *Biological Dosimetry*, Eisert, W. G. and Mendelsohn, M. L., Eds., Springer-Verlag, Berlin-Heidelberg, 1984, 3.
23. **Bauchinger, M.,** Cytogenetic effects in human lymphocytes as a dosimetry system, in *Biological Dosimetry*, Eisert, W. G. and Mendelsohn, M. L., Eds., Springer-Verlag, Berlin-Heidelberg, 1984, 15.

24. **DuFrain, R. J., Littlefield, L. G., Joiner, E. E., and Frome, E. L.,** *In vitro* human cytogenetic dose-response systems, in *The Medical Basis of Radiation Accident Preparedness,* Hubner, K. F. and Fry, S. A., Eds., Elsevier/North Holland, New York 1980, 357.

25. **Littlefield, L. G.,** The analysis of radiation-induced chromosome lesions in lymphocytes as a biological method for dose estimation, Proc. NATO Working Group Meeting Assessment of Injury from Ionizing Radiation in Warfare, Armed Forces Radiobiology Research Institute, 1982, 351.

26. Biological dosimetry: Chromosomal aberration analysis for dose assessment, Tech. Rep. Ser. 260, International Atomic Energy Agency, Vienna, 1986.

27. **Zakharov, A. and Egolina, N.,** Differential spirialization along mammalian mitotic chromosomes. I. BrdU-revealed differentiation in Chinese hamster chromosomes, *Chromosoma,* 38, 341, 1972.

28. **Perry, P. and Wolff, S.,** New Giemsa method for the differential staining of sister chromatids, *Nature,* 251, 156, 1974.

29. **Scott, D. and Lyons, C. Y.,** Homogeneous sensitivity of human peripheral blood lymphocytes to radiation-induced chromosome damage, *Nature,* 278, 756, 1979.

30. **Buckton, K. and Pike, M.,** Time in culture. An important variable in studying the *in vivo* radiation-induced chromosome damage in man, *Int. J. Rad. Biol.,* 8, 439, 1964.

31. **Heddle, J., Evans, H., and Scott, D.,** Sampling time and the complexity of the human leukocyte culture system, in *Human Radiation Cytogenetics,* Vol. 6, North-Holland, Amsterdam, 1967.

32. **Dewey, W. C., Furman, S. C., and Miller, H. H.,** Comparison of lethality and chromosomal damage induced by X-rays in synchronized chinese hamster cells *in vitro, Radiat. Res.,* 43, 561, 1970.

33. **Carrano, A. V.,** Chromosome aberrations and radiation-induced cell death. II. Predicted and observed cell survival, *Mutat. Res.,* 17, 355, 1973.

34. **Lloyd, D. C., Purrott, R. J., Dolphins, G. W., Bolton, D., and Edwards, A. A.,** The relationship between chromosome aberrations and low LET radiation dose to human lymphocytes, *Int. J. Radiat. Biol.,* 28, 75, 1975.

35. **Bauchinger, M., Schmid, E., and Braselmann, H.,** Cell survival and radiation induced chromosome aberrations. II. Experimental findings in human lymphocytes analysed in first and second post-irradiation metaphases, *Radiat. Environ. Biophys.,* 25, 253, 1986.

36. **Buckton, K. E.,** Chromosome aberrations in patients treated with X-irradiation for ankylosing spondylitis, in *Radiation-Induced Chromosome Damage in Man,* Ishihara, T., and Sasaki, M. S., Eds., Alan R. Liss, New York 1983, 491.

37. **Evans, H. and O'Riordan, M.,** Human peripheral blood lymphocytes for the analysis of chromosome aberrations in mutagen tests, *Mutat. Res.,* 31, 135, 1975.

38. **Bender, M., Awa, A., Brooils, A., Evans, J., Groer, P., Littlefield, G., Pereira, C., Preston, J., and Wachholz, B.,** Current status of cytogenetic procedures to detect and quantify previous exposures to radiation, *Mutat. Res.,* 196, 103, 1988.

39. **Lloyd, D. C., Purrott, R. J., and Reeder, E. J.,** The incidence of unstable chromosome aberrations in peripheral blood lymphocytes from unirradiated and occupationally exposed people, *Mutat. Res.,* 72, 523, 1980.

40. **Galloway, S. M., Berry, P. K., Nichols, W. W., Wolman, S. R., Soper, K. A., Stolley, P. D., and Archer, P.,** Chromosome aberrations in individuals occupationally exposed to ethylene oxide, and in a large control population, *Mutat. Res.,* 170, 55, 1986.

41. **Bajerska, A. and Liniecki, J.,** The influence of temperature at irradiation in vitro on the yield of chromosomal aberrations in peripheral blood lymphocytes, *Int. J. Radiat. Biol.,* 16, 483, 1969.

42. **Purrott, R. J. and Lloyd, D. C.,** The study of chromosome aberration yield in human lymphocytes as an indicator of radiation dose. I. Techniques, NRPB-R2 National Radiological Protection Board, Harwell, England, 1972.

43. **Prosser, J. S. and Stimpson, L. D.,** The influence of anoxia or oxygenation on the induction of chromosome aberrations in human lymphocytes by 15-MeV neutrons, *Mutat. Res.,* 84, 365, 1981.

44. **Prosser, J. S., White, C. M., and Edwards, A. A.,** The effect of oxygen concentration on the X-ray induction of chromosome aberrations in human lymphocytes, *Mutat. Res.,* 61, 287, 1979.

45. **Frome, E. L. and DuFrain, R. J.,** maximum likelihood estimation for cytogentic dose-response curves, *Biometrics,* 42, 73, 1986.

46. **Bajerska, A. and Liniecki, J.,** The yield of chromosomal aberrations in rabbit lymphocytes after irradiation *in vitro* and *in vivo, Mutat. Res.,* 27, 271, 1975.

47. **Clemenger, J. and Scott, D.,** A comparison of chromosome aberration yields in rabbit blood lymphocytes irradiated *in vitro* and *in vivo, Int. J. Radiat. Biol.,* 24, 487, 1973.

48. **Brewen, J. and Gengozian, N.,** Radiation-induced human chromosome aberrations. II. Human *in vitro* irradiation compared to *in vitro* and *in vivo* irradiation of marmoset leukocytes, *Mutat. Res.,* 13, 383, 1971.

49. **Buckton, K. E., Langlands, A. O., Smith, P. G., Woodcock, G. E., and Looby, P. C.,** Further studies on chromosome aberrations. Production after whole-body irradiation in man, *Int. J. Radiat. Biol.,* 19, 369, 1971.

50. **Schmid, E. and Bauchinger, M.,** Comparison of the chromosome damage and its dose response after medical whole-body exposures to ^{60}Co γ-rays and irradiation of blood, *in vitro, Int. J. Radiat. Biol.,* 26, 31, 1974.

51. **Norman, A. and Sasaki, M. S.,** Chromosome-exchange aberrations in human lymphocytes, *Int. J. Radiat. Biol.,* 11, 321, 1966.

52. **Savage, J. R. K.,** Sites of radiation induced chromosome exchanges, *Current Topics in Radiation Research,* Vol. 6, Ebert, M., and Howard, A., Eds., Elsevier, New York, 1970, 129.

53. **Edwards, A. A., Lloyd, D. C., and Purrott, R. J.,** Radiation induced chromosome aberrations and the Poisson distribution, *Radiat. Environ. Biophys.,* 16, 89, 1979.

54. **Lloyd, D. C.,** The Problems of Interpreting Aberration Yields Induced by *In Vivo* Irradiation of Lymphocytes, in *Mutagen-Induced Chromosome Damage in Man,* Evans, H. J. and Lloyd, D. C., Eds., Yale University Press, New Haven, 1978, 77.

55. **DuFrain, R. J., Littlefield, L. G., Joiner, E. E., and Frome, E. L.,** Human cytogenetic dosimetry: a dose response relationship for alpha particle radiation from americium 241, *Health Phys.,* 37, 279, 1979.

56. **Purrott, R. J., Edwards, A. A., Lloyd, D. C., and Stather, J. W.,** The induction of chromosome aberrations in human lymphocytes by *in vitro* irradiation with α-particles from plutonium-239, *Int. J. Radiat. Biol.,* 38, 277, 1980.

57. **Edwards, A. A., Purrott, R. J., Prosser, J. S., and Lloyd, D. C.,** The induction of chromosome aberrations in human lymphocytes by alpha-radiation, *Int. J. Radiat. Biol.,* 38, 83, 1980.

58. **Littlefield, L. G., Joiner, E., DuFrain, R. J., Colyer, S., and Breitenstein, B.,** Six-year cytogenetic follow-up study of an individual heavily contaminated with americium 241, in *Dosimetry, Radionuclides, and Technology,* Sect. E3-05, Broerse, J. J., Barendsen, G. W., Kal, H. G., and van der Kogel, A. J., Eds., Proc. VII Int. Cong. Radiation Research, Martinus Nijhoff, Amsterdam, 1983.

59. **Fischer, P. and Golob, E.,** Chromosome aberrations in peripheral blood cells in man following chronic irradiation from internal deposits of thorotrast, *Radiat. Res.,* 29, 505, 1966.

61. **Purrott, R. and Reeder, E.,** Chromosome aberration yields in human lymphocytes induced by fractionated doses of X-radiation, *Mutat. Res.,* 34, 437, 1976.

62. **Bauchinger, M., Schmid, E., and Dresp, J.,** Calculation of the dose-rate dependence of the dicentric yield after ^{60}CO γ-irradiation of human lymphocytes, *Int. J. Radiat. Biol. Relat. Stud. Phys. Chem. Med.,* 35, 229, 1979.

63. **Lloyd, D. C., Edwards, A. A., Prosser, J. S., and Corp, M. J.,** The dose response relationship obtained at constant irradiation times for the induction of chromosome aberrations in human lymphocytes by Cobalt-60 gamma rays, *Radiat. Environ. Biophys.,* 23, 179, 1984.

64. NCRP Report No. 64, Influence of dose and its distribution in time on dose-response relationships for low-LET radiations, National Council on Radiation Protection and Measurements, Washington, D.C., 1980.

65. **Brewen, J. G. and Luippold, H. E.,** Radiation-induced human chromosome aberrations: *in vitro* dose rate studies, *Mutat. Res.,* 12, 305, 1971.

66. **Sasaki, M. S.,** Use of lymphocyte chromosome aberrations in biological dosimetry: possibilities and limitations, in *Radiation-Induced Chromosome Damage in Man,* Ishihara, T. and Sasaki, M. S., Eds., Alan R. Liss, New York, 1983, 585.

67. Accidente por Contaminacion con Cobalto-60, CNSNS-IT-001, Direccion General de Communicacion Social, Mexico, 1984.

68. **Lea, D. E. and Catcheside, D. G.,** The mechanism of the induction by radiation of chromosome aberrations in *Tradescantia, J. Genet.,* 44, 216, 1942.

Chapter 9

ASSESSMENT AND MANAGEMENT OF LOCAL RADIATION INJURY

Fred. A. Mettler, Jr.

TABLE OF CONTENTS

I. INTRODUCTION

Although one would like to clearly differentiate whole-body exposure from local exposure, the truth is that there is usually a gradient of absorbed radiation dose in any accident (Figure 1). Those accidents in which the dose to the trunk of the body is high enough to cause systemic symptoms (acute radiation syndrome) are often classified as whole-body exposure. Those accidents in which a small area of the body is exposed to a very high dose and the rest of the body is exposed to a relatively low dose (such that symptoms are predominantly in an extremity or small area) are usually referred to as local radiation injury. Between 1944 and 1985, the radiation accident registry of the Radiation Emergency Assistance Center/Training Site in Oak Ridge, Tennessee, show that of 263 major radiation accidents, 150 involved severe local injuries, with 117 of these being from exposure to sealed radioactive sources. Most of these injuries occurred from unsafe handling of ^{192}Ir or ^{60}Co industrial radiography sources.[1]

It should be pointed out there have been some accidents, particularly in the early criticality experiences at Los Alamos Laboratories (Figures 2 and 3) and later at Chernobyl, in which patients have received significant lethal whole-body doses as well as much higher doses to the skin or extremities. Under these circumstances, the local and systemic radiation injuries may potentiate each other resulting in a significantly higher morbidity or mortality than would occur with either alone. Localized exposures to the trunk of the body in which effects primarily involve the gastrointestinal system or bone marrow are covered in Chapter 6.

Assessment of local radiation injuries can be quite complicated; however, there may be clinical changes which provide clues and useful information. Of course, a detailed history is very valuable and should be obtained as soon as possible. The longer one waits in obtaining a history, the less reliable are the facts. Temporal factors are among the most important points to be determined. Prognosis and treatment depends upon whether the exposure occurred recently or a long time ago and whether the total exposure was delivered in a matter of minutes (acute) or days or over a matter of months (chronic).

II. ACUTE LOCAL IRRADIATION

As has been mentioned earlier, most local radiation accidents involve the hand.[2,3] One reason for this is that objects which are not known to be highly radioactive are inadvertently picked up and the source often is a high level of activity. Another prime offender (causing radiation of the hands) is maintenance of machines which are radiation sources. In many incidences repairmen place their hands in or near the radiation beam not realizing the machine is on and producing radiation.

The second most common body site of local radiation injury is the thighs and buttocks.[4] Irradiation of these sites occurs predominantly from industrial radionuclide sources (Figures 4 and 5). Sometimes these are placed in the pants pockets and cause extremely high exposures to the thigh (front pocket) and buttocks (back pocket). Most of the industrial sources are ^{192}Ir or ^{60}Co and produce doses in the thousand-rad (tens of Gy) range per Curie. At 1 cm, the dose rate from these sources drops quickly and is approximately 1 to 10% of the contact dose (Table 1). Such radionuclide sources are sealed in a capsule. Part of the unusually high surface dose is due, in part, to production of electrons within the wall of the capsule. Approximate dose rates to the hand for different sealed sources are also shown in Table 1. The most frequent complaint following such accidents is a superficial feeling of irritation, tenderness, or itching within the first 7 to 14 d. There is restricted motion or stiffness sometimes noted, as well as a transient erythema and/or edema. Between 10 to 30 d, bulla formation or ulceration may begin. Treatment of the acute phases listed here is generally symptomatic and can be approached by simply maintaining cleanliness and trying to prevent infection with antibiotic ointments. Immobilization may also be useful.

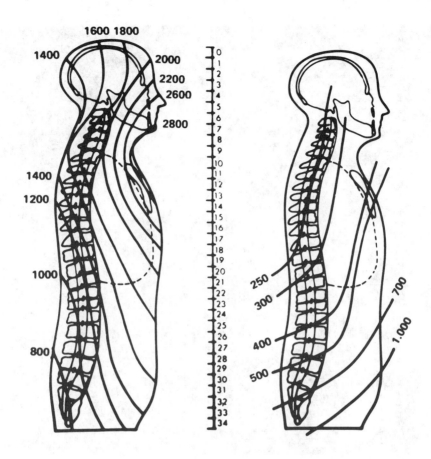

FIGURE 1. Isodose curves illustrating asymetric gradient of absorbed dose across the body in two different accidents. (From Lushbaugh, C. C., Fry, S. A., Hubner, K. F., et al., in *The Medical Basis for Radiation Accident Preparedness*, Hubner, K. F. and Fry, S. A., Eds., Elsevier, New York, 1980. With permission.)

Although such lesions are usually limited to small areas, in some instances they have been relatively large (as much as 9 cm in extent). They are rarely more than 2 cm deep and, in initial stages, there are areas of necrosis surrounded by a 2- to 4-cm-wide area of intense erythema. The principal reason that there is relatively little acute tissue effect beyond 2 to 3 cm past the area of necrosis is due to tissue attenuation and the inverse square law. Thus there is a rapid dropoff of dose with distances as small as 1 or 2 cm from the source (Figure 6). In the absence of infection, there often is not much pain and there may be spontaneous resolution of the lesion over a period of 6 to 8 weeks. Unfortunately, however, the lesion may return in 6 months to 2 years due to progressive vascular insufficiency (Figure 7). If the area does not heal, grafting may be useful to relieve pain, cover the area, and restore function.

If a local lesion is due to contact with a gamma-emitting radionuclide source, often a full thickness flap with a vascular pedicle can be utilized[4-7] (Figure 8). Management of such lesions should be individualized for each patient. In circumstances where the fingers are involved, appropriate skin grafting may not be possible and if gangrenous changes occur, amputation usually will be necessary. Most patients resist amputation of extremities until it is clear that healing will not occur through the use of conservative methods.

In addition to the typical accidents which involve hands and legs there have been a few rather bizarre incidents of local radiation injury. There has been at least one documented

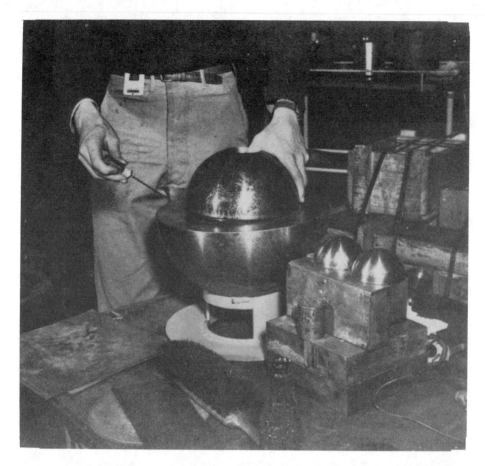

FIGURE 2.   Mock-up of early criticality accident at Los Alamos National Laboratory. Circular object represents weapons component which underwent criticality upon addition of neutron-reflecting material. Extensive exposure to hands and trunk of body followed. (From *The Medical Basis for Radiation Accident Preparedness*, Hubner, K. F. and Fry, S. A., Eds., Elsevier, New York, 1980, 22. With permission.)

successful suicide attempt utilizing an industrial radiography source. In this case, the source was held over the anterior chest wall with death occurring months later from necrosis of the anterior chest wall (Figure 9) and anterior portion of the heart.

In an incident of child abuse, industrial radioactive sources were placed in ear pieces of headphones as well as in the child's pillow. Less deliberate but equally severe radiation exposures have also occurred from linear accelerators used for radiation therapy. In several instances, a computer software malfunction (known as "malfunction 54") occurred during editing of a radiotherapeutic treatment protocol. This was responsible for several accidents in which there was an intense radiation beam approximately the size of a half dollar. In two or three incidents the absorbed dose was high enough to cause subsequent tissue necrosis and death.

A. SKIN

Skin changes are the most apparent and obvious place to begin in evaluation of the local absorbed doses to different parts of the body. There is a vast amount of literature on the effects of radiation on the skin with chronic ulceration having been reported as early as 1898.[8] Radium dermatitis and burn were described by Marie Curie and Henri Becquerel shortly thereafter. The acute skin reaction is fairly independent of various biological parameters such as skin color, type, and age of patient.[9] There is some influence on acute-radiation

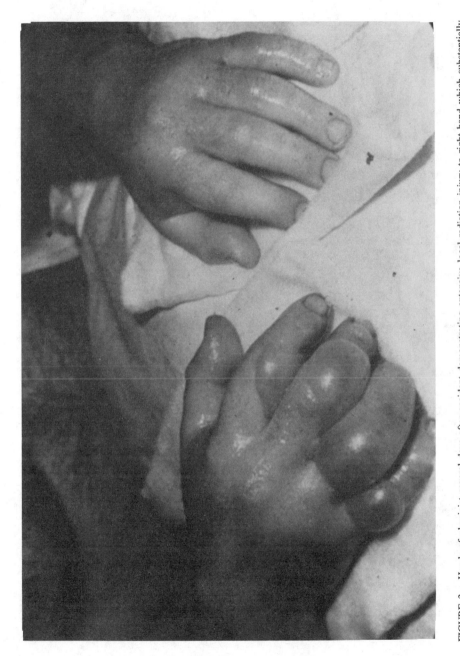

FIGURE 3. Hands of physicist several days after accident demonstrating extensive local radiation injury to right hand which substantially complicated an ultimately lethal outcome. (Courtesy of Los Alamos National Laboratory.)

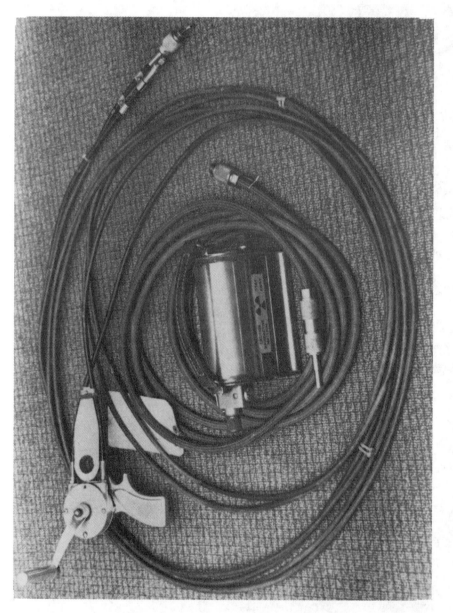

FIGURE 4.   Typical industrial radiography device. ^{192}Ir source is located in the shielded portion when the camera is not in use. For use, the crank is turned and the source is extended into the shaft for making an exposure. (From *The Medical Basis for Radiation Accident Preparedness*, Hubner, K. F. and Fry, S. A., Eds., Elsevier, New York, 1980, 273. With permission.)

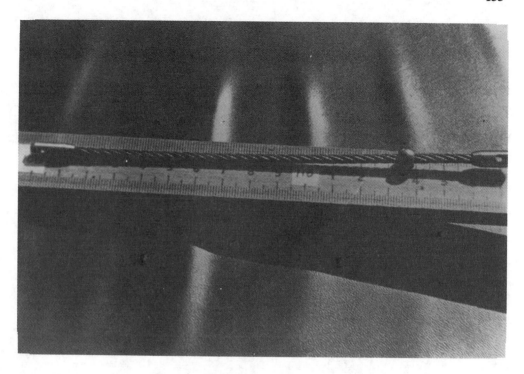

FIGURE 5. Typical ^{192}Ir industrial radiography source having been removed from shielding device. These devices may become unhooked from the cable and the camera itself. (From *The Medical Basis for Radiation Accident Preparedness*, Hubner, K. F. and Fry, S. A., Eds., Elsevier, New York, 1980, 266. With permission.)

TABLE 1
Approximate Gamma-Ray Dose Rates to the Hand for 1 Ci in a Sealed Source[a]

Nuclide	β Max (principal) MeV	γ (principal) MeV	Γ R/mCi-h at 1 cm	Surface dose rate[b] R/min	Dose rate at 1 cm tissue depth R/min	Dose rate at 3 cm tissue depth R/min
^{137}Cs	0.51, 1.2	0.662	3.26	513	28	3.7
^{60}Co	0.31	1.17, 1.33	13.00	2075	114	16.0
^{192}Ir	0.67	0.468	4.80	813	43	5.5
^{226}Ra	0.4—3.2	0.047—2.4	8.25	1310	72	9.7

[a] Industrial source housings are usually of stainless steel and for the purpose of the calculations, the activity is considered to be a point source. In considering these dose estimates, there is assumed a capsule of outside diameter 1/4 in. with a wall of stainless steel (type 304) which is 1/32 in. thick. Data from National Council on Radiation Protection and Measurements.[13]

[b] The total surface dose rate for the ^{226}Ra source is 1900 R/min based on a 45% increase due to electron production in the stainless steel wall. For other nuclides given in the table, the increase in surface dose rate due to electron production in the stainless steel wall is estimated to be 25 to 45%.

From *The Medical Basis for Radiation Accident Preparedness*, Hubner, K. F. and Fry, S. A., Eds., Elsevier, New York, 1980. With permission.

skin sensitivity with body area. The most radiosensitive areas of the skin are those which are moist and subject to friction, such as the axilla, groin, and skin folds. Additionally, the inner aspect of the neck, antecubital, and popliteal spaces also are sensitive. Less sensitive areas include the flexor surface of the extremities, the chest, the abdomen, face, and back. Least sensitive areas appear to be the nape of the neck, scalp, palms, and soles. Many of these variations in radiation sensitivity are due to the different thickness of the epidermis

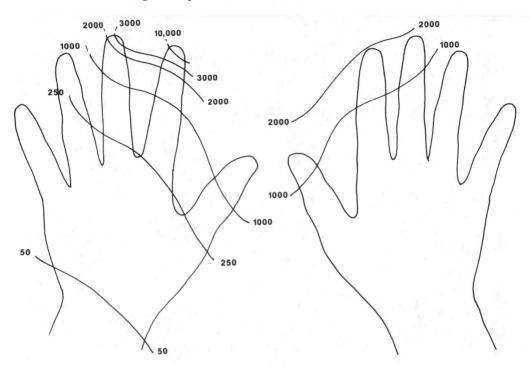

FIGURE 6.   Isodose curve showing estimated isodose curves following the handling of an 80-Ci ^{192}Ir source. (From Mettler, F. A., et al., *Clin Nucl. Med.*, 12(10), 807, 1987. With permission.)

and dermis in these areas.[10] The skin is thickest in the palms and soles, being about 0.4 mm. It is about 40 to 100 μm over most of the trunk. Damage to germinal cells in the basal layer of the epidermis is critical in the pathogenesis of erythema and desquamation (Figure 10). It is the dose to these cells that is critical in determination of the severity of the response. Desquamation is due to damage to the basal layers of cells. The basal layer is the deepest layer of the 15 layers of the skin and this is the only layer in which mitosis takes place. In the layers above this, cells do not divide, although they do differentiate. The transit time from cells dividing in the basal layer to the time when corneocytes peel off is roughly 14 d. This time period is important in expression of skin effects and healing. The germinal cells of the sensitive basal layer are about 0.1 mm deep and the dermal plexus is about 1.4 mm deep.

B. ERYTHEMA

Skin erythema, or reddening, occurs following large doses of radiation. The time at which erythema occurs depends upon the total absorbed dose, length of exposure, and the energy of the incident radiation. As with all types of exposure, the dose rate is important. If the exposure is received over a longer period of time the effect will be reduced. Skin reddening may occur one to two d after radiation, with a single dose of X-ray or gamma rays of 600 to 800 rad (6 to 8 Gy). Usually at this time there may be no symptoms of what one might usually associate with a thermal burn. The higher the radiation dose the more quickly the erythema may be identified. Erythema which appears within 2 to 3 h of an accident indicates absorbed doses in excess of 2000 rad (20 Gy). With such cases, symptoms may appear very rapidly with the onset of severe pain or a sensation of warmth. As an example of symptom dependence upon energy of the radiation, threshold erythema occurs following 300 rad (3 Gy) of 100 keV X-ray but only after 600 to 1000 rad (6 to 10 Gy) of 1000 keV X-ray.

Early erythema is presumably due to release of vasoactive amines and is similar in

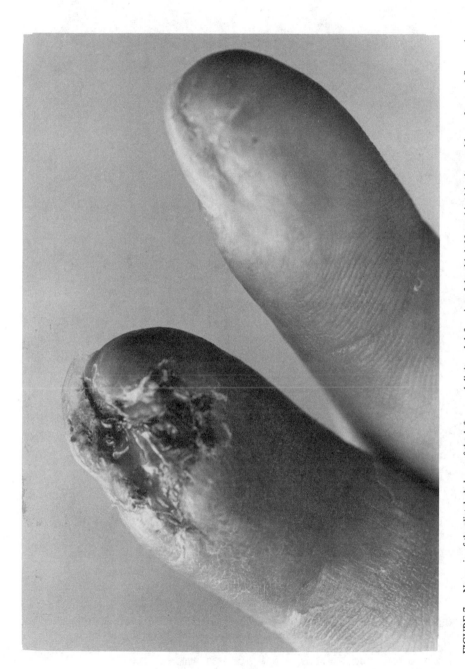

FIGURE 7. Necrosis of the distal phalanx of the left second digit and deformity of the third. Note skin thinning and loss of normal fingerprint pattern; however, the skin several centimeters from the point of contact is essentially normal. Pictures obtained 18 months after the accident. (From Mettler, F. A., et al., *Clin. Nucl. Med.*, 12(10), 806, 1987. With permission.)

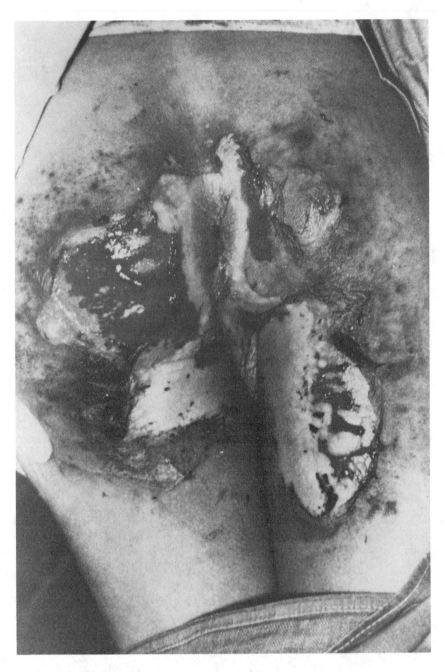

A

FIGURE 8.   Acute changes with necrosis of the buttock following an industrial radiography accident in which the source was not recognized as being radioactive and was placed in a pocket (A). Full thickness grafting (B) was performed. (From *The Medical Basis of Radiation Accident Preparedness*, Hubner, K. F. and Fry, S. A., Eds., Elsevier, New York, 1980. With permission.)

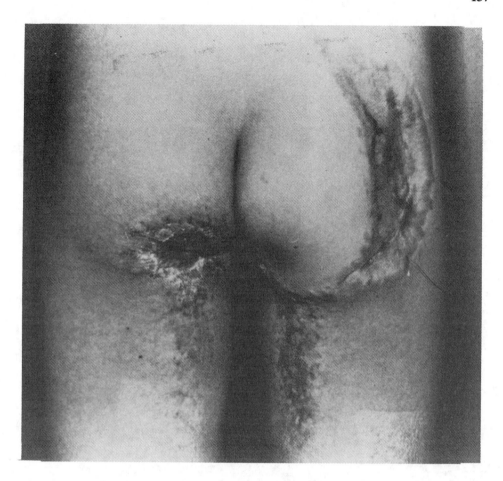

FIGURE 8B.

appearance to a first-degree thermal burn. Erythema may increase during the first week but usually fades during the second week. It then may return 2 to 3 weeks after the initial insult and last for 20 to 30 d. The second phase of erythema is thought to be due to vessel damage and an increase in blood flow. A third wave of erythema has occasionally been reported at 2 to 4 months. Initial skin findings similar to a second-degree thermal burn followed in 1 to 2 weeks by formation of blisters are indicative of a more severe type of skin injury (transepidermal). Patients with such injuries initially experience erythema, pain, swelling, or tingling. Healing usually will progress if infection does not occur.

C. DESQUAMATION

The threshold for desquamation is approximately 1,000 rad (10 Gy) with dry desquamation occurring between 1000 and 1500 rad (10 to 15 Gy) to the basal layer. At doses in this range, by the time the desquamation occurs (about 14 d), the basal layer underneath has been repaired and the epidermis remains relatively intact. At doses in excess of 1500 rad (15 Gy) to the basal layer, at the time desquamation occurs, the basal layer has not recovered and there is a transudate of plasma producing moist desquamation. With doses of radiation in the range of 2000 to 4000 rad (25 to 40 Gy) a more significant bullous-type, moist desquamation may occur. In this situation small blisters may coalesce and then rupture.

D. NECROSIS

If the absorbed dose to the basal layer is high enough, blisters may be formed beneath

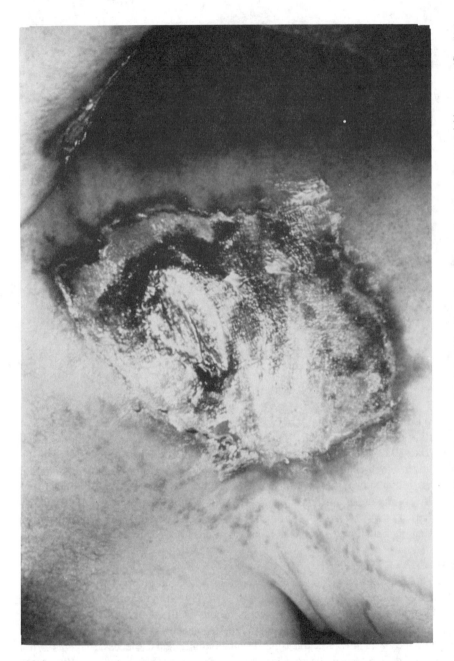

FIGURE 9. Chest wall necrosis following placement of an industrial radiography source on chest in an apparent suicide attempt. (Courtesy of Dr. W. H. Gordon.)

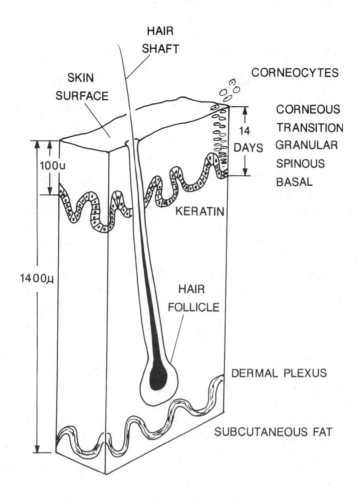

FIGURE 10. Diagrammatic representation of the structure of the dermis.

the basal cell layer. The appearance is very similar to a third-degree thermal burn (referred to as a *full thickness radiation burn*) and is often followed by necrosis. Skin tolerance to radiation depends significantly on the area of tissue irradiated. As the area of skin becomes smaller, the dose required to produce necrosis increases. If more than several cm are involved, skin grafting may be necessary, although damage to the underlying circulation is of primary importance in the late stages of healing.

E. CLINICAL DOSIMETRY

Even though the actual "dose" to the skin is rarely known, skin lesions due to radiation are reasonably well understood. Clinical examination is often the only method which is available for evaluation of local radiation injuries since it is unusual for a film badge or a dosimeter to be worn near the site of the injury. Acute radiation effects upon the skin are classed in Table 2.

In most cases, radiation burns can be distinguished from thermal burns, since with radiation burn the causative agent is often not perceptible and the ensuing damage is not immediately apparent. The latent period ranging from hours to weeks in the development or evolution of the burn is also rather unique to radiation injury.

Edema may occur with acute local radiation and may correspond to the exposed area but occasionally is noted beyond the exposed area. Edema may be seen within a few hours,

TABLE 2
Skin Reactions from Acute Radiation Dose

Erythema (first-degree burn)	$D_{50} = 600$ rad (6 Gy)
Transepithelial injury (second-degree burn)	$D_{50} = 2000$ rad (20 Gy)
Dermal necrosis (third-degree burn)	$D_{50} = 6000$ rad (60 Gy)

Note: D_{50} refers to the absorbed dose necessary to cause the effect in 50% of persons exposed.

but may not appear for up to 20 d following exposure. As with skin erythema, the higher the absorbed dose, the earlier the edema may be seen.

Fractionated exposure with irradiation of the skin, either in fractions or as low-dose continuous irradiation, shows different acute effects. With fractionation of a dose an increased dose can be tolerated. For each additional day during which the exposure occurs, about an 8% increase in dose is needed to achieve a given effect. In one clinical study of desquamation in humans, it was observed that a 1300-rad single dose was sufficient to produce the effect, but 2200 rad (22 Gy) was needed when the dose was spread out over 3 d or more. With continuous irradiation in dose rates of about 35 to 100 rad (0.35 to 1 Gy) per day, the dose rate is sufficiently low to allow for almost full repair and few if any acute effects are seen.

F. TREATMENT OF SKIN INJURIES

Treatment of skin injuries depends upon the total dose and penetration of the radiation. Mild erythema indicates that little if any treatment will be necessary; however, it is important under such circumstances to avoid further irritation of the skin by exposure to abrasive decontamination efforts, cauterizing, irritating solutions, or even exposure to the sun. With slightly higher doses causing dry desquamation, the skin may become itchy and a bland lotion with loose fitting clothes may be adequate. Some authors[12] have suggested application of a 1% aqueous solution of gentian violet, although the patients usually object to this because of the purple color. Other authors have suggested the use of antibiotic or cortisone-containing powders or sprays. In general, ointments are avoided.[13,14]

Severe radiation injury of the skin is likely to be accompanied by significant pain. Since this may be a long process, use of analgesics which are nonaddicting is recommended. Subcutaneous injury is often important in the ultimate management of radiation dermatitis. The depth-dose curve (varying dose at different depths) is dependent upon the nature of the incident radiation. Unfortunately this is often not well known at the time of the accident. With low-energy beta radiation, there is very rapid falloff of dose at increasing depths; however, with energetic beta radiation or with penetrating electromagnetic radiation, damage to the subcutaneous tissues including nerve endings, hair follicles, and small blood vessels may cause significant additional damage.

Ultimate necrosis of the skin may require split-thickness skin grafting, full-thickness grafting or even amputation. The clinical judgment involved in such decisions is difficult, due to the slow progression of these lesions. If an operation is performed too early, additional necrosis may occur. If amputation is performed too late, the patient will suffer more than necessary. Ultimately, the assessment of the underlying vascularity is the most important factor. Methods which have been suggested to assess the vascular status include arteriography, radionuclide perfusion studies, and thermography.

It is known that the underlying vacular lesions of both thermal and radiation burns can be exacerbated by physical trauma, histamine, prostaglandins, and arachidonic acid derivatives. Administration of an antiprostaglandin drug and topical application of a thromboxane inhibitor, anticoagulants, and antifibrotic drugs have all been suggested.[13,14] At this point the efficacy of such treatment remains in the research stage.

Late skin reactions are usually a function of scarring and limitation of underlying vascularity. After doses sufficient to cause moist desquamation, atrophy of the skin appears in 3 months and, although it may continue somewhat, it is usually stabilized by the 4th year. Such atrophic skin is very susceptible to breakdown from minimal trauma. Subclinical microscopic changes have been found in dermal blood vessels after 1000 to 3000 rad (10 to 30 Gy) from occupational exposure over 8 to 25 years. These vascular changes can be found, even though no other signs of skin damage can be detected.[15]

III. BETA IRRADIATION

Up to this point in the chapter we have primarily focused upon the radiation dose to the basal layer of skin and we have assumed that the radiation has been relatively penetrating (e.g., X-ray or gamma ray) with the surface and basal layer dose being almost identical. With beta radiation the situation can be very different. Radiation with beta emitters may cause significant skin reactions which are difficult to evaluate and may have a substantially different prognosis than more penetrating types of radiation. The reason for this is that beta radiation may be rapidly attenuated, giving a very different absorbed dose on the surface from that 1 or 2 mm deep in tissue. Hopewell[15] has reported a study in which the skin surface was given 4000 rad (40 Gy) from a ^{90}Sr (E = 0.93 MeV) applicator and compared it with injury from 13,000 rad (130 Gy) from ^{170}Tm (E = 0.31 MeV). With ^{90}Sr a significant amount of dermal necrosis occurred while with the thulium no dermal necrosis occurred. The reason for this is that with the less energetic beta from thulium, only 10% or less reaches as deep as the dermal plexus. With ^{90}Sr on the other hand, the dose to the dermal plexus is approximately 50% of the surface dose. For practical purposes, it is very important to know the energy of the radiation causing the injury because there may be significant differences in terms of ultimate outcome.

In the accident at Chernobyl, one of the major medical problems experienced by the patients were widespread and substantial skin reactions (Figure 11). Many experienced dry and/or moist desquamation over 90% of their bodies. This was presumably due to the beta and low-energy gamma dose from the fission cloud which was present in the reactor building. These ''burns'' significantly complicated the patient's treatment. In these patients there was immunodepression associated with the bone marrow injury from highly penetrating radiation and the areas of skin desquamation afforded a convenient but unfortunate avenue for sepsis.

The healing of conventional wounds or thermal burns in the first several days is not significantly affected by concurrent whole body radiation exposure; however, deterioration and impairment of healing can occur within weeks as a result of the radiation-induced immunosuppression.[16] In view of delayed wound healing that will occur at 2 to 4 weeks, in a radiation accident it often becomes necessary to close conventional wounds as soon as possible. With thermal burns, primary surgical treatment supplemented by high doses of antibiotics is probably optimal therapy. Unfortunately, at Chernobyl there were many patients with extensive beta burns, and these radiation beta burns really did not present as a focus of infection until the moist desquamation and dermal necrosis had begun at 2 to 4 weeks. This was at the same time that the bone marrow depression from penetrating radiation occurred. For such extensive beta burns, the only real treatment is a sterile environment, covering with artificial skin-like materials and use of antibiotics. Primary surgical treatment is often not possible.

It should be noted that alpha-emitting radionuclides pose no particular hazard if the skin is intact. Alpha particles are unable to penetrate the cornified layer of the epidermis. They only represent a hazard if there is skin contamination which is soluble and passes through the skin to become an internal contamination hazard. Pure gamma-emitting radionuclides rarely pose a problem in terms of skin effects since the penetrating capability of most gamma

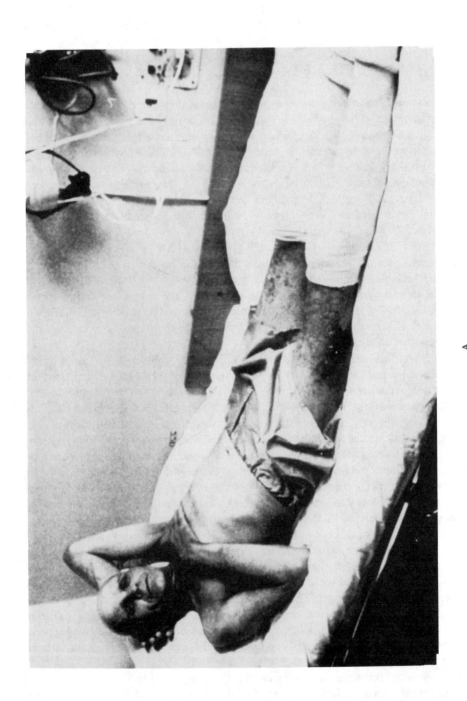

A

FIGURE 11.   Beta burns on the legs of a Chernobyl victim. (Courtesy of Dr. A. M. Davis.)

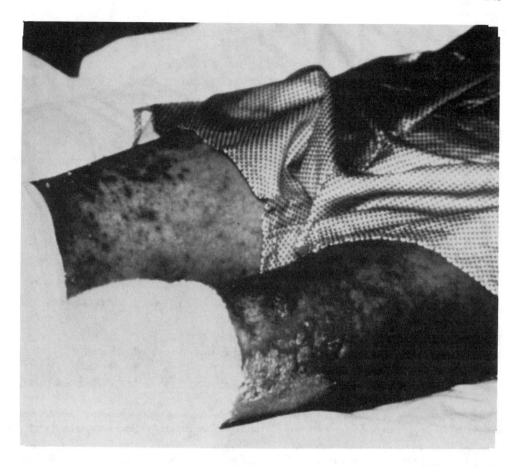

FIGURE 11B.

rays is such that the viability of the organism as a whole becomes the critically important issue due to radiation injury of sensitive structures such as bone marrow.

A. PIGMENTATION

Pigmentation is a relatively common phenomenon after skin irradiation. The sequence of pigmentation effects is variable among patients. Most patients demonstrate gradual hyperpigmentation. The increased pigmentation is felt to be caused by a radiation-induced increase in activity of melanocytes. Depigmentation may occur if the radiation dose has been high enough to destroy the melanocytes. By 1 year, the skin usually demonstrates its final appearance which may include diffuse telangectasia, suppression of sebaceous gland activity, skin atrophy, fibrosis, and limitation of motion. It should be pointed out that the radiation-induced skin pigmentation varies considerably over the body and is influenced to a minimal extent by age.

B. ALOPECIA

Alopecia or epilation (loss of hair) is another usual parameter for evaluation of actual absorbed dose received by various portions of the body. The threshold for damage to hair follicles is lower than for skin erythema. Temporary alopecia occurs after single acute doses of 300 to 500 rad (3 to 5 Gy). About 3 weeks postexposure, a single dose of 700 rad may cause permanent hair loss with the period for hair loss to occur being <3 weeks (Figure 12). Not all body areas have the same radiation alopecia sensitivity. The scalp and beard

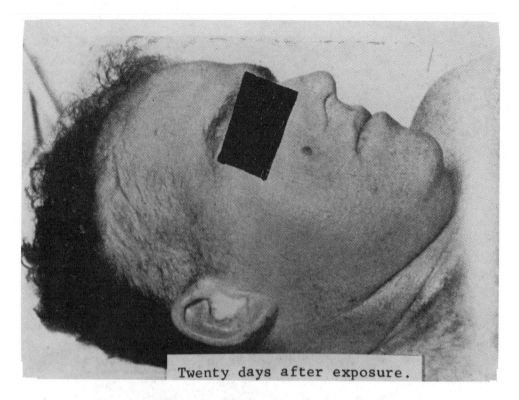

Twenty days after exposure.

FIGURE 12.   Epilation, or hair loss, over the right temporal region following radiation exposure. This indicates
the portion of the head receiving the dose in excess of 300 rad (3 Gy). (Courtesy of Los Alamos National Laboratory.)

are most sensitive, with chest wall, axillary, abdominal, eyebrow, eyelash, and pubic hair
being less sensitive, respectively. Hair follicles of children are more sensitive than those of
adults. Hair that has regrown may be finer and slower growing than original hair and also
might be a slightly different color.

In some accidental situations (such as Chernobyl) where there is desquamation due to
beta radiation, the dose to the basal layer (100 μm deep) of the epidermis can be estimated
by the degree of desquamation. If there is early regrowth of the hair or no hair loss at all,
the dose to the base of the hair follicle can be estimated. The base of the follicle is usually
located in the middle of the dermis (400 to 1000 μm), thus an absorbed dose at this level
can be estimated. With this information in hand, the depth-dose curve in tissue can be
estimated and the energy of the incident radiation inferred. In circumstances in which there
has been moist desquamation of the skin and permanent alopecia the radiation involved must
either have been a very high dose or substantially penetrating.

Several authors have pointed out that in low dose ranges (from 50 to 500 rad) even
when alopecia does not occur there is still a decrease in the diameter of the hair shaft and
this decrease is linearly related to absorbed dose.[17,18] Unfortunately, most of the work that
has been performed in this respect has been on animals and actual human data at this point
is not available.

C. HEMATOLOGIC STATUS

Assessment of the hematologic status of an acutely exposed individual by obtaining an
immediate and serial complete blood counts (CBC) is extremely important. This should be
done every 12 h for a period of at least 48 h so that an assessment of the absolute lymphocyte
count can give an estimate of potential bone marrow and gastrointestinal involvement. Of
course, whole-body radiation in excess of 100 rad (1 Gy) results in the hematopoietic

syndrome (see Chapter 8). Characteristically, the major changes in the bone marrow which may occur are an almost immediate depression of the small lymphocytes and subsequent leukopenia and thrombocytopenia approximately 30 d after exposure.

The major difference in marrow response between localized and generalized radiation injury is that in cases in which the bone marrow is irradiated heavily locally, subsequent marrow regeneration of the irradiated site may occur more quickly by repopulation from other areas. Some experience with radiation therapy is applicable to situations which may occur in an accident in which there is a relatively inhomogeneous distribution of bone marrow dose. If either the pelvis or thoracic bone marrow is irradiated in a radiation therapy treatment scheme, the lymphocyte value often falls to 40% of its original value. The eosinophil count may change depending on the site of irradiation. Pelvic irradiation tends to elevate the eosinophil count whereas treatment of the upper abdomen and thorax may cause a decrease in the relative eosinophil count. In situations in which there has been a high-level acute exposure, the distribution of the dose on the body surface may be evident if there is associated erythema of the skin. If present, this can give a clue as to the status of the underlying bone marrow in the different areas. Another method of assessing inhomogeneous exposure and its effect on the marrow is to perform a nuclear medicine bone marrow scan utilizing any one of a number of colloidal radiopharmaceuticals.

In cases in which the radiation exposure has been very high to an extremity the hematologic response basically reflects the absorbed dose to the trunk of the body, since bone marrow in adults is restricted to the pelvis and axial skeleton. Only a very minimal amount of bone marrow is present in the proximal humerus and femurs, and there is essentially no active marrow present distally in the appendicular skeleton.

D. CHROMOSOMAL ABERRATIONS

Assessment of chromosomal aberrations in peripheral lymphocytes serves as a biologic dosimeter (see Chapter 8). The value of this method is excellent, particularly when the exposure is uniform and whole body. It is of much more limited value in the assessment of partial-body or nonuniform exposures or in cases of internal contamination. The study is done by the culturing of peripheral lymphocytes and subsequent evaluation of the chromosomes for the formation of dicentrics. The dose-response curve for formation of the dicentrics depends upon the nature of the incident radiation. Fission neutrons, for example, are much more efficient at producing dicentrics/rad than are low energy X-rays. The induction of the chromosome aberrations is generally described by a Poisson distribution. This means that the number of lymphocytes which have more than one dicentric is relatively low. Overrepresentation of cells with two or three chromosomal dicentrics with respect to the cells having only a single dicentric should raise the suspicion of nonuniform external radiation exposure or internal contamination with alpha-emitting radionuclides.

E. GONADS

Permanent sterility is not a problem following whole-body uniform radiation exposure. The reason for this is that absorbed doses of 500 to 900 rad (5 to 9 Gy) to the gonads are required to produce permanent sterility and if these dose levels are whole-body, hematopoietic depression and gastrointestinal injury usually cause death. There have been several accidents in which highly radioactive sources were placed in the pocket and at least one case of child abuse in which the child was essentially castrated through use of radioactive source.[19] Temporary sterility can occur in males with doses as low as 50 rad (0.5 Gy) and permanent sterility certainly is a possibility in accidental partial-body exposure in which the source is located close to the pelvis.

A reduction in spermatogonia can be seen with absorbed doses as low as 8 rad (80 mGy). A reduction in sperm count may not be evident until 30 or 60 d after exposure. The ultimate degree and duration of depletion depends upon the magnitude of the dose received. While there is a distressingly variable number of reports in the literature about the actual dose-response curve, the consensus appears to be that temporary sterility in males may occur with single doses ranging from 150 to 400 rad (1.5 to 4.0 Gy) and with fractionated doses of 10 to 200 rad (0.1 to 2 Gy). Permanent sterility occurs with single doses in the range of 500 to 950 rad (5.0 to 9.5 Gy) and with fractionated doses of 200 to 600 rad (2 to 6 Gy). Sterility may be temporary, but exist for a matter of years. Five individuals having received doses of 230 to 370 rad (2.3 to 3.7 Gy) in an Oak Ridge criticality accident were aspermic for 4 months and hypospermic for 21 months. At least one of these individuals had "sterility" for several years and subsequently had a normal offspring.[20]

In an accident in Japan, one individual had a sperm count that was almost normal (greater than fifty million sperm/ml) 2 months after the accident and then showed total spermia at 6 months with moderate recovery of the sperm count about 2 years later. The estimated absorbed dose to the testicle was 175 rad (1.75 Gy). In another accident (in California), an individual carried an iridium source in his hip pocket for 45 min with a resultant estimated gonadal dose of 60 to 150 rad (0.6 to 1.5 Gy). On day 155 after exposure there were fewer than 0.5 million sperm/ml of semen. In most of these cases, there may be abnormalities in the spermatozoa, but libido and potency are usually unimpaired. This is due to the relative resistance of the Leydig cells to radiation damage.[21] In females, temporary sterility or reduced fertility is seen after single doses of 65 to 400 rad (0.65 to 4.0 Gy) or fractionated doses of 300 to 1700 rad (3 to 17 Gy). Permanent sterility occurs after single doses of 320 to 1000 rad (3.2 to 10 Gy) and after fractionated doses of 200 to 1200 rad (2 to 12 Gy).

F. EYE

Evaluation of the eye is important in terms of both acute and chronic effects. Most of the tissue around the eye has the same sensitivity as skin since areas such as the conjuctiva are composed of epithelial cells. In the acute period, there may be erythema and, if the dose is high enough as well, dry or moist desquamation. Fractionated doses of 2000 rad (20 Gy) can cause reddening with vascular prominence and at doses of 400 rad (40 Gy) a confluent mucositis appears. The patient may also have thick secretions from the lacrimal gland during this time and may also experience photophobia. Fractionated doses in the range of 5000 rad (50 Gy) may cause a superficial punctate keratitis. It is often very difficult to assess whether the changes identified are due to radiation or simply due to an infection. Fractionated doses of over 10,000 rad (100 Gy) can cause ophthalmitis which may require ultimate enucleation. The eyebrows are quite resistent to epilation even when it occurs at other sites.

High-dose changes which can be seen in the period from 6 months to 2 years include telangiectasia in the skin or conjunctiva, possible scarring of the cornea, and radiation retinopathy. Retinopathy can be produced by fractionated doses as low as 1500 rad (15 Gy) but is more common in the 3000 to 7000 rad (30 to 70 Gy) range. Depending upon the extent of changes, the patient may ultimately progress to blindness. Optic neuropathy may occur following fractionated doses in the range of 4000 to 7000 rad (40 to 70 Gy). Both the retinopathy and neuropathy appear to be secondary to vascular damage.

Cataracts are the most frequent delayed reaction in the eye and have been identified in a number of persons involved in accidents as well as in the atomic bomb survivors. The term cataract often denotes blindness or at least impaired vision. The vast majority of "cataracts" identified in the atomic bomb survivors were nonprogressive and did not significantly impair vision. Radiation-induced cataracts are among the few lesions that are pathologically characteristic for radiation injury. Most senile cataracts begin in the anterior pole of the lens whereas radiation cataracts begin as a small dot to a posterior pole. As the opacity develops in the posterior pole and enlarges to 3 to 4 mm, a large central clear area can be identified. Ultimately the cataract may progress to the anterior pole of the lens and

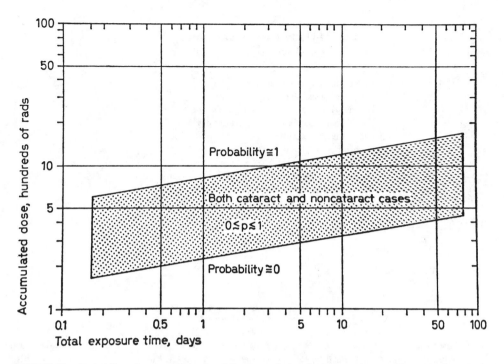

FIGURE 13.   Probability of cataract formation following radiation exposure to the eye. (From Merriam, G. R., Jr., Szechter, A., and Focht, E. F., in *Frontiers of Radiation Therapy and Oncology*, Vol. 6, S. Karger, Basel, 1972, 346. With permission.)

then it is difficult to differentiate from a senile cataract. The incidence of cataracts is dose-, time-, and age-dependent. Single doses of 200 rad (2 Gy) or fractionated doses of 400 rad (4 Gy) can result in formation of lens opacity (Figure 13). The latent period for production of cataracts from time of exposure may range from half a year to 35 years, although on the average it is 2 to 3 years. The higher the absorbed dose, the shorter is the latent period. A single dose of 750 rad (7.5 Gy) will cause cataract formation in all those exposed. A similar incidence occurs in patients who have received 1400 rad (14 Gy) over a period of 3 to 12 weeks. In situations in which there is occupational exposure over a period of years the threshold for cataract formation appears to be between 600 and 1400 rad (6 to 14 Gy). It should be noted that neutron exposure is significantly more effective in cataract production than are photons.

IV. SUMMARY

In summary, local radiation injuries involve the hands in over 90% of the cases. Depending upon the radiation source and the geometry there may be significant trunk exposure and, therefore, gastrointestinal hematological consequences as well as local injury. Assessment of the absorbed dose, length of exposure, energy, and penetrating ability of the radiation are all factors that must be assessed prior to definitive medical management. A list of items to be considered in assessment of local radiation injuries is shown in Table 3.

With consideration of these factors as well as those outlined in this chapter, it is often possible to make an intelligent estimate of the absorbed dose distribution and ultimate outcome.

TABLE 3
Items to Consider in Evaluation of
Local Radiation Injury

History and physical examination
Serial peripheral blood counts
Chromosome analysis of blood lymphocytes
Sperm counts before day 45 and after day 60
Reenactment of accident
Frequent color photos
Slit lamp exam of eyes
Radionuclide blood pool imaging and bone scan
Blood, hair, and metallic samples for neutron exposure[a]
Jeweled watches and rubies for neutron exposure.[a]

[a] See also Appendix 5.

REFERENCES

1. **Lushbaugh, C. C., Fry, S. A., Hubner, K. F., et al.,** Total body radiation: a historical review and follow-up, in *The Medical Basis for Radiation Accident Preparedness,* Hubner, K. F. and Fry, S. A., Eds., Elsevier/North Holland, New York, 1983.
2. **Saenger, E. L., Kereiakes, J. G., Wald, N., et al.,** Clinical course and dosimetry of acute hand injuries to industrial radiographers from multicurie sealed gamma sources, in *The Medical Basis for Radiation Accident Preparedness,* Hubner, K. F. and Fry, S. A., Eds., Elsevier/North Holland, New York, 1983.
3. **Hirashima, K., Sugiyama, H., Ishihara, T., et al.,** The 1971 Chiba, Japan, accident: exposure to iridium-192, in *The Medical Basis for Radiation Accident Preparedness,* Hubner, K. F. and Fry, S. A., Eds., Elsevier/North Holland, New York, 1983.
4. **Ross, J. F., Holly, F. E., Zarem, H. A., et al.,** A 1979 Los Angeles accident: exposure to iridium-192 industrial radiographic sources, in *The Medical Basis for Radiation Accident Preparedness,* Hubner, K. F. and Fry, S. A., Eds., Elsevier/North Holland, New York, 1983.
5. **Stern, T. J.,** Surgical approaches to radiation injuries of the hand, in *The Medical Basis for Radiation Accident Preparedness,* Hubner, K. F. and Fry, S. A., Eds., Elsevier/North Holland, New York, 1983.
6. **Scott, E. P.,** The 1978 and 1979 Louisiana accident: exposure to iridium-192, in *The Medical Basis for Radiation Accident Preparedness,* Hubner, K. F. and Fry, S. A., Eds., Elsevier/North Holland, New York, 1983.
7. **Jammet, H., Gongora, R., Jockey, P., et al.,** A 1978 Algerian accident: acute local exposure to children, in *The Medical Basis for Radiation Accident Preparedness,* Hubner, K. F. and Fry, S. A., Eds., Elsevier/North Holland, New York, 1983.
8. **Gassmann, A.,** Zur Histologie der Ronggenulcera, *Forschr. Gep. Ronggenstrahlen,* 2, 199, 1898.
9. **Mettler, F. A. and Moseley, R. D.,** *Medical Effects of Ionizing Radiation,* Grune & Stratton, Orlando, 1985.
10. **Trot, K.,** What can the experience of radiation therapy teach us about accidents? *Br. J. Radiol.,* Suppl. 19, 28, 1986.
11. **Karcher, K. H.,** Akute lokale Veranderungen bei Teilkorperbestrahlung und Deren Behandlung, in *Strahlenschutzkurs Fur Ermachtigge Arzte-Spezialkurs,* Stieve, F. E. and Mohle, G., Eds., Hildegard Hoffmann, Berlin, 1979.
12. **Stieve, F. E.,** Experiences with accidents and consequences for treatment, *Br. J. Radiol.,* Suppl. 19, 18, 1986.
13. **Guskova, A. K.,** Basic principles. The treatment of local radiation injuries, *Br. J. Radiol.,* Suppl. 19, 122, 1986.
14. **Leny, U., Schuttman, W., Arndt, D., et al.,** Late effects of ionizing on the human skin after occupational exposure, in *Late Biological Effects of Ionizing Radiation,* Vol. 1, IAEA publ. STI/PUB/489, International Atomic Energy Agency, Vienna, 1978, 321.
15. **Hopewell, J. W.,** Mechanisms of the action of radiation on skin and underlying tissues, *Br. J. Radiol.,* (Suppl. 19), 39, 1986.

16. **Messerschmidt, O.,** Whole body irradiation plus skin wound; animal experiments on combined injuries, *Br. J. Radiol.,* Suppl. 19, 64, 1986.
17. **Potten, C. S.,** Biological dosimetry of local radiation accidents of skin: possible cystological and viro-chemical methods, *Br. J. Radiol.,* Suppl. 19, 82, 1986.
18. **Sieber, V. K. and Wells, J.,** The use of plucked hairs as a biological dosimeter, *Br. J. Radiol.,* Suppl. 19, 92, 1986.
19. **Collins, V. P. and Gaulden, M. E.,** A case of child abuse by radiation exposure, in *The Medical Basis For Radiation Accident Preparedness,* Hubner, K. F. and Fry, S. A., Eds., Elsevier/North Holland, New York, 1986, 197.
20. **Andrew, G. A., Hubner, K. F., Fry, S. A., et al.,** Report of twenty-one year medical follow-up of survivors of the Oak Ridge Y-12 accident, in *The Medical Basis of Radiation Accident Preparedness,* Hubner, K. F. and Fry, S. A., Eds., Elsevier/North Holland, New York, 1980.
21. **Ross, J. F., Holly, F. E., and Zarem, H. A.,** 1979 Los Angeles accident: exposure to iridium-192 industrial radiographic source, in *The Medical Basis of Radiation Accident Preparedness,* Hubner, K. F. and Fry, S. A., Eds., Elsevier/North Holland, New York, 1980.

Chapter 10

EVALUATION AND TREATMENT OF PERSONS EXPOSED TO INTERNALLY DEPOSITED RADIONUCLIDES

George L. Voelz

TABLE OF CONTENTS

I. INTRODUCTION

How does a physician become aware that his patient(s) may have an internal exposure to radioactive material? Usually someone tells him. This someone may be the patient who suspects or knows that he or she has been in a contaminated area or accident. Or it may be a radiation monitor who is familiar with details of the accident. Or perhaps the state policeman who recognizes a radioactive hazard sign posted on a truck involved in an accident.

However the issue is raised, the physician is faced with finding means to evaluate the exposure. Medical history can develop preliminary details of the accident or situation, but signs and symptoms from an exposure are highly unlikely unless some corrosive or irritant chemical exposure is also present. There may be traumatic injuries that need attention. The usual clinical laboratory tests are not helpful in determining exposure and only a few radioactivity measurements may be available at the time the first decisions must be made.

Is treatment necessary? Is effective treatment available? These are the physician's questions to answer. If possible, early telephone consultation with a radiation specialist may be helpful.

This chapter focuses on the evaluation and treatment of internally deposited radionuclides from a clinical standpoint. Background information to assist physicians in the medical management of these cases is provided.

II. INITIAL PRIORITIES

The first priority in the care of the patient is to attend to any life-threatening condition. Attention to vital functions and control of severe hemorrhaging take priority. The presence of potential radioactive contamination should not deter the nature or rapidity of medical care. Even if radiation levels are not known and survey instruments are not immediately available, proceed with lifesaving assistance. Wear gloves and wrap the patient in a sheet or blanket if radioactive contamination is suspected to be a problem; this is done to reduce the spread of contamination. Accidental contamination levels are almost never a serious hazard to personnel for the time required to perform lifesaving measures. High level radioactive contamination, such as that which occurred to the Chernobyl firemen and rescue personnel, will not be encountered without immediate recognition of the occurrence of an extraordinary accident. Hospital personnel will be alerted to such unusual high-contamination accidents.

As soon as is practical, a determination should be made as to the presence or absence of loose or transportable radioactive contamination on clothing and skin. If present, clothing removal and skin decontamination should be performed. Skin decontamination, usually only requiring washing with detergent and water, reduces exposure and helps prevent contamination of other persons and the facilities. Emergency plans for management of a radioactively contaminated patient should include written decontamination procedures.[1]

Another priority is to assess the potential of an internal deposition of radioactive material. An important first step is to take a preliminary history on facts concerning the accident. Table 1 lists questions and subject areas that will assist in taking this history from the patient and other knowledgeable persons who may be available.

One of the more serious constraints on the physician is the limited time available for making a treatment decision. For maximum effectiveness, most treatments must begin within an hour or two after exposure. With each additional hour, the effectiveness of most treatment regimens is reduced. Thus an early decision based on meager and often confused, information is necessary. If the accident occurred in a university or industry setting, the best information can probably be obtained from a health physicist, radiation safety officer, or occupational physician familiar with the facility and accident details.

TABLE 1
Medical History Questions for Radioactivity-Contaminated Persons

When did the accident occur? What are the circumstances of the accident and what are the most likely pathways for exposure? How much radioactive material is involved potentially?

What injuries have occurred? What potential medical problems may be present besides the radionuclide contamination?

Are toxic or corrosive chemicals involved in addition to the radionuclides? Have any treatments been given for these?

What radionuclides now contaminate the patient? Where? What are the radiation measurements at the surface?

What information is available about the chemistry of the compounds containing the radionuclides? Soluble or insoluble? Any information about probable particle size?

What radioactivity measurements have been made at the site of the accident, e.g., air monitors, smears, fixed radiation monitors, nasal smear counts, and skin contamination levels?

What decontamination efforts, if any, have already been attempted? What success?

Have any therapeutic measures, such as blocking agents or isotopic dilution been given?

Was the victim also exposed to penetrating radiation? If so, what has been learned from processing personal dosimeters, e.g., film badge, thermoluminescent dosimeter, or pocket ionization chamber? If not yet known, when is the information expected?

Has clothing removed at the site of accident been saved in case the contamination still present on it is needed for radiation energy spectrum analysis and particle size studies?

What excreta have been collected? Who has the samples? What analyses are planned? When will they be done?

Note: These questions can be used by the attending physician at the hospital for obtaining historical information to assist in the early management of radioactively contaminated persons. The best information in industrial cases can probably be obtained from plant personnel, such as the health physicist or occupational physician familiar with the plant and accident details.

III. INITIAL EVALUATION

Essential information needed to make immediate treatment decisions for possible internal exposure to radioactive material is identification of the radionuclide(s) involved, general level of potential exposure, and mode of potential intake. There may be few, if any, radioactivity measurements available at this early time. In industrial cases, this information should be available from a radiation safety officer at the facility along with general information about the nature of the accident. One should also find out if the patient may have received significant external radiation exposure.

The physician should determine the specific hazards and characteristics of the principal radionuclide(s) present in the exposure. Appendix 4 is a table containing information on selected radionuclides for use in early evaluation of an accidental exposure. The metabolic behavior or radionuclides must be understood. This subject is discussed briefly in the next section entitled Biokinetic Models and Dosimetry.

For decontamination work, it is usually adequate to know simply whether one is dealing with a "beta-gamma" emitter or an "alpha" emitter. The key point is to ensure that the survey instrumentation being used can detect the radiation in question. For treatment decisions, it is necessary to know the exact nuclide(s) involved in order to determine its radiological and chemical properties, metabolic behavior, and the available treatment regimens. If the contaminating radionuclide(s) cannot be identified with confidence by available information, samples of the contamination should be identified by gamma and/or alpha spectroscopy.

Information available to appraise the extent of internal exposure will be limited at the early time, 1 to 4 h after exposure, when treatment decisions should be made. Exposure judgments as crude as simply being considered low or high will be developed from the limited information. At this time one will have an idea of the level of skin and clothing contamination, which is some indication of how much radioactivity is present. If the accident occurred in a facility where measurements are made, there should be contamination levels (floor, bench tops, equipment, etc.) and possibly air concentration levels to estimate potential levels of exposure. A rough estimate of inhalation potential can be made by using air concentrations times the occupancy time by the patient (without respirator) in the room.

Nasal swab samples taken within a few minutes of the exposure can give a rough idea of inhalation potential. A sample is taken from each nostril separately using a moistened Q-tip or moistened filter paper on a swabstick. The samples are dried and counted. These samples are subject to error because the individual's nose may have been contaminated with his hands or from surrounding facial contamination. In this event, the activity will not be indicative of the potential of inhaling particulates. Furthermore, the anterior nares clears itself of particulates rapidly (half time of about 10 to 20 min); thus the sample must be taken immediately after the accident to be useful. Nose blowing or snuffling in a shower will invalidate the results. By the time the individual gets to a hospital, it is likely to be too late to obtain useful information from nasal swabs.

Nasal swabs are frequently used at facilities handling alpha emitters, such as plutonium or americium. A rule of thumb judgment is that counts over 500 dpm may indicate a significant exposure, while results less than 50 dis/min suggest no more than a possible low-order exposure. High values in one nostril with low or no activity in the other are suggestive of contamination other than by inhalation.

The above information may be all that can be collected before making timely treatment decisions. There is always a question as to how much detailed monitoring and dosimetry information is needed before treatment is begun. Once the decision to treat is made, the urgency of time is past and the detailed dosimetry studies can begin.

The more definitive means of estimating internal deposition of radionuclides are by direct whole-body counts (Figure 1), chest (lung) counts, and by excretion measurements in urine or fecal samples. Unfortunately, interpretation of direct counting is often complicated by residual surface contamination during the first hours after an accident. Whole-body counters are extremely sensitive, measuring whole-body gamma activity of 1 to 2 nCi (10^{-9} Ci) or less. With this level of sensitivity, counts registered from skin contamination can be significant even though careful decontamination has been performed. The results are often more confusing than helpful in the first day or two because the counter does not distinguish between external and internal activity. High sensitivity also limits the capacity of these counters to measure high levels of activity that might be involved in accidental exposures. Thus, even though counters may be available nearby, it is usually not useful to delay treatment decisions for such a measurement if the internal deposition is thought to be high.

An exception to the above discussion on limitations of early use of monitoring methods is for certain soluble radionuclides that can be detected in urine immediately after exposure. Notable examples are radioiodine, tritium (radioactive hydrogen), and radiocesium. Radioactivity levels present in the urine are used to calculate the uptake in the body by means of excretion models appropriate for the specific nuclide.[2] For emergency estimates, spot urine samples are taken for a rough estimate of uptake. Precautions must be taken to prevent sample contamination if there is external contamination present.

Uptake of *radioiodine* can be monitored with urine excretion measurements or by direct counts over the thyroid. Accident response usually involves thyroid counts within an hour or so of intake and, therefore, the results must be adjusted for time after exposure because the peak thyroid activity occurs from about 12 to 24 h after exposure. Measurement in urine samples has been found to be an efficacious method for detecting thyroid burdens within the first 12 h after exposure.[3] A three-compartment model, using a 4-h integration period, predicts the percent of iodine intake to be excreted via urine at the following times after a single acute exposure: 0 to 4 h, 25% of iodine excreted in urine; 4 to 8 h, 16%; 8 to 12 h, 10%; 12 to 16 h, 6.1%; 16 to 20 h, 3.8%; 20 to 24 h, 2.3%. There are large uncertainties

155

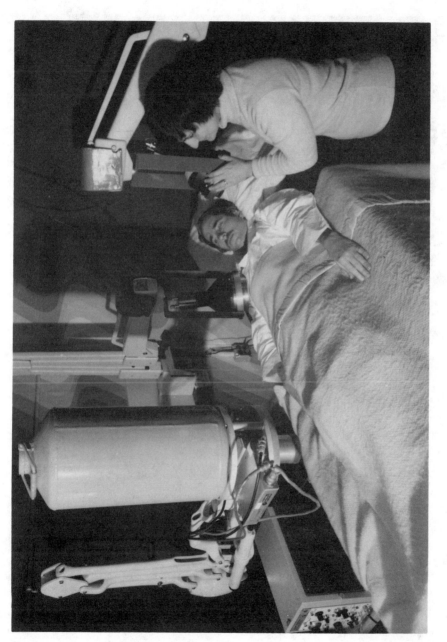

FIGURE 1. (A) This whole-body counter system simultaneously uses four radiation detectors: dual phoswich detectors over the lungs to detect low-energy photon emitters such as plutonium or americium, a planar intrinsic germanium detector (in foreground) to count the liver or other areas for similar radionuclides, and a lithium-drifted germanium detector under the subject (not seen here) to measure high-energy photon emitters (55 kev to 2 Mev) in the body. This counter room is entirely surrounded by a special 7″ steel shield to provide a low-radiation background. (B) The measurement data from the whole-body counter system is sent directly to this special data handling system which analyzes and calculates the results, prints reports, and stores the data. (Figures 1A and B courtesy of Los Alamos National Laboratory.)

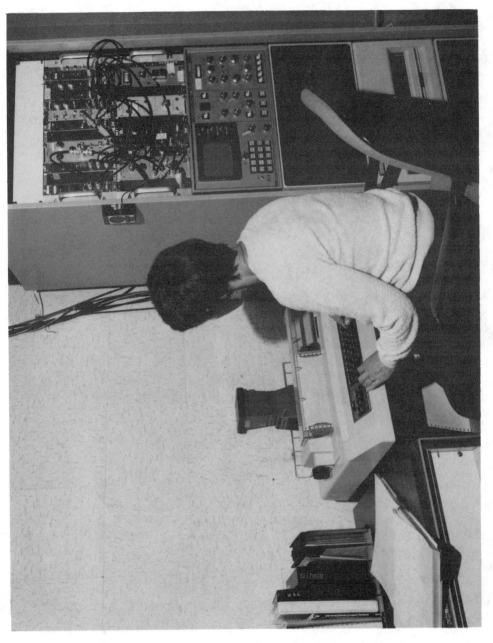

FIGURE 1B.

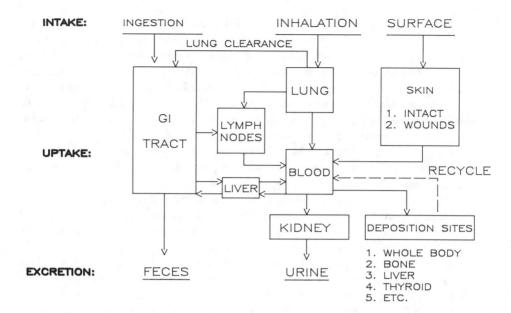

FIGURE 2.   Diagram representation of intake, metabolism, and excretion of radionuclides.

in the use of such model calculations as applied to an individual, but such estimates can be useful for early evaluation of exposures. Effective treatment of a radioiodine exposure must be done as soon as possible, preferably in the first hour. The above data indicate that a single urine sample taken early will be useful for a rough estimate of the uptake of iodine. The first voiding after the uptake can have a falsely low value because of dilution with urine excreted by the kidney prior to exposure.

Tritium is a weak beta emitter that is not detectable by normal survey instruments or by whole body counting. Detection of exposure is by urine samples, which show excretion immediately after exposure. Usually the first voiding after exposure is not used because dilution by preexposure urine results in a falsely low reading. The sample is counted by liquid scintillation techniques. A conservative rough rule of thumb, based on the peak urine concentration after a single acute exposure, is that 1 μCi/l of tritium equates to a total integrated whole-body dose of about 10 mrem (100 μSv) in the average person if not treated by forcing fluids.

Radiocesiums, [134]Cs and ^{137}Cs, are an example of gamma emitters that can be detected by whole-body counting techniques or by urine excretion. Whole-body counting in the first few hours may be complicated by the presence of external contamination. Careful collection of a urine sample will prevent contamination of the sample. Measurement by gamma spectroscopy will identify the activity due to the cesium nuclides. For interpretation, about 1% of the cesium activity in the body per day will be excreted in urine during the first 3 d after a single acute intake of soluble cesium.

It is helpful to have some reference materials at hand during an emergency that describe various radionuclides and their physical and biological properties. Such information may be located in the reports listed in References 1, 2, and 4.

IV. BIOKINETIC MODELS AND DOSIMETRY

The success of the initial evaluation described above is dependent on the physician's knowledge of the modes of uptake, metabolism, excretion, and dosimetry of the involved radionuclide. Figure 2 is a diagrammatic representation of the routes of intake, internal metabolic transfers, and routes of excretion.

The gastrointestinal tract, respiratory tract, and skin are the organ systems through which radionuclides usually enter the body. The nuclide(s), if soluble in body fluids, will be absorbed in the extracellular fluids (lymph fluid and blood) of these entry organs. Distribution to other organs is made via blood in accordance to the biochemical properties of the particular nuclide. The radioactivity within the systemic circulation and associated internal distribution to organs is termed the *systemic deposition* or *burden*. There is a continual recycling of the radionuclide deposited in various organs. The recycled material is circulated via blood, some fraction is excreted, and the rest is redeposited in organs.

The rates of transfer of the radionuclide between entry organs, blood, and deposition organs are determined primarily by the biochemical properties of the radionuclide. Some ingested or inhaled radioactive particles may include radionuclides contained within a matrix of stable compounds. Absorption is determined by the matrix, which may have solubility characteristics quite different from that expected for the radionuclides. This is usually noticed when the matrix is less soluble than the radionuclide and thus the systemic uptake from the lung or gastrointestinal tract is slower or less than expected.

The principal excretion pathways from the body are through urine and feces. Lesser paths are by perspiration and sometimes by exhalation. Concentration of the radionuclide in urine is related to the concentration present in the blood. Fecal excretion has two components: (1) insoluble material from direct ingestion or lung clearance passing unabsorbed through the gastrointestinal tract and (2) excreted systemic material via bile and gastrointestinal secretions.

In developing models of the behavior of radionuclides in man, transfer functions with time are determined for absorption, retention, and excretion of each element. Usually separate models are used for routes of entry from the respiratory tract and the gastrointestinal tract and for retention and excretion of elements after absorption. Standard models have been recommended and published by the International Commission on Radiological Protection (ICRP)[5,6] for calculating allowable limits of intake for workers.

Uptake from the gastrointestinal tract depends upon the chemical characteristics of the element. The absorption of many radionuclides is small, 10% or less. Small gastrointestinal uptake is found for radionuclides of chromium, manganese, iron, cobalt, zirconium, ruthenium, silver, antimony, cerium, mercury, uranium, plutonium, americium, curium, and californium. Elements with higher absorption from the gastrointestinal tract are radium (20%), strontium (30%), and phosphorus (80%); three elements (tritium, iodine, and cesium) are completely absorbed.

For the portion of radioactive material that is not absorbed by the gastrointestinal tract, the highest radiation dose will be delivered to the lower large intestine because of the longer residence time in this segment of the tract. In the ICRP models, mean residence time to traverse the gastrointestinal tract is taken to be 1/24 d for stomach, 4/24 for small intestine, 13/24 for upper large intestine, and 24/24 for lower large intestine.

The simple schematic drawing on radionuclide uptake (Figure 2) indicates that material inhaled into the lung can be transferred in three ways: (1) lung clearance to the gastrointestinal tract by means of the mucociliary escalator of the tracheobronchial tree and swallowing, (2) systemic absorption and distribution through extracellular (blood) fluids, and (3) particulate transfer to lymph nodes by phagocytic cells. The transfer rates are influenced primarily by the chemical characteristics of the inhaled material and the particle sizes. Completely soluble material, such as tritium or iodine, will transfer immediately to blood. Lung clearance of less soluble particulates depends on the rate of solubility in respiratory fluids and particle clearance rates.

In the ICRP compartmental lung model,[6] the respiratory system is divided into three regions: nasopharyngeal, tracheobronchial, and pulmonary. Deposition of inhaled particles is assumed to vary with the aerodynamic properties of the aerosol as shown graphically in

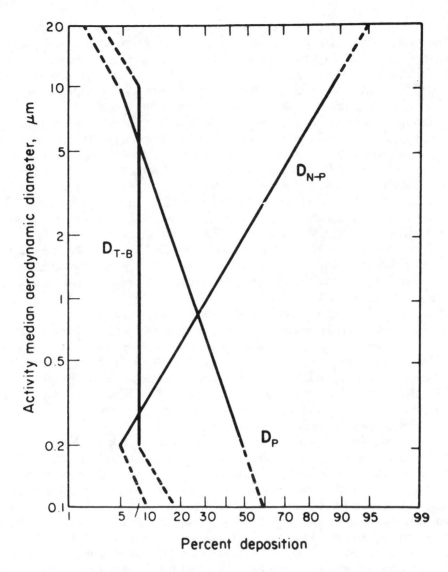

FIGURE 3. Deposition of dust in respiratory tract for different particle sizes. N-P refers to nasopharyngeal region, T-B to tracheobronchial, and P to pulmonary or alveolar areas.

Figure 3. Inspection of the graph shows that large particles (>5 μm) are mostly deposited in the nasopharyngeal section. Deposition in the pulmonary region, i.e., respiratory bronchioles, alveolar ducts, and alveoli increases with decreasing particle size. For particles below 1 μm, the major deposition occurs in the pulmonary region. General knowledge of particle size involved in an inhalation exposure may suggest whether deposition is primarily below the tracheobronchial region or not. For example, inhalation of radioactive particles from mechanical type operations (filing, sawing, lathe work, explosions without fire) are likely to be of a large particle size and, therefore, are likely to be deposited in the nasopharyngeal and tracheobronchial regions. If so, one might see significant lung clearance (sometimes essentially 100%) of insoluble particles occur within the first few days. A high proportion of the fine particles from a fume, fire, or smoke are more likely to be deposited below the ciliated portion of the respiratory tract. In this case, relatively little lung clearance may occur.

In the ICRP model,[6] the chemical character of particles is classified according to the relative biological clearance time expected from the pulmonary region for particles with an activity median aerodynamic diameter of 1 μm. The three classes are termed *D* (half-time in days), *W* (weeks), or *Y* (years). The half-time for D compounds are assumed to be <10 d; W compounds, 10 to 100 d; Y compounds, >100 d. The model assumes specific transfer fractions for the chemical classes from the three compartments of the respiratory tract into extracellular fluids, gastrointestinal tract, and tracheobronchial lymph nodes.

A unique characteristic of relatively insoluble (Y compound) particles inhaled into the lung is the nonuniform distribution of radiation dose that occurs (Figure 4). This is especially true of alpha emitters, because the range of alpha particles is only about 50 μm in tissue, or about 4 to 5 cell diameters. Nonuniform doses around particles has been the subject of much discussion as to whether this phenomenon produces an elevated risk of lung cancer. A committee of the National Council on Radiation Protection and Measurements (NCRP)[7] concluded, based on a substantial body of experimental animal data, that there is no greater hazard from particulate plutonium doses in the lung than from the same amount of plutonium more uniformly distributed throughout the lung. The NCRP concluded that averaging the dose from particulate alpha-emitting radionuclides over the entire lung is a defensible procedure. Nonuniform dose distribution by alpha emitters also occurs in other organs, i.e., skin (wounds), lymph nodes, and bone.

After uptake into the systemic circulation, radionuclides are distributed to organs/tissues depending on their elemental biochemical properties. The ICRP models assume distribution and retention in the organs/tissues in accordance with functions described in Publication 30.[6] These retention functions are expressed as sums of exponentials which take account implicitly of all transfers within the body. The reader is directed to the references for the details. Table 6 in Appendix 4 indicates a critical organ for various radionuclides. This designation is a simple but limited method for indicating the organ expected to receive the highest dose or having the most significant potential biological effect.

Systemic excretion of a portion of the absorbed radionuclides occurs through urine and feces. The models assume certain fractions through each route as being appropriate.

This discussion of models is presented to give an appreciation of the complexities of the metabolism of radionuclides and to summarize some fundamental information needed to evaluate exposures to internal emitters. It should be noted that the models rely on many assumptions regarding uptake, absorption, organ distribution, and excretion. Medical decisions to treat or not to treat a patient after an exposure will be made on limited information as previously discussed. The models are primarily used for radiation protection purposes, such as calculating allowable limits of intake. They are not intended to be used to calculate doses from internal emitters for *individual* cases, although they are often used to give an approximation of dose if more specific factors or measurements are not available. The ICRP also recommends that they not be used out of context, such as for the basis of cancer risk estimates or for calculation of doses to members of a population.

V. TREATMENT

Reduction of internally deposited radionuclides can be accomplished by means of two general processes: (1) reduction of absorption and internal uptake and (2) enhanced elimination or excretion of absorbed radionuclides. Both are achieved more effectively when treatment is begun at the earliest time after exposure.

Skin decontamination and wound management are used to reduce uptake via the skin. Other chapters in this book should be consulted for discussion of these topics.

A. REDUCTION OF GASTROINTESTINAL ABSORPTION

Gastrointestinal absorption can be reduced either by removing radioactive materials before absorption can occur or by blocking uptake by use of drugs. The main considerations are summarized:

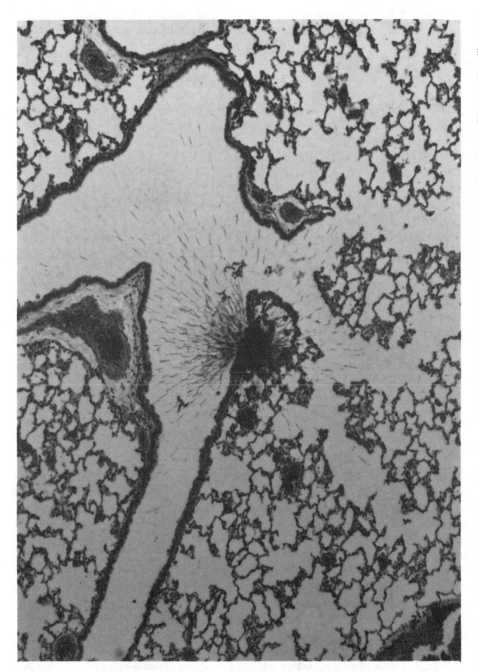

FIGURE 4. Autoradiograph of alpha particles from a plutonium particle deposited on the epithelial lining of an airway of hamster lung illustrates nonuniform radiation dose distribution within lung. Animal studies have not demonstrated an increased cancer risk from such non-uniform dose distribution compared to a uniform dose involving all cells in the tissue. (Courtesy of Los Alamos National Laboratory.)

1. Stomach lavage. A nasogastric or gastric tube may be used to empty the stomach in the unusual cirumstance where a large quantity of radionuclide is present in the stomach.
2. Emetics. Stomach lavage is often the procedure of choice, but may not always be successful. Apomorphine hydrochloride or ipecac are the most likely emetic drugs to consider in such cases.
3. Purgatives. Selection of a purgative to speed the elimination of gastrointestinal tract contents depends largely on the speed of action. An exposure of concern would be relatively insoluble radionuclides that may remain for many hours in the colon and rectum, and could be removed promptly with treatment. A phosphosoda enema will empty the colon in a few minutes and should be a primary consideration. Purgative drugs taken orally, such as biscodyl, castor oil, or phenolphthalein, require several hours before taking effect, but they have faster action than others. Some purgatives may have special advantages because they produce a less soluble compound of certain radionuclides. Magnesium sulfate is a saline cathartic that can produce relatively insoluble sulfates with some radionuclides, e.g., radium.
4. Ion exchange resins. Strong cation or anion exchange resins can produce toxic side effects and are generally not recommended. While no studies are noted in the literature on the use of activated charcoal in cases of radionuclide intake, it would seem to be a potentially useful procedure to reduce uptake.
5. Prussian Blue. In animals, ferric ferrocyanide (Prussian Blue) has been found effective in accelerating the removal of cesium, thallium, and rubidium through feces.[2] Prussian Blue is not absorbed from the gastrointestinal tract and has low toxicity. It is not available for pharmaceutical use in the U.S. nor is it approved for drug use by the Food and Drug Administration (FDA) without special permission. In situations in which use as any emergency drug is possible, the advance preparation of a pure supply and approval for its use should be obtained as part of medical emergency preparedness. One to three grams of Prussian Blue given 3 times per day from several days up to 3 weeks is well tolerated in adults. In man, the compound has reduced the biological half-time of ^{137}Cs to one third of the normal value.
6. Aluminum-containing antacids. These are effective agents in reducing intestinal uptake of strontium. A single oral dose of 100 ml aluminum phosphate gel given immediately after ingestion of radioactive strontium will decrease absorption by about 85%. A single dose of aluminum hydroxide, 60 to 100 ml, given immediately after exposure will reduce uptake by about 50%. Both drugs are nontoxic and well tolerated.
7. Barium sulfate. This highly insoluble salt is used as an X-ray contrast agent for gastrointestinal tract examinations. Except for constipation, no adverse effects have been observed. In an emergency response to a radionuclide ingestion, the principal indication for use of barium sulfate is as an immediate antidote for ingested strontium and radium. Formation of insoluble sulfates of these elements will decrease their intestinal absorption.

B. BLOCKING AND DILUTING AGENTS

A blocking agent saturates a specific tissue with a selected stable element and thereby reduces the uptake of a radionuclide usually taken up by that tissue. Isotopic dilution is achieved by the administration of large quantities of a selected stable element (compound), which lessens the organ uptake of radionuclide due to the dilution factor. Displacement therapy is a special form of isotopic dilution in which a stable element of a different atomic number successfully competes with the radionuclide for uptake in an organ. Some of the more practical examples of these agents are summarized.

1. Iodides

The early use of stable iodide can reduce uptake of radioiodine in the thyroid. A dose of 390 mg of potassium iodide (300 mg iodide) achieves maximal blocking. Administration of a single dose of stable iodide within the first few minutes after exposure to radioiodine may limit uptake to about 1 or 2% compared with the normal 12 to 20% uptake. Only about half of the uptake is blocked if the iodide administration is delayed 6 h and little effect can be achieved if delayed as much as 12 h. Daily administration of potassium iodide (KI) is recommended for about 7 to 14 d to prevent recycling of the radioiodine into the thyroid. The above dose schedule is recommended for individual exposures,[1] but for general public use in emergencies a lower dose of 130-mg KI (100 mg iodide) has been recommended.[8] Reported adverse reactions from daily 300-mg doses of iodide suggest a reaction rate of about 1 to 10/10,000,000.[8] Incidence of adverse reactions are related to dose and length of administration. After iodine administration given usually for several weeks or longer, the reported iodine-induced reactions include thyrotoxicosis, iodide goiter, hypothyroidism with goiter, iodide parotitis, acneform skin eruptions, and even less frequent systemic manifestations (fever, arthralgia, inflammatory joint involvement, etc.). Because these reactions reverse in a few days after discontinuing the drug, monitoring for reactions need not be continued beyond a few days after the last iodide administration. The side-effects problem is thought to be negligible for the dose schedules discussed here.

2. Strontium

Stable strontium is useful as a diluting agent for radiostrontium. It is available as tablets (strontium lactate, 300 mg, to be given 2 to 5 times daily) or intravenous solutions (strontium gluconate, 600 mg strontium per day infused with 500 ml 5% glucose in water over 4 h). The tablets are well tolerated if given with meals and are nontoxic at this dosage. It can be given daily for several weeks.

3. Phosphate

Phosphate can be used to decrease the intestinal absorption of radioactive strontium. It may also be useful as a diluting agent in case of medical misadministration of ^{32}P. Oral phosphates can be given in inorganic (sodium or potassium phosphate) and organic forms (sodium glycerophosphate). Vomiting, diarrhea, or both may occur from phosphate administration in doses exceeding 2 g/d. Phosphate can be used as a saline cathartic. Intravenous administration of phosphate is unlikely for treatment of radionuclide uptake. It must be done cautiously because rapid administration can cause severe hypotension, renal failure, and myocardial infarction. Serum calcium and electrocardiograms must be monitored during such infusion.

4. Forced Fluids

A high level of fluid intake by mouth will increase tritium excretion proportionately. The half-time of tritium in the body can be reduced from the normal 10 or 12 d to 6 d or less by forcing at least 3 to 4 l to 10 l or more of fluid per day. Continue forcing to tolerance for at least 1 week or until further dose reduction is judged not to be necessary. The dose may be reduced by a factor of 2 or more by careful management.

5. Calcium

Orally and intravenously administered calcium increases the urinary excretion of radioactive strontium and calcium.

C. MOBILIZING AGENTS

Mobilizing agents are compounds that increase a natural turnover process, thereby inducing a release of some forms of radioisotopes from body tissues. This results in an enhanced rate of elimination from the body and a reduced biological half-time. These agents are more effective given soon after exposure, but some still produce an effect if given within about 2 weeks.

1. Antithyroid Drugs

The treatment of choice for reducing the dose from radioiodine is to block the thyroid by administration of an iodide as discussed above. If time since exposure is 12 h or more, the use of iodide has limited effectiveness because the radioiodine is already deposited in the thyroid. In this situation the use of an antithyroid drug, such as propylthiouracil or methimazole, may be considered. These drugs interfere with the oxidation of the iodide ion and block the formation of hormone. The response to these drugs is greatly reduced if the thyroid already has an ample supply of stable iodine, such as when stable iodide has already been administered. The risk of side effects is much higher than with stable iodides. About 2 to 8% of patients on these drugs develop a maculopapular rash, which does not usually require discontinuation of the drug. Much rarer but serious side effects are hepatocellular damage, vasculitis, and agranulocytosis (in about 0.2% of patients). These side effects are usually reversible on discontinuance of the drug. The effective half-time of ^{131}I was reduced about 25% using methimazole in several human volunteers when given several days after radioiodine administration;[9] thus, the reduction of radiation dose is not likely to be great if treatment is started as late as several days after exposure.

2. Ammonium Chloride

This acidifying salt given orally (1 to 2 g four times a day) is effective in mobilizing radiostrontium deposited in the body. Its effectivesness can be enhanced by simultaneous use of i.v. calcium gluconate, 500 mg calcium in 500 ml 5% glucose in water over 4 h on 3 to 6 consecutive days. An estimated reduction in the body burden of radiostrontium between 40 to 75% may be obtained if started soon after exposure. Ammonium chloride frequently causes gastric irritation, nausea, and vomiting, and should not be used in persons with serious liver disease.

3. Diuretics

The value of diuretics is untested for treatment of internal radionuclide deposition. Enhanced excretion of sodium, chloride, potassium bicarbonate, magnesium, and water in the urine occurs with induced diuresis. Some corresponding radionuclides that could be involved in radiation accidents are ^{22}Na, ^{24}Na, ^{38}Cl, ^{42}K, and ^{3}H.

4. Expectorants and Inhalants

Studies on the effect of these agents on inhaled radioactive particles are disappointing. None provides effective action that would be dependable or particularly useful in treating persons after inhalation of radioactive particles.

5. Parathyroid Extract

Injections of parathyroid hormone promote urinary excretion of phosphorus and have been used effectively to treat an overdose of radiophosphorus.

D. CHELATING AGENTS

A number of chemical compounds enhance the elimination of metals from the body by chelation, a process by which organic compounds exchange less firmly bonded ions for other inorganic ions to form a relatively stable nonionized ring complex. This soluble complex is excreted readily by the kidney. The excretion of certain radionuclides can be increased by means of a properly selected and administered chelating agent. Chelation therapy is most effective when it is begun as soon as possible after exposure because it works only on the metallic ions in extracellular fluids and not on those already incorporated in cells.

The principal drug used for treatment of radionuclides is known as DTPA, an acronym of its chemical name, diethylenetriaminepentaacetic acid. It is approved as an investigational new drug (IND) by the FDA in two forms, calcium DTPA and zinc DTPA, for the chelation of plutonium, berkelium, californium, americium, and curium. In addition to these transuranium metals, DTPA is also an effective chelator for some rare earths (cerium, yttrium, lanthanum, promethium, and scandium) and some transition metals (zirconium and niobium). The FDA approval of DTPA covers its use only for the above-listed transuranium metals; special permission would be needed for use in exposures to radioactive rare earths or other radionuclides.

Animal studies indicate that the ZnDTPA form is less toxic than CaDTPA in some situations. ZnDTPA is recommended for long-term treatment and for use in pregnant women. CaDTPA is more effective than ZnDTPA in rats when it is given promptly after exposure to transuranium metals. For this reason, CaDTPA is the preferred form to use during the first day or two of treatment.

No serious toxicity has resulted in man with either ZnDTPA or CaDTPA when used in recommended doses. In high doses in animals, toxicity has occurred from CaDTPA due to chelation and excretion of trace metals, such as zinc and manganese. Doses in animals at levels 200 times or more that used in humans produce severe lesions of the kidneys, intestinal mucosa, and liver in animals. Teratogenesis and fetal death occur in mice when similarly high doses are given throughout gestation.

For plutonium exposures, the effectiveness of DTPA chelation is highly dependent on the chemical form of the plutonium. Soluble forms, such as the nitrate, are taken up into extracellular fluids quickly where chelation can take place. Data from persons treated with CaDTPA within about 3 h of exposure indicate that about 60 to 70% of soluble plutonium is removed compared to untreated persons. This is true for both inhalation and contaminated wounds. Insoluble plutonium forms, such as high-fired oxides, are absorbed into the extracellular fluids slowly over many months. In this case the plutonium concentration in extracellular fluid is minute and chelation does not enhance excretion significantly.

The recommended dose for either ZnDTPA or CaDTPA is a single 1-g dose per day. The dose should not be fractionated, i.e., given in multiple doses per day. It can given either intravenously or by aerosol inhalation. The usual procedure for i.v. administration has been to dilute 1 g DTPA in 250 ml normal saline or 5% glucose in water and given over a period of about 30 min. An alternate procedure, using 1 g diluted in 10 or 20 ml normal saline and injected i.v. over a period of five min is preferred by some physicians. In either case, care should be taken to avoid extravasation from the vein. Aerosol administration is done with 1 g CaDTPA placed in a nebulizer and the contents inhaled over 15 to 20 min. ZnDTPA is less well suited than CaDTPA for aerosol administration because of its metallic taste. It is prudent not to use the inhalation route in persons with preexisting pulmonary disease.

Clinical urinalysis should be performed and be normal prior to each treatment. Potential contraindications to use of the drug are significant leukopenia, thrombocytopenia, or serious kidney dysfunction.

DTPA is not available commercially. Physicians with a potential need of these drugs should contact Oak Ridge Associated Universities, Radiation Emergency Assistance Center/ Training Site (REAC/TS) Center, Oak Ridge, TN, 37831-0117. A treatment protocol and followup reports are required under the terms of the IND agreement.

E. LUNG LAVAGE

Inhalation of radioactive particles is a common mode of intake from occupational exposures. If the particles are insoluble, a large proportion of the radioactive material is retained for many months or years in the lung. Chelation therapy is not effective in these cases.

TABLE 2
Treatment Summary of Selected Internal Radioactive Contaminants

Contaminant	Procedure	Medication	Comment
Americium	Wound excision	DTPA	See Transuranic elements
Californium	Wound excision	DTPA	See Transuranic elements
Cerium		DTPA	See Rare earths
Cesium		Prussian Blue	
Curium	Wound excision	DTPA	See Transuranic elements
Hydrogens (tritium)		Water	Force fluids to tolerance
Insoluble Particles			
Ingested	Stomach lavage		
Inhaled	Lung lavage	Purgatives	If acute effects expected
Iodine		KI or NaI	
Lanthanum		DTPA	See Rare earths
Mercury		Penicillamine	
Phosphorus		Phosphates	Aluminum-containing antacid for ingestion
Plutonium	Wound excision	DTPA	See Transuranic elements
Rare earths		DTPA	Special FDA approval needed for this use
Strontium		Strontium/Calcium Oral ammonium chloride	Aluminum-containing antacid for ingestion
Transuranic elements		DTPA	1 g/d i.v. or by aerosol
Zinc		Ca DTPA	Special FDA approval needed for this use

In dog studies, lavage of the tracheobronchial tree removes about 25 to 50% of inhaled insoluble particles.[10-12] The procedure requires placement of an endotracheal tube into the trachea and major bronchi under a general anesthesia. The airways are lavaged with isotonic saline. Experimentally, five lavages were performed on both right and left lung, ten total, starting in the first week after exposure and doing one lavage from three days to a week apart. Radiation pneumonitis and early deaths occurred in only 25% of treated dogs in contrast to death of all untreated dogs. In baboons, 60 to 90% of the lung burdens of plutonium oxide was removed by ten pulmonary lavages.[13]

Use of this treatment requires a careful risk-benefit assessment. The risk lies primarily in the administration of a general anesthetic. The mortality risk appears to be 0.2% or higher for each lavage. This procedure risk is immediate, whereas radiation-induced cancer risk to the lung will be years later. The use of this procedure should, therefore, be limited to cases in which lung doses from insoluble particles of alpha emitters are sufficiently high to produce acute radiation damage.

F. TREATMENT SUMMARY

The treatments listed above summarize the main procedures and drugs available to treat internally deposited radionuclides. A quick reference in their use for selected radionuclides are listed in Table 2.

VI. BASIS FOR TREATMENT DECISIONS

The decision on whether or not to treat a person exposed to internal radionuclides is a subjective judgment. Organ doses from internal emitters are hardly ever so high as to cause acute radiation effects. An exception to this statement is on exceptionally rare occasions when medical misadministrations (unintended high dose) of therapeutic levels of radio-nuclides have occurred. In any event, if exposure to internal contamination is high enough for such concerns there will be no problem making the decision to treat, but rather on deciding how to treat most effectively.

The usual treatment decision will involve concerns about the risk of a late health effect (carcinogenesis) occurring later in life. Our understanding of the dose/effect relationship due to radiation is limited, especially at low dose rates. Therefore, decisions will often be based on anticipated, but poorly understood, risk. The need for a medical treatment decision at the earliest time possible after exposure makes an assessment of risk even more tenuous.

There are few studies or data that address the question as to whether current treatment effectively reduces health effects due to internal radionuclides. The benefits of treatment are assumed to be present based on reduction of the quantity of radionuclide deposited in the body or organs. Thus, the benefits of treatment are understood even less well than our imperfect understanding of radiation risk at low dose and low-dose rates. The decision for treatment is often based simply to achieve an ''as low as readily achievable'' internal burden or dose.

The physician will usually not have good dose estimates at the time of decision. If the radionuclide is of a type that a direct *in vivo* measurement can be made, without serious contributions from external contamination, an estimate of the quantity present in the body (organ) may be possible. In this event, a quick assessment of organ dose can be calculated. Table 6 in Appendix 4 lists 50-year committed dose equivalent estimates from various radionuclides in critical organs.

One way of judging the seriousness of a radiation dose, in terms of late effects, is comparing with doses that are known to cause excess cancers in humans. In epidemiologic studies of exposed human populations, excess cancer incidence is usually not statistically evident unless doses of 50 rad (0.5 Gy) or more are present. Bone marrow and thyroid are more radiosensitive for late effects than other organs and one may wish to reduce potential doses to these organs by an additional factor of 5.

Another way of judging is to recognize that occupational radiation protection guidelines restrict exposures to the whole body, bone marrow, and gonads to 5 rem (50 mSv) per year. The new guideline for other organs and tissues is 50 rem (0.5 Sv) per year. Guidelines for limited areas of skin (forearms) and bone are also 50 rem (0.5 Sv) per year.

By these comparisons, it appears that doses less than about 5 to 50 rem (50 mSv to 0.5 Sv), depending on the organ systems involved, would be a point of diminishing benefits for treatment of internal contamination. Fortunately, for many of the treatments discussed above, the risk of treatment is slight to negligible. If the treatment risk is small, one may proceed even if the potential benefits appear to be limited. The physician must make this judgment concerning the possible ultimate benefit vs. the potential harm or side-effects of the therapy — a type of judgment common to all medical practice.

There are other considerations in the treatment decision that are important. Probably the most important is the age of the persons involved. Children have longer life expectancy and greater radiosensitivity which increase the potential benefits of treatment for them compared to an older person. Likewise, one may treat a young adult more aggressively than older individuals. A second consideration of importance is the general health of the individual. Persons with a significant health risk already from other disease will probably benefit less from treatment of internal radionuclides than a healthy person of the same age simply on the basis of shortened life expectancy.

With proper use of currently available treatment, it is possible to reduce the dose from some radionuclides taken internally by factors of about 2 to 10. The goal of reducing dose is a worthy objective. That health effects do result from internal emitters has been amply demonstrated in radium dial painters, uranium miners, thorotrast-injected persons, and the Marshallese Islanders exposed to radioiodines in fallout. However, in all these cases there were high exposures that were orders of magnitude above those permitted by the regulatory guidelines applied to the radiation worker. The point is that the physician must keep in perspective the benefits and risks of treatment in each situation. The fact that the decision must be made very early after exposure places the physician at a great disadvantage. For treatment that involves essentially no risk, errors of therapy omission are likely to be more serious than those of commission.

REFERENCES

1. Management of persons accidentally contaminated with radionuclides, NCRP No. 65 National Council on Radiation Protection and Measurements Publications, Bethesda, MD, 1979.
2. Use of bioassay procedures for assessment of internal radionuclide deposition, NCRP Rep. No. 87, National Council on Radiation Protection and Measurements Publications, Bethesda, MD, 1987.
3. **Broga, D. W., Berk, H. W., and Sharpe, A. R., Jr.,** Efficacy of radioiodine urinalysis, *Health Phys.,* 50, 629, 1986.
4. Manual on early medical treatment of possible radiation injury, IAEA Saf. Ser. No. 47, International Atomic Energy Agency, Vienna, 1978.
5. Individual monitoring for intakes of radionuclides by workers: design and interpretation, International Commission on Radiologic Protection (ICRP) Report, Publ. 54, *Ann. ICRP,* 19(1-3), 1988.
6. Limits for intakes of radionuclides by workers, *Ann. ICRP,* Publ. 30, 2(3/4); 4(3/4); 6(2/3); Suppl. and index, 1979—1982.
7. Alpha-emitting particles in lungs, Rep. No. 46, National Council on Radiation Protection and Measurements Publications, Bethesda, MD, 1975.
8. Protection of the thyroid gland in the event of releases of radioiodine, Rep. No. 55, National Council on Radiation Protection and Measurements Publications, Bethesda, MD, 1977.
9. **Tanaka, S., Mochizuki, Y., Yabumoto, E., Iinuma, T. A., Kumatori, T., Yamane, T., Akiyama, T., and Matsusaka, N.,** Protection of thyroid gland and total body from radiation delivered by radioactive iodine, in *Diagnosis and Treatment of Deposited Radionuclides,* Kornberg, H. H. and Norwood, W. D., Eds., Excerpta Medica Foundation, Amsterdam, 1968, 298.
10. **Pfleger, R. C., Wilson, A. J., and McClellan, R. O.,** Pulmonary lavage as a therapeutic measure for removing inhaled "insoluble" materials from the lung, *Health Phys.,* 16, 758, 1969.
11. **Boecker, B. B., Muggenbury, B. A., McClellan, R. O., et al.,** Removal of ^{144}Ce in fused clay particles from the beagle dog by bronchopulmonry lavage, *Health Phys.,* 26, 605, 1974.
12. **Muggenburg, B. A., Mauderly, J. L., Boecker, B. B., et al.,** Prevention of radiation pneumonitis from inhaled cerium-144 by lung lavage in beagle dogs, *Am. Rev. Resp. Dis.,* 111, 795, 1975.
13. **Nolibe, D., Nenot, J. C., Metevier, H., et al.,** Traitement des inhalations accidentelles d'oxyde de plutonium par lavage pulmonaire *in vivo,* in *Diagnosis and Treatment of Incorporated Radionuclides,* IAEA Publ. STI/PUB/411 International Atomic Energy Agency, Vienna, 1976, 373.

Chapter 11

HOSPITAL PREPARATION AND DRILLS

Fred A. Mettler, Jr. and Jonathan C. Marshall

TABLE OF CONTENTS

I. INTRODUCTION

Preparation of a hospital to be able to handle a radiation accident is often regarded as a very complex and difficult task. In fact, it is actually quite simple. One might ask why a hospital should have a protocol to deal with radiation accidents since they occur very infrequently. Historically, hospitals located near nuclear facilities, whether commercial reactors, other industrial sites or universities, have a reasonably predictable chance of seeing a patient involved in a radiation accident. On the average, such hospitals will treat at least one seriously injured and radioactively contaminated patient every 2 to 4 years. The reason for presentation of most patients is a medical or surgical emergency such as myocardial infarction, hypotension, thermal steam burns, or trauma with resultant fracture, etc. As might be expected, many of the patients come to the hospital during the evening or night shift. Whatever preparations have been made, there needs to be certainty that the designated procedures can be carried out with limited staffing.

In the 1970s as nuclear reactors were becoming more common, it was suggested that regional centers should be set up to handle radiation accidents. Presently, there are over fifteen hospitals in the U.S. which have designated themselves as "radiation accident centers". Such self-designation is mostly in terms of preparation since only one or two of these hospitals have ever treated a patient involved in a radiation accident. Experience during the decade has indicated that immediate local medical and surgical support is critical and regional support is less important.

One change from the original planning which has occurred is that rarely is a dedicated room with fixed equipment kept ready for radiation accidents. Many of the early designs of hospital facilities for radiation accidents had a permanently installed decontamination table top in a dedicated room. There was often rigid plumbing with drainage to a specific holding tank for radioactive materials. In some instances, these facilities were located in or near the autopsy room rather than near the emergency room.

Another major change has been that the radiation aspects of the case have become secondary, and trauma, thermal burns, and myocardial infarctions have become the primary medical concern. Thus the patients must be able to be treated in the area where life support equipment exists and appropriate supplies are nearby. Most hospitals at this point, therefore, will handle radiation accidents in a designated area of the emergency room itself. This has the added advantage that the ER personnel are familiar with where their supplies are located. Now most hospitals maintain equipment which is not fixed and therefore can be readily moved, not only to the emergency room but to other parts of the hospital (in case a radioactive spill occurs within the hospital).

Most hospital plans regarding radiation accidents have assumed the possibility of 1 to 5 severely injured and contaminated patients from some industrial or research facility. We now know from the experience at Three Mile Island and Chernobyl the hospitals also need to be prepared to be able to evaluate large numbers of the public for radioactive contamination. Many people living near a nuclear facility which has had release of radioactivity will come to the hospital even though they are not injured just to check whether they have become contaminated with radioactive materials. Unless specific arrangements are made, these persons usually will come to the emergency room and possibly in very large numbers. Any plan therefore must include several people with monitoring equipment who can make such evaluations, keep appropriate records, and still leave the emergency room capable of handling severely traumatized patients.

II. COMMUNICATIONS

Communication undoubtedly is one of the most important aspects of preparation for a radiation accident. Early in the plan-writing process the hospital should develop some idea of the various facilities in their area that handle radiation sources and radioactive material. Once this has been done, one can predict the type of accident that may come from each facility. The facilities and ambulance personnel should be aware that, in the case of a suspected or actual radiation accident, the hospital will need advance notice in order to prepare for the patient's arrival. This information should be directed to the charge nurse in the emergency room. Directing such information to the hospital switchboard has not proven satisfactory in many experiences. The ER charge nurse should have a specific procedure manual immediately available to her/him. This manual should include a call sheet (see Appendix 1) which prompts certain questions to be asked of the caller including number of patients, type of injuries, and whether the accident is simply a case of overexposure (external irradiation) or contamination is involved or suspected. A phone in the room where the patient is to be treated is necessary. This will allow the physician in the room to communicate directly with the industrial facility and consultants as may be necessary. The Radiation Emergency Assistance Center/Training Site (REAC/TS) of Oak Ridge Associated Universities is a federally funded service which is available 24 hours a day to provide advice on handling radiation accidents. The phone number should be included in all radiation accident protocols.

III. AREA DESIGNATION

If there is a possibility of radioactive contamination, then a *Radiation Emergency Area* (REA) must be set up. The purpose of this area is to control the spread of radioactive materials. Choice of a radiation emergency area is made on the basis of several factors: (1) the area chosen must be suitable to appropriate life support and medical stabilization, (2) the area should be located close to an entrance or have an entrance directly into the treatment room from the outside (this will minimize the possibility of tracking contamination throughout the emergency room), and (3) the area should also be easily accessible to the ambulance so that an ambulance can back up close to the entrance to be utilized. Procedures should designate that the ambulance is to be roped off and watched by security or other personnel. The reason for this is that the ambulance may be contaminated.

The radiation emergency area is usually set up to have a *contaminated room* (i.e., a room which one is willing to let become contaminated while treating the patient) and a second area outside the contaminated area referred to as the *buffer zone*. This buffer zone is an area in which access is controlled by means of doors or ropes. Figure 1 shows a buffer zone. The object is to try to keep this area clean of contamination but with the realization that there may be breaks in technique which allow radioactive materials to come out of the contaminated room into the buffer room. Beyond the designated buffer zone is the clean (radiation-free) area of the hospital.

The entrance to the contaminated room, optimally, is directly from the outside of the hospital directly into the room. Thus, portions of the emergency room which have a fire exit are ideally suited to become an REA. If such an entrance is not available, it usually is not practical or economical to install an entrance specifically for radiation accidents. In the situation in which no such entrance already exists, there are two acceptable alternatives. The one most commonly utilized is to have a plastic floor covering rolled out from the REA down the hall and out the emergency room entrance. The patient is then taken from the ambulance (on the ambulance stretcher) into the treatment room. It is important to keep the ambulance personnel and the stretcher on the floor covering. This method is only practical if the hospital has had advance notice, time to put down the floor covering, and if the area chosen for the REA is not too far inside the emergency room entrance.

If there has been no advance call of patient arrival or if the REA is located at a fair distance from the emergency room entrance, the simplest alternative is to take a clean hospital

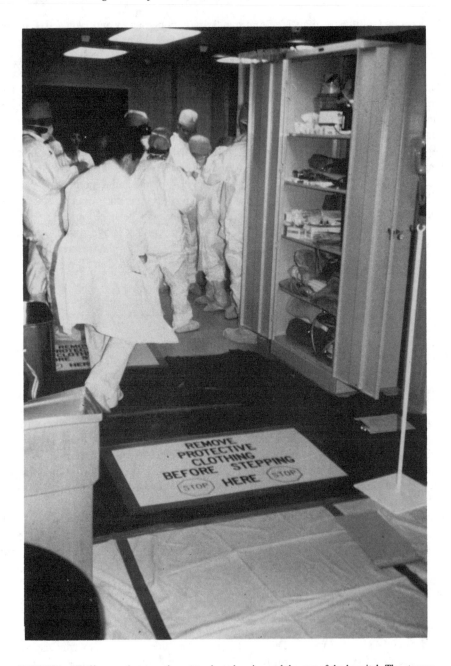

FIGURE 1.   Buffer zone between the contaminated region and the rest of the hospital. The storage cabinet with accident supplies is located in the buffer zone.

stretcher (with a sheet opened on it) out to meet the ambulance. The patient can be transferred from the ambulance stretcher onto the hospital stretcher, wrapped up in the cloth sheet, and brought into the hospital. A cloth sheet is almost always sufficient to contain the radioactive contamination. In addition, under circumstances in which the patient needs to proceed immediately to the operating room, this method can also be utilized very effectively. The only requirement for this latter technique is that the ambulance personnel must know not to bring a potentially contaminated patient to the emergency room itself but rather to ask the emergency room staff to come out to the ambulance. The use of plastic sheets to wrap the patient is generally inadvisable.

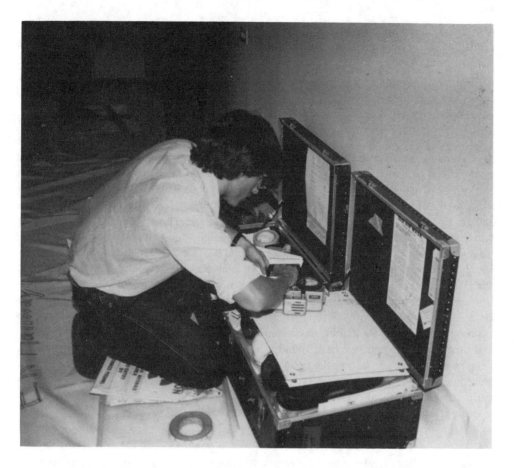

FIGURE 2.   Storage of supplies for a radiation accident — two portable trunks.

IV. SUPPLIES

Supplies needed to handle radiation accidents in general already exist in the hospital. There are a number of authors who have formulated supply lists for the radiation treatment areas of the emergency departments. A representative list may be found in Appendix 1. One of the first considerations is how to store the supplies. There are three possibilities which are often utilized. These are a closet, locker, and part or all of a large lockable box, i.e., a steamer trunk. Whichever one is utilized, however, it must be lockable. The keys to these supplies normally are kept with the narcotics key by the emergency room charge nurse. Our particular preference is for storage of the supplies in some manner by which they can be easily moved; for example, the locker or cart on wheels, or the steamer trunk. (See Figure 2.) The reason for this is that if there is an accidental spill in the hospital, the supplies can easily be moved to the site for appropriate cleanup. These supplies should be organized with an inventory list, to be checked every 6 months, and brief, explicit directions for the use of the items. This will make handling of an accident much easier if persons unfamiliar with radiation accident drills actually have to handle a contaminated and injured patient. The general category of supplies that are included are protective clothing, instrumentation and dosimeters, material for securing the area and controlling contamination, i.e., rope and signs, materials for bioassay and labeling, decontamination supplies, and a long pair of forceps to handle radioactive metallic fragments.

Various supplies which are not mentioned elsewhere in the text of this chapter include rope and radiation area signs to mark off portions of the REA. Sample taking and a decontamination kit and supplies are also needed, as well as record-keeping devices, such as pencils, paper, tape, and even a portable dictaphone. A sample inventory is listed in the Appendix 1.

V. AREA SET-UP

The REA can be set up in many different ways. The critical factor is the amount of time available between the time notification to expect such a patient is received and the actual arrival of the patient. Most areas need to be able to be set up within 15 to 20 min, although on a historical basis, one out of three or four patients will arrive at the emergency room without any prior notification. Under these circumstances, if the patient is seriously injured, area setup may have to be done while the patient is being treated. The setup may be accomplished by emergency room personnel, radiology and nuclear medicine personnel, radiation safety personnel, or the housekeeping and engineering department. The difficulty with having either the radiation safety officer or a nuclear medicine personnel in charge of this is that they are not immediately available on evening or night shifts. Most hospitals rely upon either housekeeping or the the emergency room personnel themselves to set up the area. The placement of the rope, signs, etc. can be very confusing to somebody who has never been through a training session and who is reading the procedure manual for the first time. In this regard, we have found it extremely valuable to take photographs of the setup in various stages during the course of a drill. These photographs are placed in the procedure manual so that they can be looked at to facilitate REA setup. A map of the floor space and traffic flow also is valuable.

VI. FLOOR COVERING

Mention already has been made of floor covering. Prior to patient arrival, most hospitals try to cover the floor in the contaminated room and the buffer zone. In fact, this is not necessary for treatment of the patient. The sole purpose of placing floor covering down is to make cleanup of contamination easier after the patient has been treated and left the area. There is no excuse for delaying medical treatment of a patient because there is no floor covering in place.

Several materials have been utilized for floor covering. Paper products are unacceptable since they tear easily when they become wet. Clear or black plastic has been utilized but extreme care should be taken with these materials since they become very slippery when wet. There are some plastic materials which are heavy duty and of a nonskid variety which have been successfully utilized. The most common of these is Herculite™. This is available in several different weights and colors. Probably the cheapest and most available material for floor covering is barbecue cloth. This is most commonly use for tablecloths at picnics and has a nonskid back with a plastic top. It comes in 4-ft-wide rolls and can be purchased at most fabric stores. In the interests of saving time for area preparation, many hospitals have taken the floor covering material and taped it together so that it fits the floor plan of a certain room and can simply be unfolded. All of the materials mentioned need to be taped down at the edges, as shown in Figure 1, to avoid tripping.

VII. VENTILATION

Ventilation in the REA is always a matter of concern. Some institutions have installed high-speed exhaust fans with respirable particle filters. In fact, most residual radioactive contamination usually is not in the form of easily respirable particles, but rather heavy and large particles similar to dirt. The primary reason that surgical masks are worn during treatment of radioactively contaminated patients is not to prevent inhalation of the contamination but rather to keep the hands of doctors and nurses away from their faces (thus preventing oral contamination). In spite of the fact that such residual radioactive contamination on patients is not easily airborne, it is still a wise idea to cover the exhaust duct of the hospital ventilation system from the REA with a piece of plastic and masking or duct tape. While this has little effect from a scientific viewpoint, it provides a great amount of reassurance to patients and staff in other portions of the hospital who do not understand that X-rays, gamma rays, etc., are not carried along by air currents. A particular caveat to be kept in mind is the special instance in which contamination involves transuranic elements such as plutonium or americium. Under these circumstances, if there is a lot of contamination, respiratory protection may be necessary. Respirators usually are only necessary in hospitals near weapons or very large research facilities. Arrangements to bring appropriate respiratory protection with the patient should be made prior to an accident.

VIII. PATIENT DECONTAMINATION

Decontamination of the patient may pose a problem in terms of disposing of the water utilized. Certainly, if the patient only has a minor traumatic injury, he probably should have been kept at the facility where the contamination occurred, decontaminated there, and then brought to the emergency room as a "clean" patient. A patient who has been brought to the emergency room and is severely traumatized obviously will be unable to stand up in a shower. Over the last ten years, decontamination table tops for supine patients have been developed and are available from several manufacturers (see Appendix 1). Often these are lightweight tables which have straps supporting the patient in the supine position and allow the patient to be washed off and the water collected from a drain in the table (see Figure 3). A shower head is sometimes used but there should be a mixing valve to assure that the water may be adjusted to lukewarm rather than being simply hot or cold. Some hospitals have installed fixed plumbing for these purposes (see Figure 4). In our hospital, we use a garden hose attached to a faucet with a shower head since this is much cheaper, disposable, and may be used at any location in the hospital. If a decontamination table top is available, there must be a mechanism for water drainage and collection. Decontamination table tops should have seatbelt-type straps so that they can be firmly affixed to a standard stretcher.

Specific consideration must be given to contaminated patients who present to emergency rooms and have suspected myocardial infarctions. In such circumstances, it is not wise to place such patients on metallic tables (such as a morgue table) or even on a metallic decontamination table, since the patient may need electrical defibrillation. If no decontamination table top is available, simple removal of the outer clothing will generally remove 70 to 90% of all surface contamination. The residual contamination will most likely, then, be on the exposed portions of the patient such as the hands, face, neck, and hair. These can easily be washed with a regular washcloth and a basin. During this time, the patient can be kept on a standard emergency room stretcher.

IX. SHIELDING

Shielding may provide some protection from radiation. This may be in the form of lead bricks, lead aprons, or leaded glass. Unfortunately, experience has demonstrated that shielding is only of limited value in most radiation accidents. Lead aprons are the item that most radiologists and emergency room physicians feel are necessary. However, lead aprons of the type available in radiology departments are predominantly useful for low-energy X-rays (about 30 keV). Most radionuclides involved in accidents have energies which range from

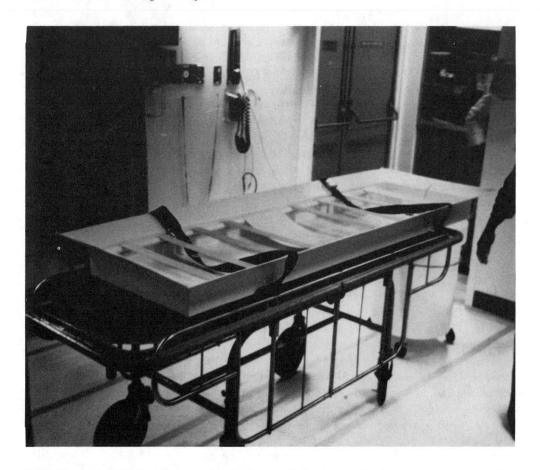

FIGURE 3.   Decontamination table top can be affixed to a regular hospital stretcher. Drainage may be through a hole and attached hose at one end into a large bucket, but for radiation protection purposes, smaller containers are better.

100 keV to over 1000 keV. Thus, in most of the circumstances, one or even two lead aprons do not provide a significant shielding.

Previously, many REAs were designed to include heavy lead shielding which could be placed about the patient. Often these lead shields weighed hundreds of pounds and were not only cumbersome but also top-heavy, so that sometimes they presented more of a danger to the patient than protection to the medical staff. Under most accident circumstances in management of a patient at a hospital, radiation protection for medical staff is best obtained by (1) increasing the distance form the radiation source and (2) spending less time near the radiation source. There is one circumstance in which shielding is important. If a radioactive metallic fragment has been removed from the patient, a lead container (such as may be found in nuclear medicine departments) should be used for placement of the item (see Figure 5). Most nuclear medicine departments also have lead bricks which can be obtained as necessary for special shielding purposes. Another item which is useful for radiation protection purposes is a clock. This should be clearly visible in the REA. With this, the radiation safety officer or radiation technician can keep tract of the amount of time various individuals have spent in the radiation area.

X. PROTECTIVE CLOTHING

Protective clothing should be utilized in handling contaminated patients. "Protective" clothing is somewhat of a misnomer, since it does not actually protect the wearer from

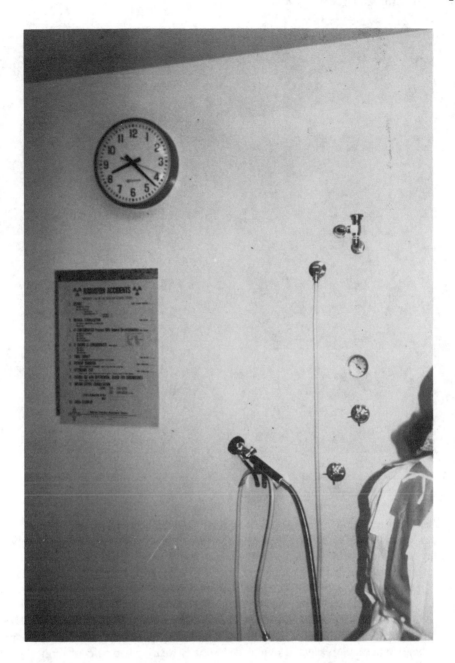

FIGURE 4. Permanent plumbing installed for decontamination with a shower head and mixing valve as well as a temperature gauge. A simpler, less expensive way is to use a rubber hose hooked to a standard faucet. Also note the clock and radiation accident poster.

penetrating radiation. Protective clothing usually consists of plastic or water-repellant gowns, jumpsuits, etc., which do not provide significant attenuation of either gamma rays or beta rays. The reason the clothing is termed protective is that it prevents radioactive contamination present on the patient from getting onto the skin of the attendants. If contamination gets on the protective clothing, it can be removed by removing the clothing.

Protective clothing that is utilized at hospitals ranges from full anticontamination gear (coveralls and hoods) to more limited and easily accessible items such as surgical scrub

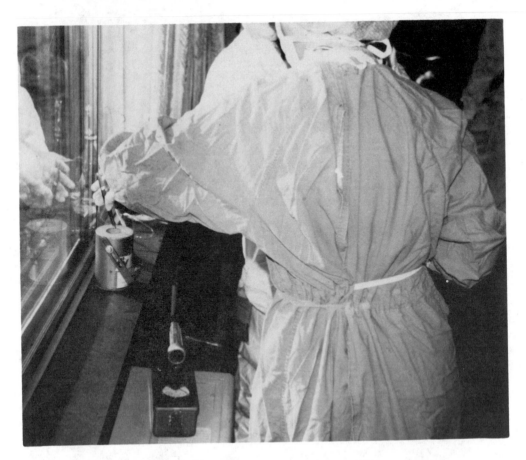

FIGURE 5. Lead container (pig) used for placement of highly radioactive fragments. Notice also that forceps are being used to handle radioactive material.

gowns and plastic aprons. Figure 6 illustrates an individual in protective clothing. The jumpsuits or coveralls with hoods provide somewhat more coverage, although they are generally very hot to wear and difficult to get out of at the end of the procedure. Presently most hospitals utilize either water-repellant jumpsuits or gowns. A surgical mask is always used to reduce the possibility of hand-oral contamination. A surgical cap is also recommended, particularly for women who have long hair. Gloves are also necessary. The best gloves to utilize are surgical gloves, since it is often necessary to handle wounds, begin intravenous lines, etc. While heavier gloves may not rip as easily, they are often more cumbersome. Some authors have recommended initially wearing two pairs of surgical gloves so that, it the outer pair becomes contaminated, it can simply be removed. This is not absolutely necessary since if only one pair of gloves is worn and it becomes contaminated it simply can be changed.

Plastic shoe covers are always utilized. Paper booties (as can be found in operating room) are insufficient since they often become wet and disintegrate. If the plastic shoe covers have a relatively high ankle portion, this should be secured with tape.

XI. INSTRUMENTATION

Radiation instrumentation and dosimeters are also necessary. The instrumentation should include as a minimum a Geiger counter. This should preferably be able to operate on batteries as well as on standard electrical current. A Geiger counter really is only utilized to determine

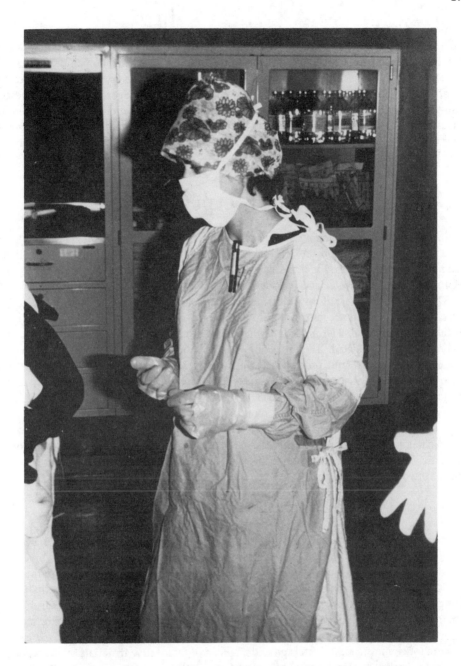

FIGURE 6. Protective clothing. This garb is designed to keep radioactive contamination from getting on the attending personnel. Surgical gloves are somewhat less cumbersome than those seen in this picture. Also note easy accessibility of pen dosimeter on collar.

whether contamination is present and, if so, where. If very high levels of contamination are present, such that there might be a medical hazard to attendants, the radiation exposure may exceed the capability of the meter and thus a higher range exposure meter is also useful. Many Geiger counters have a maximum exposure capability of about 100 mR/h.

Personnel dosimeters are necessary to determine the dose of radiation received by an individual attendant during the course of accident management. There are three forms of dosimeters which are utilized. The first is a pen dosimeter which is basically a small ionization chamber. This is set to zero or has had a baseline reading taken prior to being worn and it is placed on the outside of the collar of the individual. These dosimeters have the advantage of being instantaneously readable. At any time during the accident, the pen dosimeter may be held up to the light and the radiation exposure read. While very convenient, these do not provide a permanent record and are not as accurate as film badges or thermoluminescent dosimeters (TLDs). These latter two items are familiar to most radiologists and often to the nurses as well. These are worn underneath the protective clothing and provide a very accurate record of the dose actually received. Unfortunately, they cannot be read immediately and must be processed. It is important not to let them get contaminated prior to their processing or the dose indicated will be erroneously high. (See Chapter 18.)

XII. PROCEDURES

In spite of all the planning that is done and the procedures which are written, the management of the patient needs to be able to proceed even with a physician and/or nurses who have never participated in a drill or read the procedure manual in this regard. It is often helpful to make up a poster and include it with the supplies.

The procedure for handling a radiation accident should be written out, with copies kept in the emergency room and radiation safety office, as well as in the Radiology and Nuclear Medicine Departments. The procedures should be kept on word processors so they can be easily and quickly updated. The procedure manual should include a distribution list as well as table of contents. Sample procedures for a hospital which can be easily adapted are found in the Appendix 1. Many of these procedures are difficult to utilize during the course of an accident; a very good innovation has been implemented by the staff of Brigham and Women's Hospital in Boston, which includes a section in the procedure manual with a summary of individual duties for each person involved in the accident management. During the course of an actual accident it is simply necessary to tear the appropriate page out of the book for that individual and hand them the page. This should describe the substance of their particular duties in two or three paragraphs.

XIII. SECURITY

An often overlooked area in management of these accidents is the need for security as well as the news media aspects. The security personnel should be intimately involved, not only to direct the ambulance to the appropriate entrance, but to be able to secure the entire area in the event of a contaminated patient. A radiation accident of any size merits intense news media coverage. News media continuously scan and monitor ambulance transmissions and, in some accidents, the reporters have actually gotten to the hospital ahead of the patients. Reporters will often cross REA boundaries to be able to talk to the patient and get a story. Under these circumstances, there is potential spread of radioactive materials by the reporters. In order to circumvent this, hospital administration should be notified when there is a radiation accident. This should allow an area to be set up from which information can be given to the reporters as it becomes available. At the same time, security should be keeping the reporters out of the radiation emergency area.

XIV. DRILLS

Drills are essential to adequately prepare for handling radiation accidents. The purpose of the drill is twofold. First, to assure that the procedures which have been written are in fact functional, and also to provide training for the personnel. Radiation accidents, as has been mentioned in earlier chapters, are very uncommon and, therefore, unless drills are held it is unlikely that management of such patients will be optimal or even acceptable. We find that these drills should be held at least on an annual basis, and we often include the drill as part of the annual radiation disaster drill for the hospital. It is useful to inject as much realism as possible in the drill by going through the entire procedure with protective clothing and a simulated patient. We videotape our drills and then edit them down to a 12- to 15-min tape with audio dubbing to explain each of the steps involved. These tapes are then made available to the emergency room for training during the course of the year. As new emergency room physicians and their nursing staff are hired during the course of the year, these tapes can be used to provide a relatively short but efficient training experience. At the end of each drill a critique should be held, at which time each of the deficiencies where questions were raised can be addressed. Reports derived from the critiques and accidents suggested are normally forwarded to the radiation safety office and the disaster control committee.

XV. SUMMARY

In summary, effective management of radiation accidents requires a large amount of preparation and thought. In addition, training of the staff is absolutely essential. This is best accomplished through annual drills, but also may be accomplished through the use of videotapes. The critical points to be remembered in the handling of such accidents and in writing the procedures is that treatment of non-radiation-related injuries and medical stabilization are paramount. The second point is that it is important to be able to distinguish between a patient who has been irradiated from an external radiation source and one who is contaminated with radioactive materials. The handling of these two types of accidents is entirely different and this distinction needs to be made early. All of the items outlined in this chapter concern the care of the severely injured and radioactively contaminated.

Chapter 12

EMERGENCY ROOM MANAGEMENT OF RADIATION ACCIDENTS

Robert Rosenberg and Fred A. Mettler, Jr.

TABLE OF CONTENTS

I. INTRODUCTION

The treatment of radioactively contaminated patients is a rare occurrence. The techniques for management of radioactive contamination are also applicable to handling contamination with other toxic substances and, with appropriate modifications, may therefore be used in those circumstances. This chapter is concerned with emergency room management of accidents involving a limited number of radioactively contaminated and medically injured patients. Such circumstances may happen in transportation accidents of radioactive materials, accidents in a medical or research laboratory, or small accidents at nuclear power stations. There are four different kinds of radiation accident patients (see Figure 7, Chapter 1).

A. WHOLE-BODY IRRADIATION ONLY

These persons are not radioactive; however, they may have received very large doses of radiation from an external source. Radiation overexposure is primarily a medical disease and the patient is managed in regular hospital or emergency room without modification. Accidents of this sort occur from irradiation by radioactive industrial sources or accelerators.

B. INTERNAL CONTAMINATION ONLY

This could be secondary to inhalation ingestion or wounds involving radioactive materials. This may be from an industrial accident, a very severe misadministration of nuclear medicine materials, or even bizarre circumstances such as attempted suicides. If there is no concurrent external contamination, these patients again may be treated in routine medical or emergency rooms; however, vomitus, urine, or feces may be contaminated and must be handled with care.

C. A HIGHLY RADIOACTIVE METALLIC SOURCE IMBEDDED WITHIN A PATIENT

Such accidents are exceedingly rare, but warrant a special classification. Since activated pieces of metal can have very high specific radioactivity there may be a significant exposure hazard to treatment personnel. Dose rates from such fragments may be as high as 50 R/h very close to the object. Such accidents could occur from an explosion in the reactor of a nuclear power plant.

D. EXTERNAL CONTAMINATION WITH OR WITHOUT INTERNAL CONTAMINATION

This accident may occur as the result of a transportation accident, a nuclear power plant accident, or a spill in a nuclear medicine facility. When serious injury accompanies the contamination, this group requires special precautions to avoid spread of the radioactive contamination to the environment and to medical personnel, and to minimize or prevent internal contamination of the patient.

These patients may need emergency treatment of their injuries concurrently with their radiation dosimetry and decontamination. It must be emphatically noted that radioactive contamination (whether internal or external) is never immediately life-threatening and, therefore, decontamination should never take precedence over significant medical or surgical injuries. It is, however, important to minimize the internal contamination if at all possible.

One can then give general objectives in approximate order of importance for the emergency room management of seriously injured and contaminated patients.

1. First aid and resuscitation
2. Medical stabilization
3. Definitive treatment, if possible, of serious injuries

4. Prevention/minimization of internal contamination
5. Assessment of external contamination and decontamination
6. Treatment of other minor injuries
7. Containment of the contamination to the treatment area and prevention of contamination of other personnel
8. Minimization of external radiation to treatment personnel
9. Assessment of internal contamination
10. Treatment of internal contamination (this could be concurrent with many of the above)
11. Assessment of local radiation injuries/radiation burns
12. Careful long-term followup of patient with significant whole-body irradiation or internal contamination
13. Careful counseling of patient about expected longterm effects and risks

II. DECONTAMINATION

The theory of decontamination is relatively simple. Most radioactive contamination on intact skin behaves like loose dirt and may be removed by routine washing. The effectiveness of decontamination procedures is easily monitored by a Geiger counter. Radionuclides *on the intact skin* surface rarely, if ever, cause a high enough gamma radiation dose to be a hazard to the patient or to medical staff. Even large amounts of fresh fission contamination on a patient are unlikely to cause dose rates of more than 1 rad/h. To date, the highest recorded absorbed dose in the U.S. to a medical person treating patients from a commercial reactor has been 14 mrem (0.14 mSv). The intact skin is a very effective barrier to internal contamination. Internal contamination may be a hazard depending upon activity and residence time within parts of the body. Since the main hazard of external contamination is the possibility of internal contamination, external contamination procedures are designed to (1) minimize or prevent internal contamination and (2) decrease the external contamination which is present. All efforts are made to clean the contamination from the skin, which usually is in the form of loose radioactive dirt, but occasionally may be fixed or imbedded in the skin. The skin barrier must be preserved so that procedures such as shaving or harsh scrubbing are not done. If hair needs to be removed, clipping is effective. Warm water, not hot, is used for washing so that a hyperemia is not induced which may increase absorption of any contaminants through the skin. Cold water is not used since it would tend to close skin pores and trap radioactive contamination. Decontamination is done by progressive cleansing, starting with mild agents such as soap and water and working up to somewhat more involved procedures (Figure 1 and 2). The decontamination end point is reached when:

1. No further decrease occurs as determined by monitoring
2. The contamination is considered low enough to no longer be a significant hazard, i.e., twice background levels
3. When further decontamination would be more harmful than helpful

The latter is particularly important in contaminated wounds where debridement might result in permanent or potential deficits in areas such as hands or face. (See Chapter 13.)

III. RADIATION EMERGENCY TEAM DUTIES

The duties of the members of a radiation emergency team are as follows:

A. MAINTENANCE

It is essential to have the necessary equipment such as gowns, gloves, monitoring devices, and protective floor sheeting transported to the appropriate area and assembled. These persons

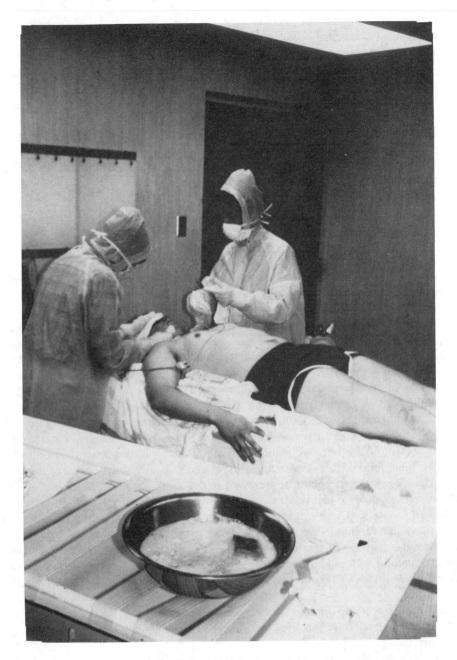

FIGURE 1.   Decontamination of a patient suspected of having a myocardial infarction as well as radioactive contamination. Note the patient has not been placed on a metallic decontamination table top and is easily being decontaminated utilizing soap, water, and washcloths.

should also consider closing off the ventilation of the area as well as placing appropriate warning ropes and signs.

B. SECURITY PERSONNEL
The radiation area may well be contaminated and must be isolated and protected from visitors. Security may be necessary to direct the ambulance to a designated site or special entrance to the treatment area.

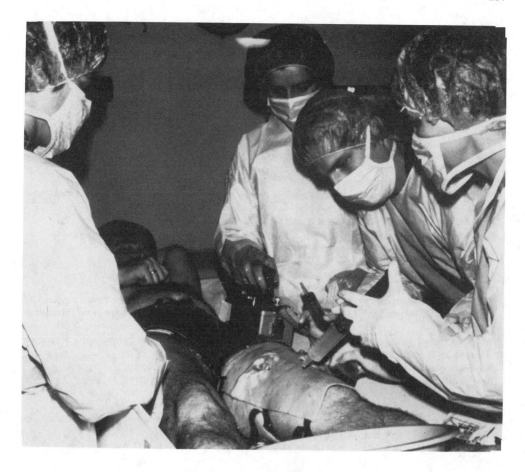

FIGURE 2. Decontamination of a wound utilizing irrigation. The wound shown here is a moulage and this is a practice drill.

C. PHYSICIAN

At least one emergency physician should be present in the decontamination room to deal with the acute medical emergencies. Other medical specialists may be needed as dictated by the other injuries in the case. A medical check list of useful information to be obtained is given in Table 1.

D. TECHNICAL PERSONNEL

A radiation technician, nuclear medicine technologist, or health physicist must ensure the monitoring instruments are operating properly and assign, collect, and distribute the personnel dosimeters. This individual should perform surveys to determine the extent and magnitude of radioactive contamination.

E. NURSING PERSONNEL

At least two nurses will be needed inside the decontamination room, one for direct patient care and decontamination, and the other assisting with transfer of equipment in and out of the room, labeling the specimens, etc. Additionally, a third nurse who controls the buffer zone of the decontamination suite is required. This is usually the busiest and one of the most important positions. One other person is required to bring equipment as needed to and from the radiation emergency area (REA) from the rest of the hospital. If possible, another person generally in or near the buffer zone, whose job is solely to monitor everything leaving the room for possible contamination, should be available.

TABLE 1
Medical Information Check List

These can be used by the attending physician at the hospital for obtaining historical information to assist in the early management of radioactively contaminated persons.

Circumstances of the accident
  When did the accident occur and what are the circumstances of the accident?
  What are the most likely pathways for exposure?
  How much radioactive material is involved potentially?
  What injuries have occurred?
  What potential medical problems may be present besides the radionuclide contamination?
  What radioactivity measurements have been made at the site of the accident, e.g., air monitors, smears, fixed
    radiation monitors, nasal smear counts, and skin contamination levels?
  Are toxic or corrosive chemicals involved in addition to the radionuclides?
  Have any treatments been given for these?

Present status of the patient
  What radionuclides now contaminate the patient?
  Where and what are the radiation measurements at the surface?
  Was the patient also exposed to penetrating radiation? If so, what has been learned from processing personal
    dosimeters, e.g., film badge, TLD, or pocket ionization chamber? If not yet known, when is the information
    expected?
  What information is available about the chemistry of the compounds containing the radionuclides? Soluble or
    insoluble? Any information about probable particle size?
  What decontamination efforts, if any, have already been attempted? With what success?
  Have any therapeutic measures, such as blocking agents or isotopic dilution been given?

Followup of patient
  Has clothing removed at the site of accident been saved in case the contamination still present on it is needed
    for radiation energy spectrum analysis and particle size studies?
  What excreta have been collected? Who has the samples? What analyses are planned? When will they be done?

F. PUBLIC RELATIONS/ADMINISTRATOR

Since radiation accidents are of intense public and media interest, one can expect reporters and photographers to arrive in droves. The hospital administration needs to be prepared to deal with such individuals, as well as to keep a liaison with the company where the accident occurred.

An optimum team would therefore include the following:

1. One physician
2. One buffer zone nurse
3. Two nurses in the decontamination room
4. One "gofor" person outside the decontamination room
5. Two survey personnel; one inside the room, one outside

IV. RADIATION ACCIDENT MANAGEMENT EXAMPLE

In order to give a clear understanding of the workings of an emergency room during a radiation accident, a scenario and the handling of such an accident will be given. The scenario involves a small chemical explosion at a nearby nuclear power plant, causing a serious physical trauma and radioactive contamination to worker A. Another (B) is contaminated and has minor injuries and other workers (C and D) have skin contamination only.

The initial response in any accident would be emergency personnel arriving at the scene. In any industrial scene, this would be the first aid team and/or security personnel. Notification would be made to the control room of the power plant (or, outside of the power plant, to police personnel). Immediately, first aid should be given to the two injured as required and the area cordoned off. An ambulance is called as soon as significant injuries are identified. If the site of the accident is in a high enough radiation field (>30 to 50 R/h) the patients should be carefully moved to a nearby lower radiation field area. The hospital should also be notified to begin preparation of the REA. It is essential that the ambulance be given specific instructions as to where to enter the plant and where to park. Ambulance personnel should be given dosimeters, be accompanied by security guards from the main plant gate, and be instructed on how they are to dress. Gowns, surgical gloves, and boot covers are usually adequate. It is particularly critical to avoid contamination of the ambulance by parking upwind if there are fumes or a fire. The ambulance personnel will perform the usual medical stabilization, make an assessment of the injuries, and again notify the hospital. Specifically, notification should be given to the emergency room of the number of victims, the nature of the injuries, and whether or not patients are or are suspected to be contaminated.

At this point triage is important. Workers C and D, who only have skin contamination, should probably be kept at the plant and decontaminated. There are several reasons for this. First, plant personnel usually are much more familiar with decontamination procedures than are emergency room personnel. Second, if all four workers are taken to the hospital, the ambulance will be needlessly crowded and the activities at the hospital REA may be more confused than necessary. Worker B, who has minor injuries and surface contamination, can be taken to the plant's first aid room and have decontamination done as well. If some wound contamination persists, this worker can have the wound covered and be driven to the hospital in a private automobile. Only worker A, who is seriously injured, needs to be transported to the hospital while still contaminated. If time permits, initial decontamination may be done in the ambulance. This involves careful removal of outer clothes and washing contaminated areas (usually face and hands). The ambulance then transports the patient to the emergency treatment area. Since the entrance to the REA may not be the usual emergency room entrance, the ambulance personnel must be so informed. It is useful for security personnel to be stationed at appropriate locations to direct them.

When the hospital emergency room receives the *notification* of the accident, it puts its radiation accident plan into action. This requires coordination of several different groups as already outlined.

It takes approximately 20 to 30 min to set up an average decontamination suite for one or two patients. When the ambulance arrives, the patients are conducted into the treatment area. If there is not an outside door to the treatment room, there are several ways to move the patients without spreading contamination. One way is to lay nonskid plastic sheeting down the hallways over which the ambulance stretcher may be wheeled (Figure 3). It is also possible, if the victim's injuries are not too serious, to transfer the patient from the possibly contaminated stretcher in the ambulance onto a clean stretcher with the patient wrapped in clean blankets or sheets. The patient can then be transported down the usual hallways with the contamination contained inside the sheet.

Upon arrival, the usual medical assessment should be performed to insure that the patient is, in fact, medically stable. This is likely to include routine blood work, physical exam and history. If IVs are needed, they should be started, preferably in areas that are uncontaminated; however, IVs or central lines, if necessary, could be started through regions that are possibly or known to be contaminated if the area is routinely cleansed. Again, external contamination is not immediately life-threatening and should not be allowed to seriously interfere with emergency or resuscitative medical procedures. If, by chance, a patient is routinely admitted to the emergency room and radioactive contamination is subsequently discovered, the following steps should be taken:

1.   Continue attending to the patient's medical needs

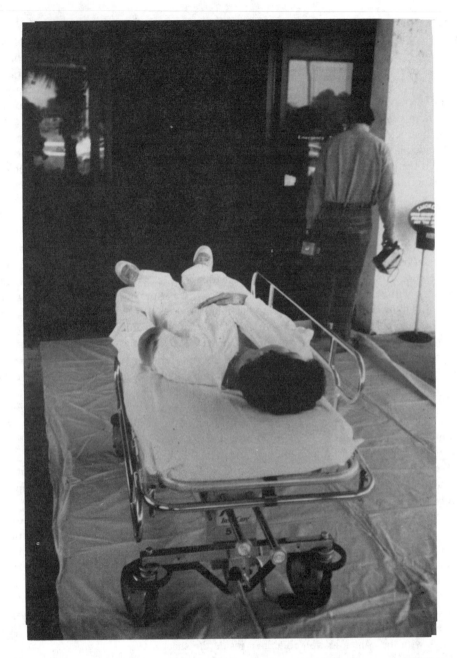

FIGURE 3.   Contaminated and injured patient being wheeled into an emergency room through the only entrance. The area has been covered. An alternative is to transfer the patient to a clean hospital stretcher out by the ambulance and not cover the ground.

2.   Secure entire area where victim and attending staff have been
3.   Do not allow anyone or anything to leave area until cleared by the radiation safety officer
4.   Establish control lines and prevent the spread of contamination
5.   Completely assess patient's radiologic status
6.   Personnel should remove contaminated clothing before exiting area, they should be surveyed, shower, dress in clean clothing, and be resurveyed before leaving area

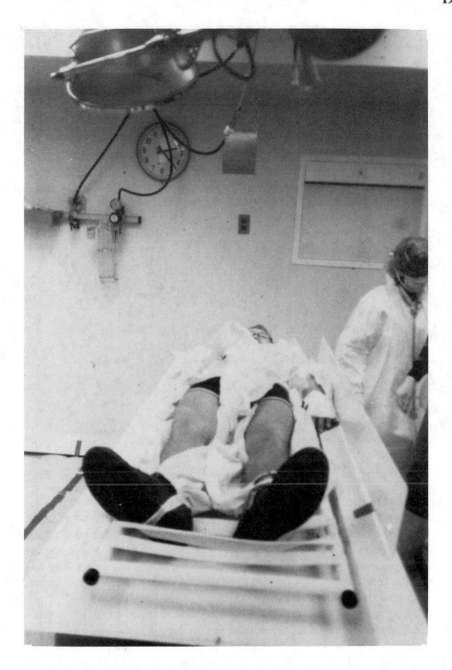

FIGURE 4. After medical stabilization, cutting, folding back, and removal of clothing will remove most external contamination.

With appropriate notification, and the patient medically stabilized, initial decontamination of the patient should be started. The most effective step, which may be done in the ambulance on the way to the hospital, involves the removal of all external clothing. This is likely to remove over 90% of the contamination with the exception of the hands, face and other exposed skin areas. This should be carefully accomplished to avoid contamination of clean skin from the dirty clothing, and to keep the contamination contained. This procedure is most easily accomplished by carefully and correctly cutting off the clothes. The cuts are best made in the midline along the leg, the arms, in the middle of the chest, and abdomen

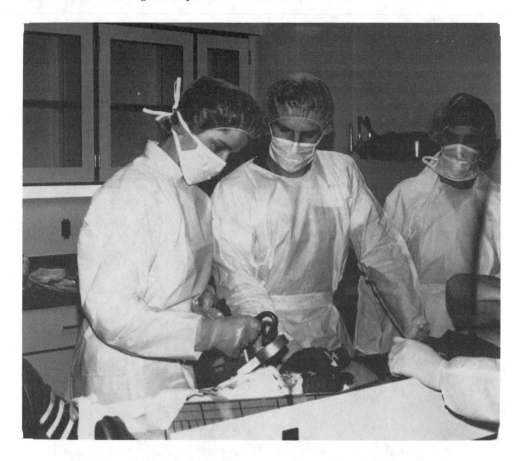

FIGURE 5.   Monitoring of an open wound to assess possible level of contamination.

of the clothes (Figure 4). The clothes are then carefully folded back away from the skin so that any dislodged contamination will not fall on the patient, but will tend to fall away from him. The clothes can then be folded inside on themselves and removed from the patient. Shoes and/or boots should also be removed if possible as this will also remove a large amount of contamination. If the clothes are heavily contaminated, they should be placed in a plastic bag and removed to a far corner of the decontamination suite so as not to affect the background reading of the patient.

Following removal of the clothing, the patient should again be carefully monitored from head to toe (including the back, if possible) and the locations and readings of any contamination remaining on the patient's skin should be carefully recorded. Swabs should be made of these contaminated areas, and the site and time must be recorded (Figure 5). The distance of the probe to the patient should be a standard distance of approximately one inch. This is essential for comparison with subsequent readings, which will be made to determine the effectiveness of decontamination. If there are sufficient personnel, decontamination and removal of clothing could be done concurrently with medical assessment and stabilization.

If contamination on skin persists, there are several items that should be considered prior to the use of more aggressive scrubbing or the use of stronger decontaminating agents. Often the persistent counts may come from contamination which is in skin folds of the ears, about the nose, etc. It also may be the result of radioactive material under or next to the fingernails. Thus, before more aggressive tactics are employed, a careful washing of these areas should be performed. A second point to remember is that not all counts on an instrument may be coming from skin contamination. They may in fact be coming from internal contamination

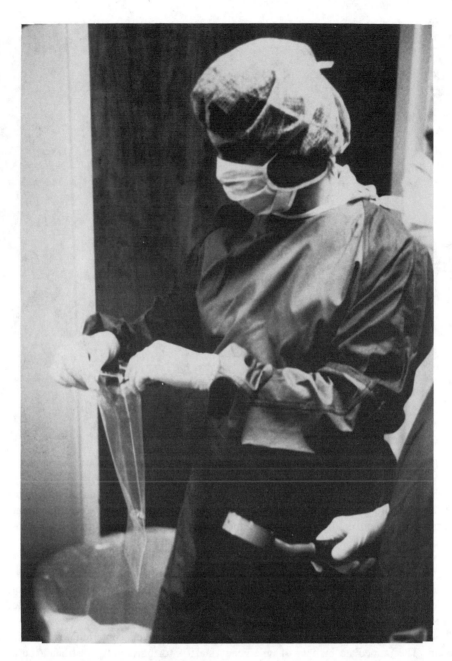

FIGURE 6.   An example of anticontamination clothing which is usually worn. Samples of skin swipes, debrided tissue, nasal swabs, etc. are all bagged and labeled for later analysis.

such as inhaled or ingested materials or even radioiodine in the thyroid or contamination of the Geiger counter probe.

Internal contamination should be assessed at a minimum by swabs of the nares and mouth. Internal contamination should be suspected if nasal or oral swabs show contamination although, since oral and nasal contamination may be rapidly cleared, negative swab readings should not be construed as an indication that internal contamination is not present. All swabs should be placed in a bag and labeled (Figure 6). The swabs can be counted either on a Geiger counter or in nuclear medicine. Nasogastric suction should be considered if there is

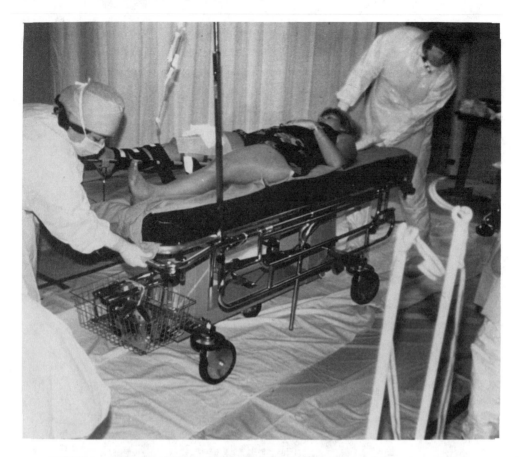

FIGURE 7.   Stabilized and decontaminated patient leaving REA after transfer to a clean stretcher.

the serious possibility of recently swallowed radioactive materials. All excreta, such as urine, feces, etc., should be collected, labeled by site and time and examined for contamination. Contamination found in any of these documents internal contamination, and the samples may be analyzed for the isotopes and compounds involved.

If there are open wounds and they are free of contamination, they should be covered with a water-proof dressing such as Op-cite™ to prevent cross-contamination. Contaminated wounds may be cleaned by gentle scrubbing with a surgical sponge and irrigation. Debridement for removal of contamination should be carefully considered before it is performed as outlined in Chapter 13.

Emergency management of thermal burns that are radioactively contaminated is a difficult problem. The immediate instinct of emergency staff is to thoroughly wash such burns to remove the contamination. This should not be done for several resons. If the thermal burn is extensive, any washing will place the patient in grave danger of hypothermia and hypotension. Even if the thermal burn is localized, scrubbing may remove marginally viable skin and make the burn treatment much more difficult. Usually, gentle rinsing of local burns is all that is necessary initially. The burn is then covered and over the next few days the exudate will lift out a lot of the contamination into the dressings.

When the patient is stable and clean, he can be moved from the room. "Clean" would suggest a contamination level at or below twice background level although, depending upon the region of contamination, more or less may be tolerated. When the patient is clean, he should be transported carefully to a clean table or stretcher for removal from the room (Figure 7). When this is done the personnel should have on clean gloves. The appropriate procedure for removal is to roll in a new stretcher over a clean plastic sheet parallel to the patient's decontamination table. The patient is then transferred to the clean stretcher. The clean patient is then wheeled out of the room. The patient, stretcher, all supplies, the IV bags, and everything leaving the room must be monitored to prevent the spread of contamination outside the REA.

At this point, it is only the personnel who will have to carefully deglove and degown as they exit the room. This involves a progressive removal of the outer toward the inner garments, leaving all possibly contaminated articles in the REA. The personnel are then monitored, particularly the feet, as they exit the room to be sure that they are not contaminated. The usual approach is removal of the outer pair of gloves, followed by the mask and/or hat. Aprons are removed, followed by the external surgical gown which is carefully removed from the outside keeping the contamination off the personnel. Finally, the booties are removed one at a time with the person then stepping from the room toward the outside one foot at a time and, while leaning back in the room, the gloves are then removed one at a time (Figure 8).

The pen-reading dosimeter and film badge thermoluminescent dosimeter (TLD) should be given to the radiation safety officer for recording and processing, if necessary. Be sure that the proper name is affixed to the dosimeter or film badge. Once all the personnel have left, one now has simply a contaminated room. This is usually cleaned up by the persons responsible for the contamination, such as the power plant or the transportation company. It is essential that the contaminated waste be properly disposed of.

V. SPECIFIC PROBLEMS

The psychological aspects of the patient are all too often forgotten in the emergency management of such patients. Certainly, the emergency room is a strange enough environment for most patients. This feeling, coupled with the appearance of frightened medical staff all suited up in gowns, etc. is even more unsettling to the patient. If we now add the patient's own fears about radiation effects, we have the makings of a genuine psychiatric consult. A calm and reassuring attitude of all concerned is essential not only in management of the patient, but of the family, news media, and hospital administrator. Careful discussion with the patient about the short- and long-term effects of the radiation are almost as essential as the decontamination. This should include the reassurance that the patient is not a hazard to their friends and families.

Often questions arise as to how to perform certain medical procedures in a decontamination suite. This list is not exhaustive, and neither are the explanations; however, they do give a good indication as to how these procedures may be easily and efficiently performed.

A. BLOOD

Blood can and should be taken for the usual routine diagnostic tests. If possible, venipunctures, including i.v. lines, should be performed outside the areas of known contamination. If this in not feasible, then the selected area should be cleansed in the usual fashion and the venipuncture performed. The puncture does not usually introduce significant contamination into the patient. The blood products should then be monitored before leaving the suite. If contamination is identified on the blood tubes, it is most likely to be contamination on the surface as significant contamination of the blood is unlikely. This surface contamination may then be cleaned off.

B. EKGs

The easiest method of performing an EKG if necessary is to leave the EKG cart outside the room in a clean area and only introduce into the room one set of EKG leads. These are

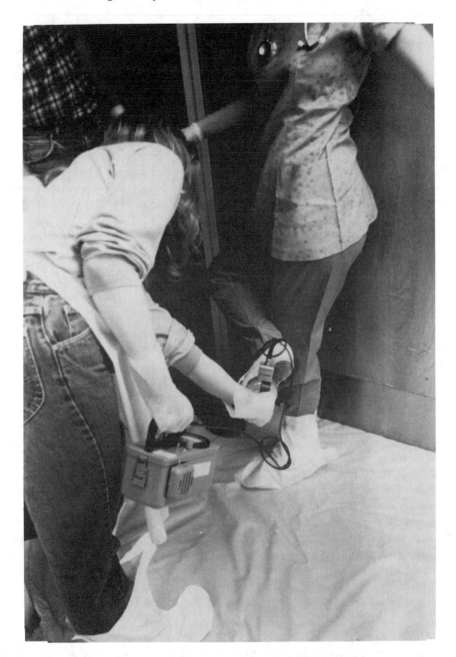

FIGURE 8.   Monitoring of individual medical staff leaving REA.

attached to the patient and a clean end is left attached to the EKG machine. The procedure is performed and the EKG leads can then be left in the room for decontamination or disposal, with the machine now being free to be used elsewhere in the hospital.

C. X-RAYS

Routine portable X-rays can be performed. Again, the X-ray machine can be left outside the decontamination room and only the head of the machine projected into the room (Figure 9). The patient should be wheeled on the stretcher toward the edge of the room and then the X-rays can be performed of the chest, abdomen, or extremities as needed. The film, of

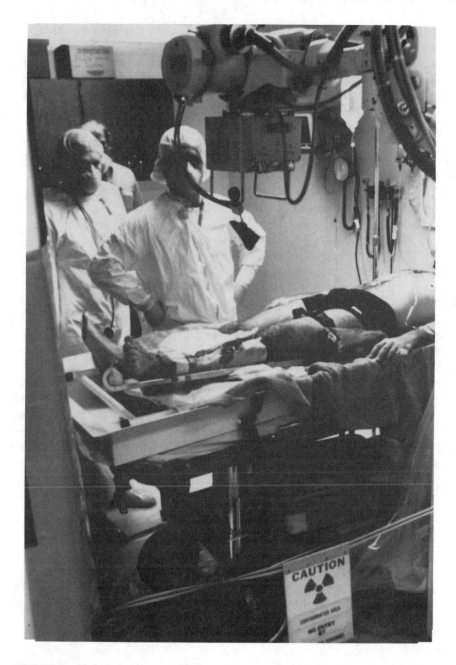

FIGURE 9. Method of taking a portable X-ray with the machine remaining in the noncontaminated buffer zone.

course, must be moved into and then out of the room. This can be done most easily by placing the clean cassette inside a plastic bag, which is then placed under the patient as required. The cassette with the bag is then handed out toward the outside of the room, the clean cassette inside the bag removed and the contaminated bag left within the decontamination suite. The X-ray machine, not being contaminated, is now free to be removed.

D. SURGICAL EMERGENCIES

Under the worst case, a patient with a surgical emergency could be moved to the operating room while still contaminated and have the emergency surgery performed. During surgery, a minimization of internal contamination should be attempted; however, any life-threatening emergency requiring immediate surgery should not be deterred or deferred by the presence of external contamination. In this case, the operating room would be contaminated and would need to be decontaminated prior to use by other patients. One could assess the presence and level of contamination in this room with a careful survey using a Geiger counter.

E. HIGH-LEVEL SOURCE OR METAL FRAGMENTS IN PATIENT

It is possible for small, highly radioactive metal fragments to be embedded in the patient. Because they may have a very high dose rate at their surface, it is essential that they be handled with forceps or pick-ups to avoid possible radiation burns to personnel. A lead "pig" from nuclear medicine is useful to shield personnel from these fragments once they are removed (Figure 5, Chapter 11).

VI. SUMMARY

Emergency room management of radioactively contaminated patients who have an associated medical injury requiring immediate attention must be handled with care. Radioactive contamination of the skin of a worker is not a medical emergency and is usually dealt with at the plant. Effective preplanning and on-the-scene triage will allow the seriously injured and contaminated patients to get the medical care they need with a minimum of confusion and interference. Immediate medical and surgical priorties always take precedence over radiation injuries and radioactive contamination.

Probably the most difficult aspect of emergency management is the rarity of such accidents and hence the unfamiliarity of the medical staff with the appropriate procedures. The simplest answer to these problems is preplanning, having a simple and workable procedure and finally having 24-h access to experts. The Radiation Emergency Assistance Center/Training Site of Oak Ridge Associated Universities offers such assistance on a 24-h basis at (615) 481-1000, extension 1502, or Beeper 241.

REFERENCES

1. **Leonard, R. B. and Ricks, R. C.,** Emergency department radiation accident protocol, *Ann. Emer. Med.,* 9, 462, 1980.
2. Management of Persons Accidentally Contaminated With Radionuclides, NCRP Rep. No. 65, National Council on Radiation Protection and Measurements, Washington, D.C., 1980.
3. **Jankowski, C. B.,** Radiation emergency, *Am. J. Nurs.,* 82, 90, 1982.

Chapter 13

MANAGEMENT OF SKIN AND WOUND CONTAMINATION

George A. Poda

TABLE OF CONTENTS

I. INTRODUCTION

Since one seldom incurs radioactive contaminated injury without some external body contamination, it may be expeditious to briefly review external decontamination in preparation for treating the injuries that might occur. Good judgment is essential in determining decontamination priorities.[1] Since some radioactive materials are corrosive or toxic because of their chemical properties, medical attention might have to be directed first to a nonradiological problem if radioactive materials were shipped as acids, fluorides (uranium hexafluoride—UF_6), mercury, or lead compounds. In general, contaminated wounds and body orifices are decontaminated first, followed by areas of highest contamination levels on the intact skin. The purpose of decontamination is to prevent or reduce incorporation of the material (internal contamination), to reduce the radiation dose from the contaminated site to the rest of the body, to contain the contamination, and to prevent its spread. Complete decontamination, which returns the area to a background survey reading, is not always possible because some radioactive material can remain fixed on the skin surface. Decontamination should be only as thorough as practical. Decontamination should again begin with the least aggressive method and progress to more aggressive ones.[2]

II. PLANT OR ON-SITE DECONTAMINATION

Medical, health physics, and support personnel need to work closely. It is advantageous to have a rough and ready decontamination site in the workplace itself. This needs to be nothing more than a warm water tank with a hose in an area protected from the elements and located close to the source of potential contamination. Near this area there needs to be small storage cabinet to hold simple monitoring instruments (remember to check the batteries frequently), some detergent, scrub pads (sanitary pads work best), coveralls, and perhaps some rubber or plastic gloves for helpers. Other items that are useful to prevent spread of contamination include shoe covers, protective clothing, etc. At the work site decontamination facility, the gross surface contaminant can be washed off quickly, reducing total exposure to all involved.

The next step is to remove the patient to a site designated by health physics and medical staff for definitive decontamination. The first step is to perform a survey of the patients as follows:

1. Wear appropriate protective clothing (gloves, gown, etc. as needed).
2. Use a survey meter with beta, gamma, and alpha detection capabilities.
3. Before entering the decontamination room or before patient arrival, perform an operational check of the instrument and determine the background level. Open the shield on the probe so that both beta and gamma radiations are detected.
4. Set instrument selector switch to the × 1 range or most sensitive scale of the instrument.
5. When necessary, adjust the range of the instrument by moving the selector switch. Meter readings should not be taken when the dial indicator reads in the lower 10% of the scale when on the × 100 and × 10 ranges. Turn the selector switch to the next most sensitive range to measure the exposure rate more accurately.
6. Holding the probe approximately 1 in. from the patient's skin, systematically survey the entire body from head to toe on all sides. Move the probe slowly (about 1 in./s) and pay particular attention to wounds, orifices, body folds, hairy areas, and hands.
7. An increase in count rate or exposure rate above the background indicates the presence of radioactive contamination on, in, or near the patient.
8. Document time and radiation measurements on an anatomical drawing; each subsequent survey result should be documented.

9. The use of headphones or an audible meter if available facilitates monitoring.
10. If unsure whether radioactivity is very localized (such as a single particle) or spread out, a piece of lead with a small hole in it can be used as a collimator.

Note: A patient survey can be done simultaneously with other emergency procedures, provided there is no interference with needed emergency care. Also try to determine whether the exposure was recent or some time ago, also whether a single acute exposure or a chronic one that was delivered over a matter of days, weeks, or months.

In a plant decontamination facility there needs to be a full shower to cleanse hair and skin. Contaminated body orifices, such as the mouth, nose, eyes, and ears, need special attention because absorption of radioactive material is likely to be much more rapid in these areas than through the skin.

If radioactive material has entered the oral cavity, encourage brushing the teeth with toothpaste and frequent rinsing of the mouth (a 30% hydrogen peroxide solution might be helpful). Gastric lavage can be used if radioactive materials were swallowed (rarely needed unless the substance is most soluble in acid media). Likewise, contaminated eyes should be rinsed by directing a stream of water from the inner canthus to the outer canthus of the eye to try avoiding contamination of the nasolacrimal duct. Contaminated ears require external rinsing; an ear syringe can be used. A sink is necessary for nasal douches. The simplest method is a saline bottle or bag with a connected i.v. tube. The loose end minus its needle is inserted into the nostril and gravity flow from the elevated bottle rinses the nostril as one bends over the sink. Lastly, the medical units should have the capability for definitive decontamination.

A. SKIN DECONTAMINATION

Percutaneous absorption is of concern with all types of radionuclides and, when it occurs, most chemicals pass through the epidermis rather than the sweat glands and hair follicles. The most important barrier to penetration is the horny layer. When contamination reaches the bottom of this layer, it diffuses rapidly through the rest of the epidermis and into the capillaries. The lower layers of the stratum corneum possess a sponge-like capacity to fill and empty. This process may explain why alpha contamination can sometimes "reappear" after decontamination.

Percutaneous absorption is a passive process determined by the chemical and physical properties of the contaminating substance and its interaction with the skin. Mechanical damage and hydration increase absorption (concentrated acid and alkaline burns tend to increase absorption).[3] Since each compound will have a different rate of percutaneous absorption, generalization is of little help. However, when internal contamination is a major concern, e.g., Pu, it must be assumed that percutaneous absorption can occur and therefore the integrity of the horny layer barrier should not be breached.

Contaminants may be held to the surface of the skin by electrostatic forces or surface tension. Also, chemical compounds may be formed between the contaminant and skin protein. Mechanical entrapment in the hexagonal plates of the horny layer may occur with material of small particle size. Although contamination may sometimes be extremely difficult to remove by physical or chemical means, the skin will cleanse itself, the horny layer being shed and renewed on a 14 to 15 d cycle. The turnover rate differs considerably in various areas of skin. Forehead skin appears to turn over faster, while on the back of the hand it is slower than for other parts of the body. Any damaging influence such as scrubbing reduces the renewal time. In general, most contamination is limited to the upper part of the horny layer and will therefore usually be shed in just a few days.

Regular soap and water should be tried first. Should contamination remain, detergents should be tried. If yet present, a solution of 1:4 sodium hypochlorite:water solution can be applied and rinsed off several times. Radioactive substances usually rest on the thin film of oil which covers the outer layers of the skin and the pores and hair follicles. There are a few radionuclides which can penetrate this oily layer and be absorbed through the intact skin if the contact time is long enough (e.g., iodine and tritium). Decontamination methods are based on the removal of this oily film by means of soap and detergents followed, only if necessary, by the removal of the outer horny layer of the skin itself by stronger agents. From this it will be appreciated why dry, diseased skin is so difficult to decontaminate — not only will the skin condition itself be made worse, but there is a much greater possibility of producing absorption of the radioactive material. Soaps and detergents also emulsify and dissolve contamination and are frequently all that are needed for decontamination of skin. Gentle brushing is done using a Kotex type pad, soft surgical sponge, or the use of powdered detergent. This dislodges some contamination physically held by the skin protein or removes a portion of the horny layer of the skin. Although some authors recommend use of mixtures of Tide, Calgon, carboxylmethylcellulose, and cornmeal, we feel that this produces too much skin abrasion. If contamination is yet present, a solution of 1:4 sodium hypochlorite:water can be applied and rinsed off several times. Full strength sodium hypochlorite (household bleach) has been used, but since this warms the skin it needs to be rinsed off quickly. Do not use this solution around the eyes. While chemical techniques are seldom necessary, they can be used. Some texts recommend the use of potassium permanganate (4%), a powerful oxidizing agent. Sodium acid sulfite (4%) removes the permanganate stain. This will remove a portion of the horny layer, but is messy and no better than sodium hypochlorite.

In especially stubborn cases in which the contamination seems to be localized in one or two tiny spots in the thick horny layer, such as the palms of the hands, a small high-speed abrasive wheel can be used to sand off the spot. Obviously care must be taken to prevent environmental contamination. Sticky tapes have been used successfully by some, but they tend to remove the horny layer rapidly and, if not used carefully, can lead to increased percutaneous absorption. A table of decontamination techniques with detailed instructions is presented in Table 1.

When using any of the above agents or techniques, always begin with the least irritating and proceed to stronger or more abrasive techniques only if absolutely necessary. It should be recognized in this sequence that the stronger agents are used after a certain amount of skin irritation has already occurred.

It is a common mistake to underestimate the potential for skin irritation until too late. Decontamination procedures are always carried out starting at the periphery of the contaminated area and working gently towards the center. Contaminated washings must not be allowed to run onto uncontaminated areas of the skin or into wounds or body orifices. Pads of the fingers and nails often resist all decontamination attempts. Simple sanding with fine emory cloth works well on both. Fingerprints may be removed, but this is temporary and the skin whorls regrow within a few days. If hands resist decontamination or become reddened or sore, one might try putting on a rubber glove for 8 to 16 h. The sweating from inside out does a good job of cleansing the skin.

Dermatographia or soreness of the skin is a signal to stop, as this indicates a break in the skin barrier. The physician will want to know when the decontamination effort can be safely stopped. Citing an absolute numerical level would require so many assumptions as to be misleading. The rate of the initial contamination, as least as far as absorption is concerned, depends on its physical and chemical characteristics. For these reasons, it is not realistic to set down arbitrary radiation levels that would indicate whether or not to pursue additional decontamination. Nevertheless, calculations have been made to estimate the contamination level of various radionuclides on the skin that would deliver 15 rem/year to the

TABLE 1
Decontamination of Personnel and Equipment[3]

Contaminated area	Decontaminating agent	Remarks	Maximum suggested levels contamination
Skin and hands	Mild soap and water or detergent and water If necessary, follow by soft sponge, heavy lather, and tepid water	Wash 2—3 min and monitor; do not wash over 3—4 times Use light pressure with heavy lather wash for 2 min, 3 times, rinse, and monitor; use care not to scratch or erode skin	Alpha 150 d/m/100 cm²
			Beta—Gamma Average less than 0.3 mR/h for each hand surface or 100 cm² of skin surface, using Geiger-Mueller instrument
	Apply a freshly prepared 5% solution of sodium acid sulfite (NaHSO₃)	Apply in the same manner as above; apply for not more than 2 min. The above procedure may be repeated; apply lanolin or hand cream when completed.	
Wounds (cuts and breaks in the skin)	Running tap water report to Medical Officer and Radiation Safety Officer as soon as possible.	Wash the wound with large volumes of running water immediately (within 15 sec.); spread the edges of wound to permit flushing action by the water	Keep wound contamination as low as possible
Clothing	Wash, if level permits	Use standard laundering procedures, 3% versene or citric acid may be added to wash water.	Alpha 150 d/m/100 cm²
			No area to average more than 0.1 mR/h. Geiger-Mueller ²²⁶Ra calibrated, open window measured with 30 mg/cm² thick tube wall.
	Store	To allow for decay if contamination is short lived	(If clothing is worn 100 hr/week this will give 1/10 of maximum external dose.)
	Disposal	Treat as solid waste if necessary	

basal layer if maintained to 40 h/week and 50 weeks/year. Such a case is theoretical, since contamination would remain only days to a few weeks even without interim decontamination. A rough rule of thumb can be used to convert dpm beta to cpm, i.e., dpm ÷ 10 = cpm. With ^{32}P, a persistent level of almost 180 cpm could be left on the skin and would not exceed the 15 rem/year occupational dose level to the basal layer. Levels twice as high on the forearms and five times as high on the hands will deliver doses at the current "permissible" level. It has been suggested that 10^{-4} μCi/cm² beta and 10^{-5} μCi/cm² alpha could reasonably be considered as maximum permissible levels of skin contamination. As a practical matter, working numbers used by some health physicists as upper limits on skin contamination that is especially difficult to clean are 1 mR/h beta (portable G-M meter) and 1000 dpm alpha (air proportional counter with a 60-cm² window). Much higher levels may be encountered in emergencies and the decision to cease decontamination will probably rest on evidence of the decreasing effectiveness of the decontamination efforts and/or presence of signs of excessive irritation to the skin. If high levels of activity remain on the skin, it will probably be prudent to resort to mild decontamination efforts 2 or 3 times per day rather than to a single intensive effort. Hair needs to be rinsed and washed several times. It may take as many as twenty times to become clean. If the contaminant is a liquid that embeds in the hair, one needs to consider cutting of the hair, although this is seldom necessary.

B. WOUND DECONTAMINATION

Wound contamination needs to be handled somewhat differently from skin contamination. Basic to all first aid principles, serious injuries need primary attention first, thus someone seriously injured needs to be wrapped in a sheet or some method of containment and transported to a hospital capable of handling contaminated persons. Here the staff can carefully handle the emergency expeditiously and then secondarily perform needed decontamination. Most wounds are lacerations, abrasions, puncture wounds, or burns. Any or all of these can be contaminated by radionuclide. Translocation and absorption of a contaminant from a wound to the general circulation or to regional lymph nodes is the major concern. It helps to know the type of contaminant, particularly with reference to its particle size, pH, and solubility in water. If acidic or caustic, the contaminant may coagulate proteins and actually reduce dispersion. For soluble contaminants one might consider a chelate given internally (by aerosol or intravenously) to block absorption either before or during treatment of the wound site. The methodology for chelation therapy is outlined in Chapter 10.

Health physics personnel need to perform a wound count. Should the adjacent area still be contaminated, a thin piece of lead or a vinyl lead material with a hole punched or cut in may be used. The hole should just be large enough to admit the wound site and thus will give an accurate reading, even though there is surrounding contamination present. It is mandatory to have a good count before the wound is decontaminated in order to determine if decontamination or debridement is successful. This obviously means that there needs to be monitoring of the wound performed during the attempts of decontamination and postdecontamination.

Cuts are probably the most frequently contaminated injury. If they are bleeding profusely, standard first aid measures are needed, that is, pressure dressing, etc. while en route to the medical facility. Should they be bleeding slightly, a *venous* tourniquet helps them continue slight bleeding with its decontaminating effect while the patient is en route to a decontamination area. Much of the contamination is deposited on the skin edges of the cut. At the medical facility, gentle scrubbing is usually performed. Jagged or deep cuts are often decontaminated with the use of a Water Pik™-type device. When surgical instruments become contaminated, as determined by frequent monitoring, they should be removed from the surgical field and replaced with fresh, sterile tools in order to prevent extension of contamination. The difficulties involved in detecting the contaminant, while preventing its spread, will mean that the surgical procedure may last much longer than normally expected. Many more instruments and sponges than usual will be required. When all else fails, sodium hypochlorite (dilute or up to full strength) can be used and the wound quickly rinsed. The better the decontamination, the less debridement is needed. Try to preserve the anatomy. It may be better to leave a small amount of contamination rather than to amputate a digit or damage a tendon or joint. This is especially true if the materials are expected to be relatively insoluble. These materials have a tendency to form a granuloma in roughly six months which can then be felt and easily removed. If there is a minute amount left (as evidenced by a low wound count but higher than background), touch the wound with a 12% solution or stick of silver nitrate. This provides hemostasis and also seems to bind the material in an eschar, and if the wound is either left open or only loosely closed, it allows the material to leave with the precipitated tissue. A post-operative wound count will need to be performed by the health physics personnel and followup debridement could be done later when the skin and other areas are free of contamination. When drains are used, dressings should be monitored for radioactivity. Care should be used to collect any scab when it detaches from the wound. Often appreciable contamination can be found in it when it is analyzed. When an extremity is severely contaminated and adequate decontamination is not possible, the surgeon may be faced with the decision whether or not to amputate. The conservative approach may be stated as follows: unless the extremity is so severly injured that functional recovery is unlikely, or unless the beta-gamma contamination is so severe that extensive and severe radiation-induced necrosis can be expected, amputation is rarely indicated. Long-lived alpha emitters such as plutonium may represent a potential long-range threat, but conservative treatment should be tried first and the decision to amputate postponed until the potential long-term risks are clearly defined and understood. In other words, decontaminate but do not mutilate.

Puncture wounds seem to be the next most common, and these mostly involve the hands, especially the fingers. Punctures of the finger pad are simplest to treat. There are no vital structures and it is therefore possible to inject a local anesthetic adjacent to the puncture. If necessary, finger block may be performed. The $1/4$ in. diameter ''skin biopsy punch'' is then placed over the puncture and rotated till it comes to rest on the tuft or shaft of a distal phalanx. A pair of curved eye scissors cuts out the tissue as it is held up with a pair of forceps. Such ''biopsy'' areas tend to bleed a fair amount but a silver nitrate stick rotated to touch all interior surfaces followed by a snug bandaid controls the bleeding well. Anything left behind usually comes out with the eschar. After such procedures the finger is well healed in approximately 10 d. Other sites may require more extensive microsurgical debridement, using the same principles.

Postoperative wound counts can be very confusing, being high one day and even negative on another. What does this imply? The implication is that the angle of the wound to the counter is at variance. To obviate this, it is useful to get powdered wood putty and mix it to a doughy consistency. With this spread out and placed in a pie pan, the hand can be placed in a position with the wound exposed. Thus an imprint of the hand can be produced. When the mold dries, the health physicist simply has to place the hand in the mold each day to get consistent reading and eliminate confusion.

Avulsion injuries do occur, especially in laboratories where zealous laboratory attendants try to force syringes containing radionuclides. Syringes break and cut away pieces of skin from fingers, especially along the lateral aspect of the digits. Too often the patient appears with a bloody digit and one wonders how to cover the defect cosmetically. It is useful to indoctrinate workers to hunt for and bring all tissues to the medical facility. Even though contaminated, dousing such tissues in a 1:1 solution of sodium hypochlorite and water and rinsing several times will decontaminate the avulsed tissue, which can then be applied as a cover for the defect. I usually steri-strip rather than suture these as eventually the tissue dries up and falls off, often leaving behind a nice clean area of granulation tissue which has bridged across the defect with the help of the covering offered by the avulsed tissue. This method applies to fingertips as well. Burns when contaminated are usually caused by acid solutions of a radionuclide. Except for tritium and iodine, most radionuclides do not pass through the barriers of intact skin. Once the barrier breaks down absorption can occur; this must be kept at or to a minimum. Thus, for small areas of burns either thermally or chemically caused, the usual techniques for all such are followed (application of cold to thermal burns and flushing of chemical burns). The therapy then consists of application of 12% silver nitrate solution and a loose cover. In approximately 24 h a firm eschar has formed, which has entrapped most of the radionuclide. To expedite its removal application of urease enzyme

(Panafil-White) does a good job of breaking down the eschar in 24 h so that approximately 48 or 50 h after the initial burn, one sees a clean pink and uncontaminated tissue. Depending on the depth of the burn, this usually heals quickly. The one thing to consider is the total area involved so that one does not apply too much silver. To date, areas to approximately 50 in.[2] have shown no clinical problem. With burns, a chelate or neutralizer for the radio-chemical should be given promptly. This is usually done systemically as described earlier. Acne, if contaminated, can cause some absorption as the skin barrier has been broken. The same problem occurs with rashes. Simple scrubbing with a surgical soap is usually sufficient, although sodium hydrochlorite may be used. Stubborn spots can be touched with silver nitrate. Blisters can be treated as burns if gentle scrubbing will not decontaminate the area.

Confidence, cheerfulness, and honesty need to be extended toward the patient. The person contaminated is "just plain scared", no matter what the educational level. A "gloomy Gus" personality is further frightening and no matter who says what at a later time, the initial impression almost undoubtly will remain. If you do not have the answer admit that you do not have it. Of course, total uptake of the radionuclide is the greatest worry. Initially, one can only take a far-out guess. If often takes weeks or months of wound counting and bioassy to get a figure one may use with confidence. The point is, tell the injured party just that. Give "guesstimates" if they insist, but emphasize that these are in fact guesses and can be as much as four-fold off from the correct answer. As data becomes available, let the patient know. Once one develops confidence on the part of the patient, the entire post-accident course becomes easier. Long-term wound counting and bioassay are also needed. A combination of these statistics can, in time, give a fairly accurate dose figure.

These are some clinically tried and used techniques of some 35 years experience in a nuclear fuel production plant and research laboratory. The described procedures work and they represent four-generation therapy modality and are current. It is hoped the readers of this chapter will go on to formulate and develop even better techniques.

REFERENCES

1. Management of Persons Accidentally Contaminated with Radionuclides, NCRP Rep. 65, National Council on Radiation Protection and Measurements, Washington, D.C., 1980.
2. **Poda, G. A.,** Decontamination and decorporation; the clinical experience, in *The Medical Basis for Radiation Accident Preparedness,* Hubner, K. F. and Fry, S. A., Eds., Elsevier/North Holland, New York, 1980, 327.
3. **Kusama, T., Itoh, S., and Yoshizawa, Y.,** Absorption of radionuclides through wounded skin, *Health Phys.,* 51(1), 138, 1986.

Chapter 14

LONG-TERM FOLLOWUP OF PATIENTS INVOLVED IN RADIATION ACCIDENTS

Jonathan C. Marshall and Fred A. Mettler, Jr.

TABLE OF CONTENTS

I. INTRODUCTION

Medical examination and followup of patients involved in radiation accidents is important not only for the patient and legal reasons, but also in order to identify and add useful data to the literature concerning effects of radiation on humans. There are two basic types of radiation effects which need to be considered: stochastic and nonstochastic.

Stochastic effects are those which do not appear to have a threshold for induction and which occur with increasing probability related to dose. Another characteristic of stochastic effects is that, even though the probability of induction is related to dose, the severity of the effect is not. The typical long-term stochastic effects are tumorigenesis and genetic effects. Radiation-induced cancer is a good example that can be used to elucidate the characteristics of stochastic effects. The probability that a given patient will develop a radiation-induced malignancy increases with increasing absorbed dose, but the nature, severity, and agressiveness of the maligancy is not related to dose.

Nonstochastic effects are predominantly related to cell killing. Typical examples of late nonstochastic effects include sterility, cataract formation, skin atrophy, fibrosis, and tissue breakdown. The severity of all these effects is directly related to the absorbed dose.

II. TUMOR INDUCTION

Tumor induction is the most important somatic effect of radiation doses below 100 rad (1 Gy). For both philosophical and protection purposes, one assumes there is no threshold for cancer induction, and this philosophy suggests that in theory even a small dose of radiation may have the potential of inducing a neoplasm. It must be emphasized, however, that there is a minimal amount of statistically valid data regarding human carcinogenesis at dose levels below 10 rad (0.1 Gy). All risk estimates that have been utilized are extrapolations from high-dose data.

Radiation is capable of producing benign as well as malignant neoplasms. With one or two exceptions, the risk estimates for induction of benign tumors have never been well defined; fortunately, however, they tend not to be of much clinical significance. Benign tumors have been reported following irradiation of the salivary, parotid, and parathyroid glands. A large experience after thyroid irradiation has allowed identification of benign thyroid adenomas with a risk factor approximately 4 to 12 cases annually per million persons exposed per rad (10 mGy).

In terms of developing malignant changes, it is well known that different organ systems and tissues of the body have different sensitivities. The susceptibility of different tissues to radiation-induced cancer is shown in table 1. Ascertainment of the risk per unit of radiation dose is a function of (1) the dose response and risk models utilized, (2) the age of the patient at the time of exposure, and (3) the sex of the patient. The risk factors published by the National Academy of Sciences Committee (Committee on Biological Effects of Ionizing Radiation [BEIR]) are shown in Table 2. The tissues with the highest rates of malignant induction are bone marrow, female breast, and thyroid. Due to the inclusion of breasts in this category, as well as the higher rate of induction of thyroid tumors in females as compared to males, overall risk per rad for tumor induction is significantly higher in females than males. As Table 2 also indicates, the risk of radiation-induced cancer depends strongly on age at exposure, and, in general, children appear to be more sensitive in this regard than adults.

Radiation-induced tumors are characterized by a latent period, which is the time from radiation exposure to the clinical appearance of the tumor. The latent period may be conceptualized as being comprised of at least two portions: the first is the true latent period, or interval from initiation of malignant cells to the beginning of unrestrained growth. This is

TABLE 1
Susceptibility of Different Tissues
to Radiation-Induced Cancer

High
  Bone marrow (leukemia)
  Breast (female)
  Thyroid (more common in females)
Moderate
  Bladder
  Gastrointestinal tract
  Liver
  Lung
  Lymphatic system
  Ovary
  Pancreas
  Pharynx
Low
  Bone
  Brain
  Connective tissue
  Kidney
  Larynx
  Nasal sinuses
  Salivary glands
  Skin
Very low or absent
  Cervix
  Chronic lymphatic leukemia
  Melanoma
  Prostate

From *Medical Effects of Ionizing Radiation,* Mettler, F. A. and Moseley, R. D., Eds., Grune & Stratton, New York, 1985. With permission.

then followed by a second period of tumor growth, which is the time to diagnosis or presentation. The mean latent period for various tumor types are shown in Table 3. Minimum latent periods are 2 to 3 years for leukemia, 3 to 4 years for bone cancer, and approximately 10 years for solid tumors. The existence of the latent period indicates that if followup studies are to be conducted on irradiated individuals, the studies need to be of sufficient length to extend past the latent period. As an example, if one were to design a study to followup those individuals exposed in the Chernobyl accident to identify radiation-induced malignancies, the study would need to extend for over 30 years, or past the year 2020. Similarly, if malignancies are identified before 1990 (i.e. earlier than the minimum latent period) in this population, it would be very unlikely that they were radiation-induced.

The length of the latent period depends on the age of the individual at exposure. This has been well documented for breast carcinoma. Radiation-induced tumors are often manifested with a high frequency when the individual reaches an age at which the ''normally occurring'' tumor has a high incidence. Thus, a woman exposed to radiation at age 30 may develop breast cancer at an age of 40 to 50. A female child exposed at 10 years of age will, however, have a longer latent period and may not demonstrate an excess incidence of malignancy until the age of 40.

Not all tumors, however, behave the same with regard to the latent period. For example, the length of the latent period in leukemia shortens with decreasing age of exposure.

III. RISK ESTIMATES

Relatively consistent risk estimates have been derived for tumors of the thyroid, female breast, and bone marrow. Studies of tissues which appear to be of less radiogenic sensitivity,

TABLE 2

Estimated Annual Excess Cancer[a] in 1 Million Persons per 10 mGy (rad)
(Excluding Leukemia and Bone Cancer) by Site, Sex, and Age at Exposure

Site	Age at Exposure (year)					Age-weighted average
	0—9	10—19	20—34	35—49	50+	
Males						
Thyroid	2.20	2.20	2.20	2.20	2.20	2.20
Lung	0.00	0.54	2.45	5.10	6.79	3.64
Esophagus	0.07	0.07	0.13	0.21	0.56	0.26
Stomach	0.40	0.40	0.77	1.27	3.35	1.53
Intestine	0.26	0.26	0.52	0.84	2.23	1.02
Liver	0.70	0.70	0.70	0.70	0.70	0.70
Pancreas	0.24	0.24	0.45	0.75	1.97	0.90
Urinary system	0.04	0.23	0.50	0.92	1.62	0.81
Lymphoma	0.27	0.27	0.27	0.27	0.27	0.27
Other	0.62	0.38	1.12	1.40	2.90	1.52
All sites	4.80	5.29	9.11	13.66	22.59	12.85
Females						
Thyroid	5.80	5.80	5.80	5.80	5.80	5.80
Breast	0.00	7.30	6.60	6.60	6.60	5.82
Lung	0.00	0.54	2.45	5.10	6.79	3.94
Esophagus	0.07	0.07	0.13	0.21	0.56	0.28
Stomach	0.40	0.40	0.77	1.27	3.35	1.68
Intestine	0.26	0.26	0.52	0.84	2.23	1.12
Liver	0.70	0.70	0.70	0.70	0.70	0.70
Pancreas	0.24	0.24	0.45	0.75	1.97	0.99
Urinary system	0.04	0.23	0.50	0.92	1.62	0.88
Lymphoma	0.27	0.27	0.27	0.27	0.27	0.27
Other	0.62	0.38	1.12	1.40	2.90	1.64
All Sites	8.40	16.19	19.31	23.86	32.79	23.10

[a]   Calculated for 11-30 years after exposure.

From *Medical Effects of Ionizing Radiation,* Mettler, F. A. and Moseley, R. D., Eds., Grune & Stratton, New York, 1985. With permission.

such as brain, salivary glands, bladder, and alimentary tract have yielded risk estimates which have somewhat greater uncertainty. There are, interestingly enough, some tissues which have an extremely low risk for radiogenic tumor induction, particularly adipose tissue, muscle, and prostate. The United Nations Scientific Committee on Effects of Atomic Radiation (UNSCEAR) has suggested that for whole-body irradiation, the risk factor for induction of fatal malignancies from acute high-dose radiation is approximately 4 to 7 per 1000 person Gy.[1] This means that 4 to 7 fatalities could be expected in a group of 1000 persons who were exposed to 100 rad (1 Gy) or in a group of 1000 persons, each exposed to 10 rad (0.1 Gy). Lower risk occurs if exposure is fractionated or chronic. A similar risk is quoted by the International Commission on Radiological Protection (ICRP) in its Report 26.[10] The risk for nonfatal malignancies is approximately the same. The effect of various exposures is shown in Table 4. The table also indicates the increase over the normal expectation of cancer mortality in the same population. It is clear from this table that an exposure of a population to 10 rad (0.1 Gy) will result in about a 1% increase of radiogenic cancer, as compared to the spontaneous cancer incidence.

With such figures in mind, one can begin to estimate a carcinogenic effect on the hundred thousand persons surrounding Chernobyl at the time of the accident. The average dose appears to be in the range of about 10 to 20 rad (0.1 to 0.2 Gy). If the spontaneous cancer

TABLE 3
Estimates of Latent Periods for Various
Tumors following External Irradiation

Tumor Type	Mean Latent period (year)
Brain	27
Salivary glands	20
Pharynx, larynx	24
Thyroid	20
Breast	22
Lung	25
Stomach	14
Sarcomas	12
Intestine, rectum	26
Cervix	27
Bone	10—15
Leukemia	7—10
Skin	24

From *Medical Effects of Ionizing Radiation*, Mettler, F. A. and Moseley, R. D., Eds., Grune & Stratton, New York, 1985. With permission.

TABLE 4
Estimated Excess Mortality in 1 Million Persons from All Forms of Cancer (Linear Quadratic Dose-Response Model for Low-LET radiation)

	Normal expectation	Absolute risk		Relative risk	
		Model	Excess	Model	Excess
Single exposure to 0.1 Gy (10 rads)	163,800	766	(0.47)	2,255	(1.4)
Continuous exposure to 10 mGy/year (1 rad/year for lifetime)	167,300	4,751	(2.8)	11,970	(7.2)
Continuous exposure to 10 mGy/year (1 rad/year) for ages 20—65	171,500	3,268	(1.9)	5,508	(3.2)
Continuous exposure to 10 mGy/year (1 rad/year) for ages 35—65	173,600	1,952	(1.1)	2,283	(1.3)
Continuous exposure to 10 mGy/year (1 rad/year) for ages 50—65	171,600	952	(0.55)	978	(0.57)

Note: Numbers in parentheses indicate what percentage of the normal expectation of spontaneous cancers the radiogenic excess represents.

From *Medical Effects of Ionizing Radiation,* Mettler, F. A. and Moseley, R. D., Eds., Grune & Stratton, New York, 1985. With permission.

incidence in the U.S.S.R. is comparable to the U.S., it would be expected that about 17,000 of this group would develop "spontaneously occurring cancers" during their lifetime. The absorbed radiation dose the population received from Chernobyl might increase this number by 1 or 2%, or <500 additional cancer cases. There certainly have been claims in the media that many thousands of cancer cases will be induced and the best one can say is that such claims have little or no scientific basis.

The risk estimate of 500 or so additional cancer cases in the Chernobyl population appears to be a reasonable number in light of the experience at Hiroshima and Nagasaki: approximately 80,000 Japanese survivors have now been followed up for almost 45 years

TABLE 5
Estimates of Projected Lifetime Risks From 1000 Persons Exposed to 100 rad (1 Gy) of High Dose Rate Radiation

	Risk projection model	Excess fatal cases	Years of life lost
Total population	Additive	40—50	950—1200
	Relative	70—110	950—1400
Working population	Additive	40	880
(aged 25-65 years)	Relative	80	970
Adult population	Additive	50	840
(over 25 years)	Relative	60	640

Note: Estimates are calculated from 500 males and 500 females and are based upon the Japanese population.

From United Nations Scientific Committee on the Effects of Atomic Radiation, Sources, Effects, and Risks of Ionizing Radiation, Report ot the General Assembly, United Nations, New York, 1988.

(Table 5). Approximately 24,000 have died from all causes, with 4500 of these dying from cancer. The radiation-induced excess identified (when comparison is made with other comparable cities in Japan) has been about 250 cases. The population is fairly similar in size to the Chernobyl population (80,000 vs. 100,000) and the absorbed dose is also quite similar (10 to 20 rad or 0.1 to 0.2 Gy).

One implication of the above facts is that followup of patients after exposure must be conducted for a very long time. The exact radiation risk for carcinogenesis depends upon the absorbed dose in the various tissues. For a given accident in which a patient has received a nonuniform gradient exposure across the body, risk evaluation can be quite difficult, since the dose to various tissues and individual tissue risk factors must all be calculated. Risk evaluation also will need to take into account the age and sex of the patient, since both of these factors may significantly affect the risk estimates that should be appropriately utilized.

IV. WHAT TO DO AFTER CANCER DEVELOPS

One of the inherent difficulties in following up patients after radiation accidents is that spontaneously occurring tumors will be identified. In any U.S. population, even without accidental radiation exposure, the chances of developing a spontaneous malignancy is about 32% and there is about a 17% chance that any given person will die from a malignancy. The question which has plagued legions of scientists, physicians, and attorneys over the years is how to determine whether a malignancy that has been identified in a followup study was a spontaneous tumor or a radiation-induced tumor. Certainly many individuals who have developed cancer after radiation exposure are convinced that their particular cancer was caused by radiation and will file a claim or lawsuit.

In analyzing an individual with cancer to determine the likelihood that the cancer was radiation-induced, one needs to have the following information: (1) the relative contribution of the various causes of cancer in the population group to which that individual belongs, (2) the best possible risk estimate for radiation induction of that tumor for an individual of that age and sex at exposure, (3) the probability of the individual dying from or incurring the given tumor under normal circumstances, (4) the actual risk factors incurred by that specific individual, and (5) the temporal events and modifying factors involved.

The first and simplest item to examine is whether the cancer has occurred at a time after exposure that is less than reported minimum latent period. For example, if a lung cancer occurs 2 to 3 years after an accidental exposure to radiation, there is very little chance that it is a radiation-induced tumor. A second item to be examined is whether the tumor is occurring in a tissue which is known to be of very low or negligible tumor induction, or is a tumor type that has not been reported to be radiation-induced. An example of a neoplasm which does not appear to be radiation-induced is chronic lymphocytic leukemia.

If a tumor occurs after the minimum latent period in a tissue which has been irradiated and the tumor is known to be a type induced by radiation exposure, one must next employ probability calculations. The reason for this is that there is nothing pathognomic about a radiation-induced tumor as it appears similar to spontaneously occurring tumors. A method of probability calculations for causation have been published by Bond.[3] In simplest terms, the probability of causation (P.C.) is the ratio of the excess risk imposed by radiation dose (R) to the total risk, which is the sum of the spontaneous risk plus radiation risk. The formula is as follows:

$$\text{P.C.} = \frac{R \times X}{B + (R \times X)} \times 100\%$$

where X is the absolute annual site-specific risk per rad, and where B is the spontaneous cancer rate specific for site, age, and sex. The factor B is usually ascertained from the Surveillance, Epidemiology, and End Results (SEER) data.[4]

Let us take an example to indicate how this approach is utilized. A 55-year-old black male received an accidental whole-body exposure of 10 rem (0.1 Sv). He has now presented with an adenocarcinoma of the lung. The annual incidence for this tumor type for black males of this age is 341/100,000. The radiation risk calculated from BEIR date indicates the radiation risk for 10 rem in an individual of this age and with a lung cancer is 5 in 100,000. Thus, the probability of causation is 5/346, or between a 1 and 2% chance that this tumor was radiation-induced. Additional modification of the probability could also be performed based upon the particular individual's other pertinent history, such as smoking.

V. EPIDEMIOLOGICAL STUDIES

So far tumor induction, risk factors, and causation in a specific individual have been discussed. What remains to be discussed is whether or not an epidemiologic study is warranted or feasible following a given accident and, if so, what are the requirements to assure the study is scientifically valid. The major difficulty with an epidemiological study to identify radiation carcinogenesis is the high spontaneously occurring rate of cancer and the relatively low radiation induction rate. Estimates have been made that a statistically valid epidemiological study for radiation carcinogenesis can be performed if the exposed population consists of 1000 persons who have each received a 100 rem (1 Sv) whole-body dose. A control population of 1,000 would also be needed. As the absorbed dose to individuals is reduced to 1/10 (10 rem or 0.1 Sv), the population needed for statistical validity increases dramatically. For a valid study of the effect of 10 rem per individual, a population of 100,000 exposed persons is necessary, as well as an equal number of controls. At a dose level of 1 rem (10 mSv) per person, exposed and control populations each must be about 10 million persons for a statistically valid study. Thus, it becomes very obvious that whether or not an epidemiological study is warranted depends upon the number of persons exposed and their doses.

It is clear from the above statistical constraints that after accidents such as Three Mile Island (TMI), where absorbed doses to the population were <0.1 rem per person, that for a scientifically valid study, a population of >100 million persons is necessary. It must be concluded, therefore, that any epidemiological study performed around Harrisburg or TMI is being conducted for purely political reasons and that any results, whether positive or negative, are unlikely to have any statistical validity.

Another question which needs to be answered is whether a proposed epidemiological study will actually yield new data, or the study is spending money to reaffirm risk factors that are already reasonably well known. The economics of an epidemiological study can be staggering. Since 1945 the U.S. has followed the 80,000 survivors from Hiroshima and Nagasaki. This 45-year followup has cost in excess of $2 billion dollars and has identified only 250 radiation-induced cancer cases on the background of 4,500 spontaneously occurring cancer cases.

The base (spontaneously occurring) cancer rate is also very important to ascertain when conducting an epidemiological study. One way such epidemiological studies may be done is to compare the cancer rates in an exposed population to that currently recorded, for example, in tumor registries. The difficulty with this approach is that in many places tumor registries are poorly developed and only after a radiation accident is an epidemiological study begun. At this time, tumors are vigorously sought and autopsies performed. One may find spontaneous cancers that were present all the time, but which were not recognized or recorded. If this happens, it would erroneously elevate the identified radiogenic cancer risk.

The best way to conduct studies is to have an age- and sex-matched control group who were not exposed. Under these circumstances, the cost of an epidemiological study is at least doubled, since twice as many individuals need to be followed and one needs to ascertain that the control population is in fact subject to the same risk factors during the followup period (for example, that they have similar smoking habits, etc.).

VI. FOLLOWUP SCREENING TESTS

What screening tests, if any, should be done to look for radiation-induced tumors? Again, some of these questions fall into the realm of the political and legal sphere rather than in the medical domain. While there are no firm recommendations, the following represents at least our medical opinion. We believe that screening tests and annual physicals are *not* indicated for patients involved in accidents which do not fit the Radiation Emergency Accident/Training Site (REAC/TS) definition of significant exposures as outlined in Section II in Chapter 2. The reason for this is that any tumor found is likely to have a less than 3% chance of having been radiation-induced.

When the guidelines have been exceeded, for example, whole-body dose in excess of 25 rem (0.25 Sv), patients should be followed using the Navy protocol (NAVmed). This reasonably includes an annual physical exam, complete blood count (CBC), and routine blood chemistries. An annual chest X-ray represents only an additional radiation dose of about 10 mrem (0.1 mSv).

Screening for lung cancer with annual chest radiographs, even in high-risk populations, however, has not been shown to significantly increase survival. When specific organs are involved, for example, thyroid or breast, a baseline technetium thyroid scan or mammogram may be useful, followed by annual physical examination. Routine good medical practice for a specific age group should be adhered to. For example, screening mammography in women over the age of 50 should be done whether or not the individual had ever been in a radiation accident.

VII. EVALUATION OF LONG-TERM SOMATIC EFFECTS

Significant cell killing with resultant long-term effects are extremely unusual at doses below 100 rad (1 Gy) and relatively unlikely below 300 rad (3 Gy). Thus followup of patients for long-term somatic damage usually refers to those who have received inhomogeneous or partial-body irradiation with absorbed doses in excess of 300 to 400 rad (3 to 4 Gy). The exact followup would depend on the absorbed dose level and the organ systems involved.

In the following section the most common areas affected in accidental exposure will be discussed. For other areas and central portions of the body (such as the liver) the reader is referred to the radiation therapy literature or textbooks on effects of radiation on humans.[5]

A. EYE

The eye is important in accidental exposures, since the head may be exposed to relatively high absorbed doses while the rest of the body is shielded by some structure or barrier. Tissues about the eye have the same sensitivity as the skin; however, the lens of the eye is particularly radiosensitive with subsequent production of cataracts and lenticular opacities. Cataracts are the most frequent delayed reaction in the eye and have been identified in accidentally irradiated individuals. The term "cataract" often connotes blindness; however, absorbed doses of several Grays can cause lenticular opacities which do not progress and may not even impair vision. At high doses, radiation can cause cataracts which do interfere with vision. Such cataracts are among the few lesions that are pathologically quite characteristic for radiation injury. Most senile cataracts begin in the anterior pole of the lens, whereas radiation cataracts begin as small dots in the posterior pole. This may enlarge to 3 to 4 mm and then a central clear area may be identified. Ultimately, the cataract will progress to the anterior pole of the lens and at that point it may be indistinguishable from a senile cataract.

The incidence of radiation cataracts is dose-, time-, and age-dependent. The latent period from irradiation to production of cataracts may range from half a year to 35 years, although on the average it is 2 to 3 years. The higher the absorbed dose, the shorter the latent period. The threshold for the production of cataracts following acute exposure appears to be about 200 rad (2 Gy) and a single acute dose of X-ray or gamma ray of 750 rad (7.5 Gy) will cause cataract formation in all those exposed. With chronic exposures the threshold appears to rise to approximately 400 rad (4 Gy) with the probability approaching 100% with chronic absorbed doses in excess of 2,000 rad (20 Gy). Neutrons are especially effective in formation of cataracts. In humans, no changes have been observed with neutron doses of <80 rad (0.8 Gy), but permanent loss of vision has occurred following neutron doses in the range of 200 rad (2.0 Gy).

It should be noted that followup of patients after radiation exposure may identify senile cataracts. About 15% of persons in the age range of 52 to 85 are affected by cataracts. Diabetes, diastolic hypertension, and various drugs, such as allopurinol, dilantin, corticosteroids, barbiturates, and some antidepressants are all risk factors associated with cataract formation.

Very high doses of radiation to the eyes may result in other late changes such as telangiectasia of the skin and conjunctiva. There may be deep keratitis of the cornea, retinopathy, and neuropathy, causing blindness following fractionated doses in excess of 3000 rad (30 Gy). Such effects may appear 6 to 36 months after exposure. Followup of patients with estimated absorbed doses to the eye in excess of 200 rad (2.0 Gy) should have a baseline slit lamp examination and then a semiannual examination by an ophthalmologist.

B. GONADS

Evaluation of gonadal function has been important in many accidental situations in which unsuspected but highly radioactive sources were placed in pants pockets. Both male and female gonads are very radiosensitive. One very interesting difference between irradiation of the male and female is that in the female, radiation may not only cause reduction or obliteration of gamete production, but also a decrease in production of hormones. In the male, there are few, if any, changes in hormone production. A review of the topic has been published by Lushbaugh and Ricks.[7]

The ovary demonstrates temporary sterility or reduced fertility with single doses of 150 to 600 rad (1.5 to 6.0 Gy) and with fractionated doses of 150 to 1200 rad (1.5 to 12 Gy). Permanent sterility results from single doses of 320 to 1000 rad (3.2 to 10 Gy) or higher fractionated doses. The sensitivity of the ovary is greater in older women. Following radiation exposure, there may be a fertile period before temporary radiation sterility. This temporary fertile period occurs as a result of the final maturation process of follicles that are in the late stage of development. Resumption of growth of ovarian follicles may not occur for a year or two after irradiation and, if the dose is high enough, permanent sterility and atrophy will occur, not only in the follicles, but also in interstitial gland cells and the corpora lutea.

Sterility, both temporary and permanent, has been identified following accidental testicular irradiation. Although spermatogonial cell necrosis is detected within 4 to 6 h after irradiation, the more mature cells are relatively unaffected by doses <300 rad (3 Gy). These latter cells continue to mature normally after doses <300 rad (3 Gy) and thus a normal sperm count may be maintained for approximately 45 d. After this, the sperm count begins to drop and azospermia occurs at approximately 10 weeks after doses >100 rad (1.0 Gy). Oligospermia is induced by doses as low as 15 rad (0.15 Gy). Plasma and urinary levels of follicle stimulating hormones increase after doses to the testes greater than 10 rad (0.1 Gy). Levels of urinary testosterone and plasma testosterone usually are not changed significantly. ''Sterility'' may be temporary for a matter of years before returning. Five individuals who received doses of 230 to 370 rad (2.3 to 3.7 Gy) in the Oak Ridge criticality accident were aspermic for 4 months and hypospermic for 21 months; at least one person in this accident demonstrated ''sterility'' for several years, but subsequently had a normal offspring.[8] Thus, in followup of patients with accidental irradiation of the testicle and estimated doses in excess of 15 rad (0.15 Gy), an initial sperm count and a followup sperm count at approximately 45 to 60 days postexposure should be performed. Additional counts may be necessary over a period of years in patients with estimated absorbed doses in excess of 200 rad (2.0 Gy).

VIII. EVALUATION OF EXTREMITY INJURY

The majority of radiation accidents involve local or partial-body exposure. The hand is involved in approximately 90% of such accidents. The acute effects, early evaluation and treatment have been discussed earlier in the chapter on partial-body irradiation. The purpose of this section is to discuss followup in the period beyond 30 d postexposure. The ultimate effects, of course, depend on the total absorbed dose; however, the structures involved that need to be evaluated include the skin, underlying soft tissue and muscles, vascularity, cartilage, joint spaces, and the bone.

If the initial injury is such as to produce desquamation followed by reepithelialization, delayed effects in the skin may be identified and progress slowly. In some patients the skin may demonstrate gradual hyperpigmentation; however, in blacks there may be depigmentation of the skin. By 1 year the skin usually demonstrates its final appearance and this may include diffuse telangiectasia, suppression of sebaceous gland activity, and thin, dry, semitranslucent, atrophic skin. There may be breakdown of the skin with minimal amounts of trauma due to its delicate nature and marginal vascular supply. If such breakdown occurs, healing is often delayed and there may be ulcer formation.

Even though healing of the initial desquamation may occur within 60 d postirradiation, subsequent tissue and skin breakdown may occur at 12 to 36 months. Usually this is due to progressive arteriolar narrowing, and resultant vascular insufficiency. For such patients, evaluation of the vascular status is important. This can be done by a number of methods. A popular method in France is the use of thermography, although in the U.S. other methods, such as nuclear medicine radionuclide angiogram or digital arteriography, are often employed. It may be useful in patients with local injuries to have a baseline vascular status examination within the first 6 months postexposure so that appropriate comparison can be performed later if necessary.

In general, bone, cartilage, and muscle are quite resistant to the effects of radiation. However, with the very high absorbed doses that may be incurred with extremity injuries, all of these tissues can be affected. The bone may be evaluated through the use of a radionuclide bone scan. Decreased activity in affected areas may be seen on the bone scan from 4 to 19 months after irradiation. Most of the literature in this regard is derived from radiation therapy and with fractionated doses in excess of 2000 rad (20 Gy). Decreased activity in irradiated areas may be identified in 60% of persons receiving fractionated doses in excess of 4500 rad (45 Gy). Actual bone necrosis is quite rare and normally not seen unless there are fractionated absorbed doses in excess of 6500 rad (65 Gy). Similarly, cartilage is usually able to tolerate doses in the same range. The predominant effects which are seen at somewhat lower doses occur as a result of ischemia. This will result in atrophy and fibrosis of musculature and limitation of motion. Followup of such patients, therefore, should include an analysis of the range of motion of the joints involved. Examination of the patient by an orthopedic or hand surgeon should be done every 3 months for the first year or two and then at least annually for a period of 4 to 5 years.

IX. INTERNAL CONTAMINATION ACCIDENTS

Long-term followup of patients accidentally internally contaminated with radionuclides needs to be assessed after one has information concerning the radionuclide, solubility, and the estimated absorbed dose to various organs. In contrast to exposure in other types of radiation accidents, in these patients any residual radioactive material within the body will continue to irradiate the tissues until it is excreted by some physiologic process, or it becomes stable through radioactive decay. A determination of the amount of radionuclide in the body at some early time after the accident is crucial. This is done principally through measurements of excretion, such as urine and fecal analysis, or through measurement, using a whole-body counter. For long-lived radionuclides, these measurements must be obtained for a period of months or years. The use of these measurements is subject to a number of interpretation problems, particularly the lack of knowledge regarding distribution of the radionuclide within various tissues of the body and the excretion rates from each of those tissues or organs.

There is some human data which has been summarized in NCRP Report #65.[9] Unfortunately, excretion rates of radionuclides vary from individual to individual; so one needs to individualize the calculation. The fate of inhaled radionuclides is dependent on a large number of factors, including solubility, particle size, shape, etc. Once the radionuclide and organ deposition is ascertained, appropriate studies for the function of that organ, or nearby organs, can be obtained.

X. SUMMARY

Followup of patients involved in accidental exposures should be tailored to the circumstances of the accident. The critical issues for long-term followup are divided into analysis at relatively low absorbed doses for carcinogenic effects, and such followup may take the form of epidemiologic studies that may need to be continued over a period of decades. With higher doses, direct or nonstochastic effects are important, and the exact followup scheme that should be utilized depends upon the patient, absorbed doses and tissues irradiated. In general, patients exceeding the REAC/TS guidelines for significant exposure are followed using the Navy protocol (NAVmed). Certainly, for significant exposures, appropriate medical consultation in design of the followup procedure is preferable to a routine protocol.

An annual physical examination has substantial merit if an individual has been involved in a significant radiation accident. At the time of the examination, the physician can order appropriate tests based upon clinical findings and patient symptoms. Most physicians also will take the opportunity to order a CBC, urine test, and some blood chemistries. This is done more as a matter of good preventative medicine to detect abnormalities *not* related to radiation exposure than for identification of radiation effects per se.

REFERENCES

1. United Nations Scientific Committee on the Effects of Atomic Radiation (UNSCEAR), Sources, Effects and Risks of Ionizing Radiation, Report to the General Assembly, United Nations, New York, 1988.
2. Committee on Biological Effects of Ionizing Radiation (BEIR), National Research Council, Effects on Populations of Exposure to Low Levels of Ionizing Radiation, National Academy Press, Washington D. C., 1980.
3. **Bond, V. P.,** Cancer risk attributable to radiation exposure: some practical problems, *Health Phys.*, 40, 108, 1981.
4. **Young, J. L., Jr., Percy, C. L., and Asire, A. J., Eds.** Surveillance, Epidemiology and End Results: Incidence and Mortality Data, 1972—1977, NCI Monogr. 57, NIH Publ. 81-2330, National Cancer Institute, National Institutes of Health, U.S. Government Printing Office, Washington, D.C., 1981.
5. **Mettler, F. A. and Moseley, R. D.,** *The Medical Effects of Ionizing Radiation,* Grune & Stratton, Orlando, FL, 1985.
6. **Merriam, G. R., Szechter, A., and Focht, E. F.,** The effects of ionizing radiations on the eye, *Front. Rad. Ther. Oncol.*, 6, 346, 1972.
7. **Lushbaugh, C. C. and Ricks, R. C.,** Some cytokinetic and histopathologic considerations of male and female irradiated gonadal tissues, *Front. Rad. Ther. Oncol.*, 6, 228, 1972.
8. **Andrews, G. A., Hubner, K. F., Fry, S. A., et al.,** Report of 21-year medical follow-up of survivors of the Oak Ridge Y-12 accident, in *The Medical Basis of Radiation Accident Preparedness,* Hubner, K. F. and Fry, S. A., Eds., Elsevier/North Holland, New York, 1980.
9. National Council on Radiation Protection and Measurements, Management of Persons Accidentally Contaminated with Radionuclides, NCRP Rep. 65, Washington, D.C., 1980.
10. International Commission on Radiological Protection (ICRP), Rep. No. 26, ICRP, Oxford, U.K.

Chapter 15

EVALUATION OF FETAL AND GENETIC CONSEQUENCES

Carol B. Jankowski

TABLE OF CONTENTS

I. INTRODUCTION

Accidental radiation exposure of women in their childbearing years always raises concern for both heritable genetic effects and direct developmental anomalies in embryos. If there is a possibility of pregnancy at the time of exposure, the effect on the conceptus must be given special consideration. Many women are aware of the radiosensitivity of the embryo/fetus and will be anxious about possible injury, even if the dose is quite low. This feeling is apparent even when pregnant women require medically indicated radiological examinations.

The embryo/fetus is indeed more sensitive to radiation than the adult. However, it is essential to consider all the features of any *in utero* exposure before judging the likelihood of untoward effects. The question of therapeutic abortion following accidental *in utero* radiation must be approached as knowledgeably as possible. Risk levels can be calculated and should be considered in comparison with other risks to pregnancy.

Studies as to the effects of radiation on human conceptuses are of two major types: (1) retrospective studies of moderate to high doses received accidentally or as the result of therapeutic radiation to an adjacent area and (2) large populations for whom low-dose radiation was the result of medically indicated diagnostic studies of the mother. The uncertainty of extrapolating from high dose effects to possible effects at low doses, as discussed previously in Chapter 14, is equally an issue when considering the embryo/fetus. Animal studies have contributed widely to the study of radiation effects *in utero*, but extension of this information to humans is problematic. Fetal growth and development are similar for lab animals and humans, but the radiation doses required for specific fetal responses at certain stages are not always identical.

The question of possible genetic effects following an overexposure is difficult to answer definitively because of the lack of proof thus far for *any* heritable genetic effects in humans from radiation. Extensive studies of rodents suggest a causal relationship; the link in humans is less certain.

The purpose of this chapter is to provide the information needed to advise women of the possible effects or *lack* of effects that may occur as the result of unplanned radiation exposure of their abdomen.

II. RADIOSENSITIVITY OF EMBRYONIC/FETAL CELLS

Those cells that have a high degree of mitotic activity and are undifferentiated are most susceptible to radiation.[1] When ionizing radiation, in the form of photons (gamma or X-rays) or particles (alphas, betas), impacts cells, water molecules are most likely to be ionized or excited. Electrons from water are dissociated, causing the instantaneous formation of water radicals. These radicals in turn may break sugar-phosphate bonds or alter the base rings within the DNA. However, for most cell types, it is not until the cell begins to divide that the injury to the genetic material becomes apparent as cell death, failure to divide, or other abnormality. Fortunately, the cell has the capacity to repair DNA correctly and does so most of the time.

Because embryonic/fetal cells are rapidly dividing and undifferentiated, their radiosensitivity is understandable. As the organs develop from early poorly differentiated cells, unrepaired injury or cell depletion could result in serious anomalies at birth. In addition, during most of gestation, the size of the conceptus is small, so that any radiation to the uterus would be to the total conceptus.

The most frequent effects of high dose *in utero* radiation are death, congenital anomalies, mental retardation, and growth retardation. If sufficient cells or cells crucial to life are injured, death may occur, most likely during the earliest period of pregnancy or the neonatal period. Congenital anomalies will reflect the amount of irradiation and the timing in relation to organ development. Animals irradiated on specific days of gestation may manifest anomalies of various organs corresponding to the exact stage of organ development at the time of exposure.

In humans, anomalies have been related most frequently to central nervous system (CNS) development; the most common is small head size, often with concurrent mental retardation and ocular defects. The preponderance of CNS deficiencies may be due to several factors. Human irradiations have occurred randomly during the gestation period. Whereas the period of major organogenesis in rats is 20% of their gestation, in humans it is only 5%.[2] Unlike other systems, the CNS continues to develop throughout the pregnancy and therefore has more opportunity to be affected. Abnormalities in the skeletal as well as other systems may also be present, but much less frequently.[2]

Growth retardation is thought to be related to cell depletion or deletion *in utero;* it often accompanies and may be the cause of other CNS defects.[2,3] No reduced birth weights, however, have been attributed to exposures <25 R, even in animal studies.[1] Low birth weight caused by exposure during the very early developmental period, 2 to 6 weeks, may not be permanent. Exposures during the early fetal period, however, appear to cause more permanently stunted growth. Every acknowledged report of *in utero* radiation effects in humans has described some form of CNS abnormality or growth retardation, alone or in combination with other morphological abnormalites.[2]

An association between low levels of radiation (5 R) and increased risk of childhood cancer has been suggested by several studies, although a causal relationship has not been established (see below).

Finally, there is some question as to functional disabilities being induced by radiation *in utero.* Rat studies have shown some deficiencies in motor function and learning ability tests.[4,5]

III. FACTORS TO BE CONSIDERED WHEN ASSESSING INJURY OR RISK OF INJURY

With the use of ultrasound and other recent advances in fetal testing, it is now possible to identify gross malformations that could occur following a serious overexposure to radiation. But severe accidental overexposures are *very* rare; it is far more probable that the physician will need to evaluate the pregnancy of a radiation-accident casualty involving very low to moderate exposure. He/she will need to make a calculated estimate of the risk of embryonic/fetal injury based on several parameters. Period of gestation, type of radiation, rate of exposure, and possible internal dose, as well as the external dose, must all be considered, as each affects the risk of injury.

Determining the external dose may not be easy. Even a dosimeter may not reflect accurately the uniform dose to the abdomen and will not record exactly the dose to the fetus which is protected somewhat by the mother's body. Reenactment of the accident may be necessary to make a more accurate estimate. The degree of attenuation by maternal tissue must be calculated as well. Exposure from an off-site release of radioactivity from a nuclear reactor may be even more difficult to determine, as several sources of radioactivity would need to be considered. There could be exposure from the passing radioactive cloud, from radioactivity deposited on the ground, and even some ingestion or inhalation of radionuclides. Models have been constructed that will help to assess the total dose if the woman could accurately describe her location during the period of greatest exposure. Chromosomal studies of lymphocytes might be helpful in determining the approximate level of exposure if the exposure were thought to be >20 R.

Calculation of the fetal dose from internal contamination is complex and requires consultation with experts. A fetal dose can result from exposure to a radioisotope residing in adjacent maternal organs, and, in some instances, the isotope may actively pass through the placenta into fetal tissue.

The period of gestation must be taken into consideration. Irradiation prior to implantation, 0 to 2 weeks postconception, is thought to cause either death, resulting in resorption of the conceptus, or no observable injury.[2] The totipotency of the early blastomeres allows the remaining cells to replace the injured ones.[6] Animal studies have shown reduced litter size following radiation of the uterus during this period.[4] The degree to which resorption occurs in humans is unknown.

In experimental animals, the period of major organogenesis is unquestionably the period of greatest radiosensitivity. For rats exposed to 100 R during this time, almost 100% reveal congenital anomalies of many organs; the mortality rate is close to 50% at 150 R.[2] In humans, microcephaly (>2 SD below normal) is the most common defect from irradiation during this period, although ophthalmic, skeletal, and other defects have been reported at very high doses.[3,7] Neonatal death and growth retardation also may result from sufficient irradiation in the 2- to 8-week gestation period.

The most significant and disabling impairment found among the Japanese bomb survivors irradiated *in utero* was mental retardation; correlation with radiation was most positive during gestation weeks 8 to 15.[8] This corresponds directly to the period of cerebral histogenesis during which neuroblasts divide logarithmically to form neurons and migrate from the proliferative zones to the cerebral area.[3] By 18 weeks, both the proliferation and migration essentially have been completed, and the more mature neurons are less radiosensitive.

The sensitivity of migrating neuroblasts during those crucial weeks has been suggested even among persons not classified as mentally retarded. Intelligence tests administered at 10 years to the Japanese children irradiated *in utero* ($<$ 2000 meters from the hypocenter) indicated the greatest decrease in intelligence for children in the 8- to 15-week gestation group for increasing doses over 10 rads.[9] This was true even when those diagnosed as severely retarded were excluded. Indications of even lesser degrees of impairment have been extracted from performance grades of those children so irradiated. Those exposed during weeks 8 to 15 postconception showed the greatest impairment.[10] It may be that for humans, the period of 8- to 15-weeks gestation should be considered the most crucial period because of the seriousness of this effect.[3]

High-dose radiation during the period of 16 to 25 weeks gestation may result in small body size, metal retardation, and microcephaly but with less severity.[7] Beyond 25 weeks, there appear to be few anatomical effects even for high doses. Mental retardation and lower IQ scores were not seen in children irradiated in the third trimester but the numbers were small.[8,9]

The type of radiation causing the exposure also plays a role in determining possible effects. X-rays and gamma irradiation will be the primary concern in evaluating accidental fetal exposure from external sources. If internal contamination has occurred, the beta dose also must be considered. Alpha radiation of the conceptus would be possible only if the alpha emitter was able to cross the placenta.

Studies of neutron irradiation of mice suggest the relative biological effectiveness (RBE) for neutrons is between 2 and 4, but qualitative differences in teratogenic effects from those caused by gamma radiation are not present.[11,12] There appears to be a threshold for mortality from neutron exposure, but none for major malformations.[12]

The rate of exposure and period of time over which the dose is received also will influence the effectiveness of the fetal dose and the risk of injury. If a woman receives an exposure of 25 R within 1 min, the risk of untoward effects is greater than if she were to receive that same dose spread over 100 d in increments of 1 R every 4 d. The latter sequence allows for considerable repair of DNA during the interval period. In addition, the most critical period of sensitivity for most defects is very short and only a small portion of the total dose would be received during that period.

In summary, it is very likely that the actual dose to the embryo/fetus resulting from a radiation accident or off-site release of radioactivity will be less than the original preliminary estimate. Therefore, it is essential that calculated dose estimates be as accurate as possible. This may require consultation with health or medical physicists more familiar with the parameters to be considered. Likewise, in estimating the risks of untoward effects given the dose, thought must be given to the other factors discussed, especially period of gestation and rate at which the radiation was received. If the estimated dose is sufficient to consider the possibility of a therapeutic abortion, parental input must be sought. Some parents may choose to complete the pregnancy and assume a higher risk of some untoward effect.

IV. ACTUAL EXPERIENCE – MODERATE TO HIGH-DOSE EXPOSURES (>15 R)

The risk of serious injury to the conceptus is very great for high dose *in utero* radiation. Among 26 case reports of mothers receiving 250 to 20,000 R to the abdomen for therapeutic purposes, the only infants without abnormalities were those irradiated prior to 4 weeks and after 20 weeks gestation.[7] All infants were born near or at term, although death did occur within 24 h for four subjects. The abnormal findings described related closely to gestational development during the period of exposure. The 16 conceptuses irradiated betweeen 4 to 12 weeks exhibited low birth weight, markedly stunted growth, microcephaly, mental retardation, microphthalmus, pigmentary degeneration of the retina, genital and skeletal malformations, and cataracts. Fetuses irradiated between 12 to 20 weeks gestation all exhibited small size, microcephaly and mental retardation, although generally to a milder degree than the former group. Other abnormalities were not noted in the latter group. Those infants irradiated after 20 weeks had no organ or system abnormalities, although epilation, a deficient hematopoietic system, and healed skin lesions were reported.

Infants born to Japanese mothers irradiated during the bombings in 1945 have been studied exhaustively. Almost 500 live offspring were exposed *in utero* within 2000 m of the hypocenter.[13] Four times as many infants were exposed in Hiroshima as Nagasaki.

Microcephaly and mental retardation were the outstanding findings among these infants. Small head circumference (<2 SD) was noted even among some infants in Hiroshima who received <20 rad; among those infants, the prevalence, for gestation weeks 0 to 17, was 9% (10/117); prevalence among controls out of the city was 4%, higher than might be expected, but perhaps a reflection of other environmental factors. As the *in utero* dose increased, so too did the risk of microcephaly. Of those fetuses receiving 20 to 50 rads prior to week 18, 30% (13/43) were microcephalic. It appears that at lower doses, the embryonic period was most sensitive; as the received dose increased, however, the susceptibility period was lengthened into the fetal period.[14]

The risk of mental retardation also correlated positively with dose but only in Hiroshima. Seventeen of the study children proximal to the hypocenter were diagnosed as severely mentally retarded.[8] Sample numbers are small, but the estimated risk for gestation weeks 8 to 15 increased from 3.4% at 1 to 9 rads, to 44% for those exposed to 50 to 100 rads, and to 100% for those with doses >150 rads.

Among Nagasaki infants there was no significant increase in microcephaly or mental retardation in the small number of infants exposed to <150 rads. Reexamination of the radiation quality has indicated that neutron exposure was minimal even in Hiroshima, and was *not* a significant reason for greater cerebral damage among the Hiroshima children.[15]

V. LOW-DOSE RADIATION EXPOSURE (<15 R)

Several experimental animal studies have shown measureable damage caused by exposure of <10 R *if* acute exposure occurs at the most sensitive stage for a specific effect.[6] Protracted ingestion of tritiated water by mice can cause oocyte killing at doses of 5 rads. Likewise, fetal mouse oocytes have been reduced by 50% with a 9-rad dose from external gamma radiation given at the time of greatest radiosensitivity; litter size was reduced in subsequent generations.[16] Similar results in humans would be almost impossible to document. Few experimental studies have ever attributed any observable congenital defects or conceptus death to low-dose *in utero* radiation.

There also have been case studies of pregnant women who received diagnostic X-rays to the pelvic area or therapeutic radiation to organs outside the pelvic area wherein the fetus may have received 1 to 15 rads. None has reported abnormalities in excess of the expected spontaneous rate.[17-20] Reassurance as to the lack of radiation-induced abnormalities may be given to women who might have received low doses either from an accident situation or from medically indicated X-rays.

There is, however, some indication that *in utero* diagnostic X-rays may be associated with an increased risk of childhood cancer. The association was first noted in a study of the mothers of 8000 English children who had died of cancer prior to age 15.[21] In comparison with a matched control group, the most significant factor was the increased number of cohort mothers who had received abdominal X-ray examination during the last trimester of their pregnancy. A greater number (14%) of the mothers whose children died of cancer had received X-rays as compared to 10% of the control mothers. From these numbers, the risk for developing childhood cancer was determined to be approximately 50% greater for fetuses so exposed. The reason for the X-rays in both groups of mothers was overwhelmingly for obstetrical concerns unrelated to prior illness. The increased risk appeared to be the same for both leukemia and solid tumors.

This phenomenon has not been duplicated in animal studies and confirmation from the irradiated Japanese children is not apparent, albeit open to statistical interpretation.[10,22]

There is disagreement among hypotheses explaining these findings; is there a direct causal relationship or is there an *a priori* selective factor related to maternal radiography? One report reviewing the English data has shown that among the 10% of control mothers who did receive X-rays, there were significantly more primiparas and a higher incidence of medical illnesses during the preganancy.[23] Both situations may have caused the pregnant women to have greater contact with their physician, thereby more opportunity for referral to X-ray.

Other studies have both supported the English study and disputed it;[24-26] one study reports a greater risk of cancer for children born to mothers having received abdominal radiation *prior* to conception.[27] A recent study of 32,000 twins born in Connecticut between 1930 and 1969 revealed 31 children with cancer during the first 15 years.[28] Twins were studied to avoid any bias related to the reasons for the X-rays, as it was common practice to visualize the pelvic area of mothers suspected of carrying twins. Among mothers of the 31 children, 39% had received abdominal X-rays, whereas among the matched control group only 26% of the mothers were so tested. In this study, the risk of solid tumor cancer was higher than that for leukemia, although the reported number of cases was very small. In contrast, Monson and MacMahon's study showed a lower risk for solid tumors than for leukemia.[25]

Thus, a causal relationship between low-dose diagnostic X-rays and induction of childhood cancer has been neither established nor discredited. Low-dose radiation has not been shown to increase adult cancer rates, and animal studies also are negative. With the introduction of ultrasound, few pregnant women now receive abdominal X-rays. Also, modern radiographic techniques deliver substantially lower doses for the exams in question. Prospective studies to confirm a relationship would require very large populations with extended followup.

The implications of these studies for internally emitted radiation from radionuclides of varying energies are very uncertain. Few pregnant women have received accidental, occupational, or even medically related internal doses of even 1 rad from radionuclides.

Although the association is not fully understood, the results of these studies do suggest that it is prudent to avoid unnecessary diagnostic X-ray examinations. For an accidental exposure in the 1- to 15-rad range, the risk of childhood cancer must be considered, but even a 50% increase in risk of the disease is less than the risk of untoward effects from other environmental agents, such as cigarettes and alcohol;[29,30] it certainly would not be reason for advocating termination of the pregnancy.

VI. INTERNAL DOSES FROM RADIONUCLIDES

If unsealed volatile forms of radionuclides are present during an accident, the possibility of ingestion or inhalation of isotopes must be considered. The potential dose to the conceptus is influenced by several additional factors: the specific radionuclide; its chemical form, energy, and half-life; location of the maternal target organ(s); ability of the nuclide to cross the placenta; and the metabolic pathway of the compound.

The radioiodines provide the greatest concern for fetal injury because the fetal thyroid readily absorbs radioiodine. Prior to 12 weeks gestation there is little or no fetal uptake but after this time, the uptake increases rapidly.[6] Price and Holeman have estimated that if a pregnant woman were to inhale or ingest 2 to 3 μCi ^{131}I, it would result in an uptake of 1 μCi to her thyroid.[31] The integrated dose to the fetal thyroid would be in the range of 1 to 10 rad, the dose increasing as the size of the fetal thyroid increases through birth. By week 16, dose to the fetal thyroid would be 6 rads, greater than the maternal thyroid dose. There would be some additional whole-body irradiation of the fetus, although much less than to the critical organ.

Therapeutic doses of ^{131}I have caused serious problems. One child whose mother received 9.2 mCi during weeks 10 through 15 developed features consistent with cretinism.[32] In a review of 237 women treated during pregnancy with ^{131}I for hyperthyroidism, there were six nonrelated complications in neonates and six infants found to be hypothyroid.[33] Four of these mothers had been treated after week 12 (12 to 150 mCi) and mental deficiency was also present. Another mother had received 10 mCi at 9 weeks; the infant's hypothyroid state was transient. The dose and timing information about the sixth mother was unknown. It is of interest and concern that therapeutic abortion was advised and completed for 55 of the 237 women, despite the evidence that untoward effects are uncommon.

Although external exposure to tritium is of little biological concern, prolonged internal doses from tritiated water may be hazardous because of rapid access to living cells.[6] Rat studies have shown decreased organ weights among newborns whose mothers consumed tritiated water throughout pregnancy. In rodents, fetal oocytes appeared to be very sensitive to tritium. The low-energy electrons emitted by tritium appear to have a greater RBE than external gamma rays (^{60}Co).[34] During the narrow period of greatest radiosensitivity, a dose of <5 rads from tritiated water can reduce the number of rat fetal oocytes by 50%. Tritiated thymidine has been shown to be even more effective in its effect on the developing fetal ovary.[36]

Inorganic radioactive potassium, sodium, phosphorus, and strontium can cross the placenta; phosphorus and strontium have been shown experimentally to cause embryonic pathology and death if the dose is large enough.[6,37] In mice, the placenta appears to serve somewhat as a barrier to radiocesiums when injected early in the pregnancy.[38,39]

One study of ^{239}Pu injected in pregnant rabbits (10 to 40 μCi/kg), indicates an increase in prenatal mortality and some fetal growth retardation.[40]

VII. GENETIC CONSEQUENCES

''Radiation-induced transmitted genetic effects have not been demonstrated in man.''[6]

"The estimated relative mutation risk for humans is 0.02 to 0.004/rem (or a doubling dose of 50 to 250 rem)."[6]

These two statements exemplify the controversy surrounding the issue of radiation-induced mutagenesis and chromosomal abnormalities in humans. Indeed, among the first generation or progeny of Japanese parents irradiated in 1945, and conceiving after 1947, no significant increases in genetic defects have been documented.[41] Studies of females exposed to therapeutic doses prior to conception have reported no significant increased prevalence of observable genetic defects in their offspring.[42-44] However, studies of Drosophila and of mice have documented the ability of both chronic and acute radiation to cause mutations within the genetic material.[45,46] Although experimental doses to mice generally were ≥50 rads, there appears to be a linear dose response, at least for low dose rate, with chronic exposure.[45]

Studies of spermatogonia and arrested immature oocytes, the germ cells of greatest long-term importance, indicate that in mice, oocytes are only 44% as radiosensitive as the germinal sperm cells.[45] Postspermatogonia and mature oocytes, those germ cells potentially available at the time of conception, appear to be more radiosensitive than the earlier states. This implies a need for humans to avoid conception for several months following high-dose irradiation to the gonadal area, as temporary sterility or otherwise damaged germ cells may occur.

For the single individual irradiated accidentally or even for therapeutic reasons, the long-term genetic consequences of nonsterilizing doses are unknown, but only because as yet, no data have indicated any significant positive findings.

The public health implications of large populations exposed to even small increments of radiation can only be estimated based on animal studies. The National Research Council has calculated an increase of 5 to 75 dominant effects from an additional 1 rad to parents of a million live births over a 30-year period.[6] This is in addition to the 10,000 (1%) dominant spontaneous defects known to occur. The increase in irregularly inherited disorders from the 1-rem radiation dose would be negligible in relation to those observed in 9% of the birth population.

Some radioisotopes have been shown experimentally to increase untoward genetic effects when internally deposited.[47] For example, ^{239}Pu injected in male mice is retained in the testes and has been shown to cause genetic defects. The implications for humans of internal emitters such as ^{239}Pu and other isotopes is unknown.

VIII. GUIDELINES FOR ADVISING PREGNANT WOMEN FOLLOWING ACCIDENTAL OR MEDICALLY INDICATED EXPOSURE OF THE CONCEPTUS

The National Council on Radiation Protection and Measurements (NCRP) has suggested exposure limits both for occupational and medical exposures. These guidelines can be applied to some degree to exposures received accidentally. Regarding occupational exposures, the NCRP recommends " . . . a total dose equivalent limit of 0.5 rem for the embryo/fetus. Once a pregnancy becomes known, exposure of the embryo/fetus shall be no greater than 0.05 rem in any month."[48] This limit considers both the absence of data indicating any untoward effects at this level and the concerns for women to be able to continue working in a safe environment. Only in rare instances would it be necessary for a pregnant woman to have to leave a job because this dose equivalent could not be guaranteed.

The NCRP has also provided guidance concerning medically indicated radiation of the conceptus.[49] In keeping with general radiation protection philosophy, no radiological examinations should be performed during pregnancy unless the examination is essential to the diagnosis or well-being of the patient. However, the risk of abnormality "is considered to be negligible at 5 rads or less when compared to other risks of pregnancy." Few studies, including those with fluoroscopy, give a dose to the uterus as great as 5 rads. Even if multiple exams are necessary, "the risks of malformations is significantly increased above control levels only at doses above 15 rads."[49]

IX. CONCLUSIONS

There is no disagreement as to the prudence of minimizing radiation exposure of the pregnant uterus and gonads. Occupational limits for pregnant women are purposely restrictive. Medical radiation of the embryo/fetus should be tolerated only when there is reasonable anticipation of clinical benefit and after consideration of alternatives. However, when confronted with an embryo/fetal dose already received accidentally, the physician's role is to offer accurate advice and appropriate reassurance during the continuing pregnancy. The low risk of untoward effects must be considered in relation to other risks of pregnancy generally acceptable to prospective parents. Congenital anomalies, prenatal, and perinatal deaths occur frequently even in the absence of any radiation exposure.

In most situations, the embryonic or fetal dose will be <15 rads; interruption of the pregnancy would not be warranted on a scientific basis. Both among humans and in experimental studies, untoward effects have been rare at doses below 15 rads.

With exposures in the range of 10 to 15 rads, especially during the most radiosensitive period (2 to 15 weeks postconception), counseling the expectant parents is essential. They will be anxious and may think abnormalities are a certainty following such a significant dose. It is important that they understand the derivation of the increased risk, usually an extrapolation downward from higher doses.

For uterine doses known to be greater than 15 rads, input from a medical or health physicist should be solicited to ensure that the calculated uterine dose is accurate. The decision as to whether or not to consider therapeutic abortion should be made only after reviewing all the factors with the parents-to-be. The higher the dose to the conceptus, the greater the risk of some untoward effect. Gestation age is a critical variable; if the dose was acute and occurred during the period of greatest radiosensitivity (2 to 15 weeks), parents may choose to terminate the pregnancy rather than assume the increased risk that accompanies higher doses. If exposure was late in the pregnancy, completion of the pregnancy may be the best alternative, as few serious defects have been observed beyond 25 weeks, even at doses >100 rads. It is not reasonable to set an arbitrary dose beyond which therapeutic abortion is recommended because of the many factors to be considered, not the least of which are parental wishes.

Young women whose gonads have received appreciable radiation (>15 rad) may be concerned about possible future genetic effects. Considerable reassurance can be given to them. Unless the dose to the gonads is in the therapeutic range, no human data indicate a need to proscribe future pregnancies. It would be prudent to avoid pregnancy for several months to assure that the irradiated maturing oocytes had been eliminated.

X. CONCERNS OF EMERGENCY PERSONNEL

Emergency Medical Technicians (EMT), nursing, and medical personnel may question the risk to themselves from caring for a contaminated accident victim emitting some radiation. Their concerns should be addressed in advance by didactic programs and examples from routine medical radiological practice. In most instances, the dose to staff giving hands-on care will be <50 to 100 mrem. This dose can be explained as being considerably less than most diagnostic radiological exams and about the same as a year of background radiation.

If the attending health physicist or radiation safety officer estimates higher exposures while giving emergency care, other staff could be rotated. Increasing distance from the patient whenever possible also would reduce total dose. In the hospital setting, there should be no reason for emergency staff to receive more than 125 mrem, the quarterly recommended upper limit for nonoccupational workers, during care of any conceivable accident victim. Although this figure is well below the suggested upper limit for total dose to the embryo/fetus, it is not advisable for pregnant personnel to be assigned primary care of these casualties.

REFERENCES

1. **Hall, E.J.**, *Radiobiology for the Radiologist,* 3rd ed., Harper & Row, Philadelphia, 1988.
2. **Brent, R. L.**, Radiation teratogenesis, *Teratology,* 21, 281, 1980.
3. **Mole, R. H.**, Consequences of pre-natal radiation exposure for post-natal development. A review, *Int. J. Radiat. Biol.,* 42, 1, 1982.
4. **Hoffman, D. A., Felton, R. P., and Cyr, W. H.**, Effects of Ionizing Radiation in the Developing Embryo and Fetus: a Review, HHS Publ. (FDA) No. 81-8170, Health and Human Services, U.S. Government Printing Office, Washington, D.C., 1981.
5. **Norton, S.**, Behavioral changes in preweaning and adult rats exposed prenatally to low ionizing radiation, *Toxicol. Appl. Pharmacol.,* 83, 240, 1986.
6. National Research Council, Committee on the Biological Effects of Ionizing Radiation, *The Effects on Populations of Exposure to Low Levels of Ionizing Radiation,* National Academy Press, Washington, D.C., 1980.
7. **Dekaban, A. S.**, Abnormalities in children exposed to X-radiation during various stages of gestation: tentative timetable of radiation injury to the human fetus. I, *J. Nucl. Med.,* 9, 471, 1968.
8. **Otake, M. and Schull, W.J.**, *In utero* exposure to A-bomb radiation and mental retardation; a reassessment, *Br. J. Radiol.,* 57, 409, 1984.
9. International Commission on Radiological Protection, Developmental effects of irradiation on the brain of the embryo and fetus, ICRP Pub. No. 49, Pergamon Press, Oxford, 1986.
10. **Mole, R. H.**, Irradiation of the embryo and fetus, *Br. J. Radiol.,* 60, 17, 1987.
11. **Cairnie, A. B., Grahn, D., Rayburn, H. B., Williamson, F. S., and Brown, R. J.**, Teratogenic and embryolethal effects in mice of fission-spectrum neutrons and γ-rays, *Teratology,* 10, 133, 1974.
12. **DiMayo, V., Ballardin, E., and Metalli, P.**, Comparative effects of fission neutron and X-irradiation on 7.5 day mouse embryos, *Radiat. Res.,* 87, 145, 1981.
13. **Miller, R. J. and Blot, W. J.**, Small head size after *in utero* exposure to atomic radiation, *Lancet,* 2, 784, 1972.
14. **Miller, R. J. and Mulvihill, J. J.**, Small head size after atomic irradiation, *Teratology,* 14, 355, 1976.
15. **Otake, M., Yoshimaru, H., and Schull, W. J.**, Effects of ionizing radiation on the developing human brain, *Proc. NCRP Annu. Meet.,* 9, 203, 1988.
16. **Rönnbäck, C.**, Effects on foetal ovaries after protracted, external gamma irradiation as compared with those from internal depositions, *Acta. Radiol. Oncol.,* 22, 465, 1983.
17. **Neumeister, K. and Wässer, S.**, Clinical data for radiation embryology: investigation programme 1967, Rep. 1984, *Radiat. Environ. Biophys.,* 24, 227, 1985.
18. **Becker, M. D. and Hyman, G. A.**, Management of Hodgkin's disease coexistent with pregnancy, *Radiology,* 85, 725, 1965.
19. **Covington, E. E. and Baker, A. S.**, Dosimetry of scattered radiation to the fetus, *JAMA,* 209, 414, 1969.
20. **Cohen, Y., Tatcher, M., and Robinson, E.**, Radiotherapy in pregnancy. A case report with estimation of the dose to the fetus, *Radiol. Clin. Biol.,* 42, 34, 1973.
21. **Bithell, J. F. and Stewart, A. M.**, Prenatal irradiation and childhood malignancy: a review of British data from the Oxford study, *Br. J. Cancer,* 31, 271, 1975.
22. **Jablon, S. and Kato, H.**, Childhood cancer in relation to prenatal exposure to atomic bomb radiation, *Lancet,* 2, 1000, 1970.
23. **Totter, J. R. and MacPherson, H. G.**, Do childhood cancers result from prenatal X-rays? *Health Phys.,* 40, 511, 1981.
24. **Oppenheim, B. E., Griem, M. L., and Meier, P.**, Effects of low-dose prenatal irradiation in humans: analysis of Chicago Lying-In data and comparison with other studies, *Radiat. Res.,* 57, 508, 1974.

25. **Monson, R. R. and MacMahon, B.,** Prenatal X-ray exposure and cancer in children, in *Radiation Carcinogenesis: Epidemiology and Biological Significance,* Boice, J. D., Fraumeni, J. F., Eds., Raven Press, New York, 1984.

26. **Diamond, E. L., Schmerler, H., and Lilienfeld, A. M.,** The relationship of intra-uterine radiation to subsequent mortality and development of leukemia in children, *Am. J. Epidemiol.,* 97, 283, 1973.

27. **Shiono, P. H., Chung, C. S. and Myrianthopoulos, N. C.,** Preconception radiation, intrauterine diagnostic radiation, and childhood neoplasia, *J. Nat. Canc. Inst.,* 65, 681, 1980.

28. **Harvey, E. B., Boice, J. D., Honeyman, M., and Flannary, J. T.,** Prenatal X-ray exposure and childhood cancer in twins, *N. Engl. J. Med.,* 312, 541, 1985.

29. **Shiono, P. H., Klebanoff, M. A., and Rhoads, G. G.,** Smoking and drinking during pregnancy: their effects on preterm birth, *JAMA,* 255, 82, 1986.

30. **Rosett, H. L., Weiner, L., Lee, A., Zuckerman, B., Dooling, E., and Oppenheimer, E.,** Patterns of alcohol consumption and fetal development, *Obstet. Gynecol.,* 61, 539, 1983.

31. **Price, K. W. and Holeman, G. R.,** Dynamics of maternal and fetal iodine uptake and assessing fetal thyroid absorbed dose, in *Medical Health Physics: Proc. Health Physics Society Fourteenth Mid-Year Topical Symposium,* New England and Connecticut Chapters of the Health Physics Society, Hyannis, MA, 1980.

32. **Green, H. G., Gareis, F. J., Shepard, T. H., and Kelley, V. C.,** Cretinism associated with maternal sodium iodide I-131 therapy during pregnancy, *Am. J. Dis. Child.,* 122, 247, 1971.

33. **Stoffer, S. S. and Hamburger, J. I.,** Inadvertent I-131 therapy for hyperthyroidism in the first trimester of pregnancy, *J. Nucl. Med.,* 17, 146, 1976.

34. **Dobson, R. L. and Kwan, T. C.,** The tritium RBE at low-level exposure: variation with dose, dose rate, and exposure duration. *Curr. Top. Radiat. Res. Q.,* 12, 44, 1977.

35. **Dobson, R. L., Koehler, C. G., Felton, J. S., Kwan, T. C., Wuebbles, B. J., and Jones, D. C. L.,** Vulnerability of female germ cells in developing mice and monkeys to tritium, gamma rays, and polycyclic aromatic hydrocarbons, in *Proc. Symp. Developmental Toxicology of Energy-Related Pollutants,* DOE Symp. Ser., Department of Energy, Washington, D.C., 1980.

36. **Brent, R. L.,** Radiation and other physical agents, in *Handbook of Teratology,* Vol. I, Wilson, J. G. and Frazer, F. C., Eds., Plenum Press, New York, 1977.

37. **Olsen, J. and Jonsen, J.,** Sr-90 in placentas, embryos, and foetuses of mice, evaluated by whole body autoradiography, *Acta Pharmacol. Toxicol.,* 44, 22, 1979.

38. **Wycoff, M. H.,** Distribution of Cs-134 in the conceptus of the pregnant rat, *Radiat. Res.,* 47, 628, 1971.

39. **Mahlum, D. D. and Sikov, M. R.,** Comparative metabolism of Cs-137 by adult, suckling and pre-natal rats, *Comp. Biochem. Physiol.,* 30, 169, 1969.

40. **Kelman, B. J., Sikov, M. R., and Hackett, P. L.,** Effects of monomeric Pu-239 on the fetal rabbit, *Health Phys.,* 43, 80, 1982.

41. **Schull, W. J., Otake, M., and Neel, J. V.,** Genetic effects of the atomic bombs: a reappraisal, *Science,* 213, 1220, 1981.

42. **Sarker, S. D., Beierwaltes, W. H., Gill, S. P., and Cowley, B. J.,** Subsequent fertility and birth histories of children and adolescents treated with I-131 for thyroid cancer, *J. Nucl. Med.,* 17, 460, 1976.

43. **Holmes, G. E. and Holmes, F. F.,** Pregnancy outcome of patients treated for Hodgkin's disease, *Cancer,* 41, 1317, 1978.

44. **Li, F. P., Fine, W., Jaffe, N., Holmes, G. E., and Holmes, F. F.,** Offspring of patients treated for cancer in childhood, *J. Nat. Canc. Inst.* 62, 1193, 1979.

45. **Russell, W. L.,** Mutation frequencies in female mice and the estimation of genetic hazards of radiation in women, *Proc. Nat. Acad. Sci. U.S.A.,* 74, 3523, 1977.

46. **Rönnbäck, D. and Sheridan, W.,** Induction of lethal mutations in female mice by 9 generations of γ-irradiation during foetal development, *Mutat. Res.,* 61, 275, 1979.

47. **Searle, A. G.,** Genetic effects of internal emitters in mammals, in *Radiation Research, Proc. VI International Congress Radiat. Res.,* Okada, S. et al., Eds., Japanese Association for Radiation Research, Tokyo, 1979.

48. National Council on Radiation Protection and Measurements, Review of NCRP Radiation Dose Limits for Embryo and Fetus in Occupationally Exposed Women, NCRP Rep. No. 91, June, 1987.

49. National Council on Radiation Protection and Measurements, Medical Radiation Exposure of Pregnant and Potentially Pregnant Women, NCRP Rep. No. 54, July, 1977.

Chapter 16

SPECIAL ASPECTS OF NUCLEAR POWER

Henry D. Royal

TABLE OF CONTENTS

I. INTRODUCTION

Ninety-seven nuclear power plants are now in operation in the U.S. (Figure 1, Table 1) and 281 plants are in operation in the rest of the world.[1] These reactors produce 15% of the world's electricity. In addition to power-generating nuclear reactors, there are an additional 335 operating research reactors worldwide.[2] Since Three Mile Island and Chernobyl, nuclear power plants have served as a focus for the public's concern about the safety of nuclear technology.

The safety issue is a complex one. Certainly nuclear power has not been as safe as some had expected, nor will it be as hazardous as some predict. The decision to support or oppose nuclear power must be based on an assessment of a benefit/risk ratio rather than as an assessment of risk alone. The benefit/risk ratio can reach unacceptable levels by decreasing the benefit or increasing the risk. Well-informed opposition to nuclear power is just as likely to be due to discounting the benefits as it is to inflating the risk. Nuclear opponents discount the benefits of nuclear power by suggesting that energy conservation efforts could save more energy at less cost than can be produced by nuclear power. The risk assessment is greatly inflated if one believes that any proliferation of nuclear technology indirectly increases the risk of nuclear war by providing greater access to the technology required for the production of nuclear weapons. This particular philosophy quickly leads to an anti-nuclear everything stance.

Proponents of nuclear power had promised electricity that was cheap to meter. Accidents like Three Mile Island and Chernobyl were unthinkable. A more sober view of nuclear power is that it will continue to play a role in the production of energy of the U.S. and the world for years to come. Gradually, the experience gained will dictate the future of energy sources.

Medical professionals are often caught in the middle of this debate. Radiation safety drills are absolutely necessary to develop and maintain the skills required to handle an accident involving radiation. These drills often require the cooperation of members of the medical community and the nuclear power industry. Those in the medical community who, after careful consideration, have decided that the risks of nuclear power outweigh the benefits, may feel that any cooperation with the nuclear industry is counterproductive. Upon further consideration this position can not be justified. Health care professionals have a responsibility to provide the best possible health care for all individuals. Although medical professionals oppose drunk driving, they provide the best care for drunk drivers. The best care can only be provided by gaining a thorough realistic understanding of the problems that may be encountered and by preparing for those problems. The goal of this chapter is to review the potential health consequences of accidents at nuclear power plants. In order to understand what can go wrong, the basic principles of how a nuclear power plant functions must be understood. This knowledge will help health care professionals provide better care by enabling them to better communicate with and understand the problems of those in the nuclear industry.

With these goals in mind, this chapter begins with a review of the fission process followed by a brief description of the design of nuclear power plants. Since this chapter is for the naive reader, basic and, in many cases, oversimplified principles are presented. Once this background information is consumed, the health consequences of accidents that are most likely to occur at a power plant are discussed. Finally, the potential health consequences of major accidents at nuclear power plants will be considered. In the subsequent chapter, the actual health consequences of two major accidents, Three Mile Island and Chernobyl, will be reviewed.

There are many issues related to nuclear power that this chapter will not address. Little discussion is included on the general health effects of normally operating plants. Problems

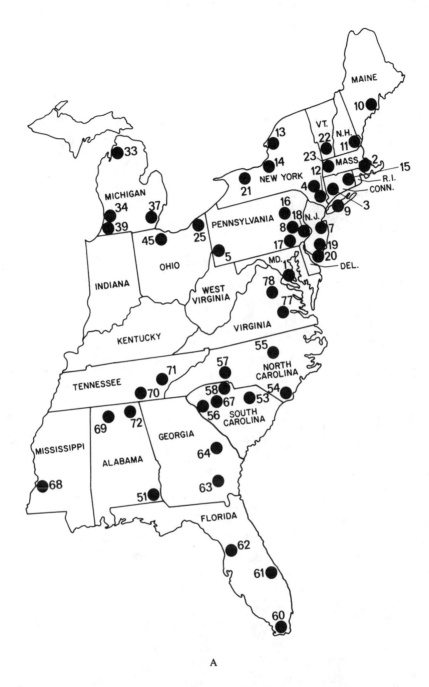

FIGURE 1. (A) Commercial nuclear power stations in the eastern U.S. The numbers on the map correspond to the map location number in Table 1. (B) Commercial nuclear power stations in the western U.S. The numbers on the map correspond to the map location number in Table 1.

related to mining uranium, decommissioning plants, and the long-term disposal of radioactive waste are also not discussed. The focus is potential mechanisms for injury and/or accidental radiation exposure/contamination at nuclear power plants.

II. NUCLEAR FISSION AND CRITICALITY

$E = mc^2$ is probably the best known equation in the world. This remarkably simple

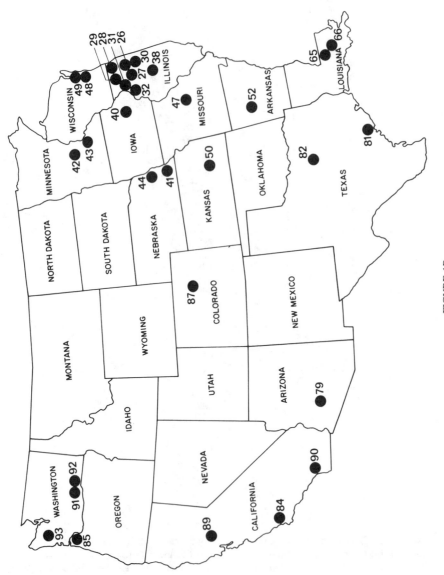

FIGURE 1B.

TABLE 1
Commercial Nuclear Power Stations in the U.S. Operable, Constructed, Under Construction, or Ordered August 1, 1987

Map location		Net MWe	Reactor supplier	Commercial operation
	Baltimore Gas & Electric Co.			
1	● Calvert Cliffs 1 (Lusby, MD)	850	C-E	5/75
	● Calvert Cliffs 2 (Lusby, MD)	850	C-E	4/77
	Boston Edison Co.			
2	● Pilgrim 1 (Plymouth, MA)	670	GE	12/72
	Connecticut Yankee Atomic Power Co.			
3	● Haddam Neck (Haddam Neck, CT)	582	W	1/68
	Consolidated Edison Co.			
4	● Indian Point 2 (Indian Point, NY)	873	W	7/74
	Duquesne Light Co.			
5	● Beaver Valley 1 (Shippingport, PA)	833	W	4/77
	○ Beaver Valley 2 (Shippingport, PA)	833	W	9/87
	GPU Nuclear Corporation			
7	● Oyster Creek 1 (Forked River, NJ)	620	GE	12/69
8	● Three Mile Island 1 (Londonderry Twp., PA)	792	B&W	9/74
	Long Island Lighting Co.			
9	□ Shoreham (Brookhaven, NY)	809	GE	Pending
	Maine Yankee Atomic Power Co.			
10	● Maine Yankee (Wiscasset, ME)	825	C-E	12/72
	New Hampshire Yankee, Inc.			
11	□ Seabrook 1 (Seabrook NH)	1150	W	Pending
	New York Power Authority			
12	● Indian Point 3 (Indian Point, NY)	965	W	8/76
13	● James A. FitzPatrick (Scriba, NY)	821	GE	7/75
	Niagara Mohawk Power Corp.			
14	● Nine Mile Point 1 (Scriba, NY)	610	GE	12/69
	○ Nine Mile Point 2 (Scriba, NY)	1080	GE	/88
	Northeast Utilities			
15	● Millstone 1 (Waterford, CT)	660	GE	12/70
	● Millstone 2 (Waterford, CT)	870	C-E	12/75
	● Millstone 3 (Waterford, CT)	1150	W	4/86
	Pennsylvania Power & Light Co.			
16	● Susquehanna 1 (Berwick, PA)	1050	GE	8/23
	● Susquehanna 2 (Berwick, PA)	1050	GE	2/85
	Philadelphia Electric Co.			
17	● Peach Bottom 2 (Peach Bottom, PA)	1065	GE	7/74
	● Peach Bottom 3 (Peach Bottom, PA)	1065	GE	12/74
18	● Limerick 1 (Pottstown, PA)	1055	GE	2/86
	○ Limerick 2 (Pottstown, PA)	1055	GE	2/90
	Public Service Electric & Gas Co.			
19	● Salem 1 (Salem, NJ)	1106	W	6/77
	● Salem 2 (Salem, NJ)	1106	W	10/81
20	● Hope Creek 1 (Salem, NJ)	1067	GE	2/87
	Rochester Gas & Electric Corp.			
21	● Robert E. Ginna (Ontario, NY)	490	W	3/70
	Vermont Yankee Nuclear Power Corp.			
22	● Vermont Yankee (Vernon, VT)	514	GE	11/72
	Yankee Atomic Electric Co.			
23	● Yankee (Rowe, MA)	175	W	6/61
	The Cleveland Electric Illuminating Co.			
25	○ Perry 1 (North Perry, OH)	1205	GE	9/87
	☑ Perry 2 (North Perry, OH)	1205	GE	Indef.
	Commonwealth Edison Company			
26	● Dresden 2 (Morris, IL)	794	GE	8/70
	● Dresden 3 (Morris, IL)	794	GE	10/71

TABLE 1 (continued)
Commercial Nuclear Power Stations in the U.S. Operable, Constructed, Under Construction, or Ordered August 1, 1987

Map location		Net MWe	Reactor supplier	Commercial operation
27	● LaSalle County 1 (Seneca, IL)	1078	GE	10/82
	● LaSalle County 2 (Seneca, IL)	1078	GE	6/84
28	● Zion 1 (Zion, IL)	1040	W	12/73
	● Zion 2 (Zion, IL)	1040	W	9/74
29	● Byron 1 (Byron, IL)	1120	W	9/85
	□ Byron 2 (Byron, IL)	1120	W	Pending
30	○ Braidwood 1 (Braidwood, IL)	1120	W	9/87
	○ Braidwood 2 (Braidwood, IL)	1120	W	9/88
31	☑ Carroll County-1 (Savanna, IL)	1120	W	Indef.
	☑ Carroll County-2 (Savanna, IL)	1120	W	Indef.
	Commonwealth Edison Co. and Iowa-Illinois Gas & Electric Co.			
32	● Quad-Cities 1 (Cordova, IL)	789	GE	8/72
	● Quad-Cities 2 (Cordova, IL)	789	GE	10/72
	Consumers Power Co.			
33	● Big Rock Point (Charlevoix, MI)	69	GE	12/62
34	● Palisades (South Haven, MI)	777	C-E	12/71
	Detroit Edison Co.			
37	○ Fermi 2 (Newport, MI)	1100	GE	9/87
	Illinois Power Co.			
38	□ Clinton 1 (Clinton, IL)	985	GE	Pending
	Indiana & Michigan Electric Co.			
39	● Donald C. Cook 1 (Bridgman, MI)	1020	W	8/75
	● Donald C. Cook 2 (Bridgman, MI)	1060	W	7/78
	Iowa Electric Light & Power Co.			
40	● Dane Arnold (Palo, IA)	538	GE	2/75
	Nebraska Public Power District			
41	● Cooper (Brownsville, NE)	778	GE	7/74
	Northern States Power Co.			
42	● Monticello (Monticello, MN)	536	GE	7/71
43	● Prairie Island 1 (Red Wing, MN)	520	W	12/73
	● Prairie Island 2 (Red Wing, MN)	520	W	12/74
	Omaha Public Power District			
44	● Fort Calhoun 1 (Fort Calhoun, NE)	486	C-E	9/73
	Toledo Edison Co.			
45	● Davis-Besse 1 (Oak Harbor, OH)	866	B&W	11/77
	Union Electric Co.			
47	● Callaway 1 (Fulton, MO)	1150	W	4/85
	Wisconsin Electric Power Co.			
48	● Point Beach 1 (Two Creeks, WI)	485	W	12/70
	● Point Beach 2 (Two Creeks, WI)	485	W	10/72
	Wisconsin Public Service Corporation			
49	● Kewaunee (Carlton, Wi)	535	W	6/74
	Wolf Creek Nuclear Operating Corporation			
50	● Wolf Creek (Burlington, KS)	1150	W	9/85
	Alabama Power Company			
51	● Joseph M. Farley 1 (Dothan, AL)	829	W	12/77
	● Joseph M. Farley 2 (Dothan, AL)	829	W	7/81
	Arkansas Power & Light Co.			
52	● Nuclear One 1 (Russellville, AR)	836	B&W	12/74
	● Nuclear One 2 (Russellville, AR)	858	C-E	3/80
	Carolina Power & Light Co.			
53	● Robinson 2 (Hartsville, SC)	665	W	3/71
54	● Brunswick 1 (Southport, NC)	790	GE	3/77
	● Brunswick 2 (Southport, NC)	790	GE	11/75
55	● Shearon Harris 1 (Newhill, NC)	900	W	5/87

TABLE 1 (continued)
Commercial Nuclear Power Stations in the U.S. Operable, Constructed,
Under Construction, or Ordered August 1, 1987

Map location		Net MWe	Reactor supplier	Commercial operation
	Duke Power Co.			
56	● Oconee 1 (Seneca, SC)	860	B&W	7/73
	● Oconee 2 (Seneca, SC)	860	B&W	9/74
	● Oconee 3 (Seneca, SC)	860	B&W	12/74
57	● McGuire 1 (Cornelius, NC)	1180	W	12/81
	● McGuire 2 (Cornelius, NC)	1800	W	3/84
58	● Catawba 1 (Clover, SC)	1145	W	6/85
	● Catawba 2 (Clover, SC)	1145	W	8/86
	Florida Power & Light Co.			
60	● Turkey Point 3 (Florida City, FL)	666	W	12/72
	● Turkey Point 4 (Florida City, FL)	666	W	9/73
61	● St. Lucie 1 (Hutchinson Island, FL)	827	C-E	12/76
	● St. Lucie 2 (Hutchinson Island, FL)	837	C-E	8/83
	Forida Power Corporation			
62	● Crystal River 3 (Red Level, FL)	825	B&W	3/77
	Georgia Power Co.			
63	● Edwin I. Hatch 1 (Baxley, GA)	810	GE	12/75
	● Edwin I. Hatch 2 (Baxley, GA)	820	GE	8/79
64	● Vogtle 1 (Waynesboro. GA)	1100	W	5/87
	○ Voglte 2 (Waynesboro, GA)	1100	W	7/89
	Gulf States Utilities Co.			
65	● River Bend 1 (St. Francisville, LA)	940	GE	6/86
	Louisiana Power & Light Co.			
66	● Waterford 3 (Taft, LA)	1104	C-E	9/85
	South Carolina Electric & Gas Co.			
67	● Virgil C. Summer 1 (Parr. SC)	900	W	1/84
	System Energy Resources, Inc. (subsidiary of Middle South Utilities)			
68	● Grand Gulf 1 (Port Gibson, MS)	1250	GE	7/85
	◨ Grand Gulf 2 (Port Gibson, MS)	1250	GE	Indef.
	Tennessee Valley Authority			
69	● Browns Ferry 1 (Decatur, AL)	1067	GE	8/74
	● Browns Ferry 2 (Decatur, AL)	1067	GE	3/75
	● Browns Ferry 3 (Decatur, AL)	1067	GE	3/77
70	● Sequoyah 1 (Daisy, TN)	1148	W	7/81
	● Sequoyah 2 (Daisy, TN)	1148	W	6/82
71	□ Watts Bar 1 (Spring City, TN)	1177	W	Pending
	□ Watts Bar 2 (Spring City, TN)	1177	W	Pending
72	○ Bellefonte 1 (Scottsboro, AL)	1213	B&W	/94
	○ Bellefonte 2 (Scottsboro, AL)	1213	B&W	/96
	Virginia Electric & Power Co.			
77	● Surry 1 (Gravel Neck, VA)	781	W	12/72
	● Surry 2 (Gravel Neck, VA)		W	5/73
78	● North Anna 1 (Mineral, VA)	893	W	6/78
	● North Anna 2 (Mineral, VA)	893	W	12/80
	Arizona Public Service Co.			
79	● Palo Verde 1 (Wintersburg, AZ)	1270	C-E	2/86
	● Palo Verde 2 (Wintersburg, AZ)	1270	C-E	9/86
	○ Palo Verde 3 (Wintersburg, AZ)	1270	C-E	10/87
	Houston Lighting & Power Company			
81	○ South Texas Project 1 (Palacios, TX)	1250	W	12/87
	○ South Texas Project 2 (Palacios, TX)	1250	W	12/89
	Texas Utilities Generation Company			
82	○ Comanche Peak 1 (Glen Rose, TX)	1150	W	3/89
	○ Comanche Peak 2 (Glen Rose, TX)	1150	W	9/89
	Pacific Gas & Electric Co.			
84	● Diablo Canyon 1 (Avila Beach, CA)	1084	W	5/85
	● Diablo Canyon 2 (Avila Beach, CA)	1106	W	3/86

TABLE 1 (continued)
Commercial Nuclear Power Stations in the U.S. Operable, Constructed,
Under Construction, or Ordered August 1, 1987

Map location		Net MWe	Reactor supplier	Commercial operation
	Portland General Electric Co.			
85	─⊏ ● Trojan (Prescott, OR)	1130	W	5/76
	Public Service Company of Colorado			
87	─⊏ ● Fort St. Vrain (Platteville, CO)	330	GA	1/79
	Sacramento Municipal Utility District			
89	─⊏ ● Rancho Seco (Clay Station, CA)	913	B&W	4/75
	Southern California Edison and San Diego Gas & Electric Co.			
	● San Onofre 1 (San Clemente, CA)	436	W	1/68
90	● San Onofre 2 (San Clemente, CA)	1100	C-E	8/83
	● San Onofre 3 (San Clemente, CA)	1100	C-E	4/84
	United States Department of Energy			
91	─⊏ ● Hanford-N (Richland, WA)	860	GE	7/66
	Washington Public Power Supply System			
	● WNP-2 (Richland, WA)	1100	GE	12/84
92	☑ WNP-1 (Richland, WA)	1250	B&W	Indef.
93	─⊏ ☑ WNP-3 (Satsop, WA)	1240	C-E	Indef.
	U.S. Total (126 units)	**116,939**		

Note: Abbreviations are as follows: B & W: Babcock & Wilcox (pressurized); C-E: Combustion Engineering (pressurized); GA: General Atomic (gas-cooled); GE: General Electric (boiling); W: Westinghouse (pressurized).

Key: ● Commercial operation
☐ Constructed
○ Under construction
☑ Indefinite

Reproduced with permission of the American Nuclear Society.

equation states that mass can be converted directly into energy. The fact that extraordinary amounts of energy can be produced by converting mass into energy is apparent even to the nonmathematician, since c^2 (the speed of light squared) is recognized to be a very large number.

Nuclear fission produces energy by converting mass into energy. During fission a nucleus splits into two smaller nuclei. The combined mass of the two smaller nuclei is less than the mass of the original nucleus. Some of the mass of the original nucleus is converted to energy. The reduction in mass of the original nucleus is very small (<1/1000 of the original mass) but the amount of energy produced is very large. The energy produced during a fission (200 MeV per fission) can be compared with the energy produced by breaking a chemical bond (burning fossil fuels). Approximately 50 million times as much energy is produced by a single fission as is produced by breaking a single chemical bond. On a larger scale, a typical large nuclear plant fissions several pounds of uranium a day. A similar size fossil fuel-burning plant would burn several thousand tons of coal. Given this potential for the production of great amounts of energy, it is easy to understand the initial great enthusiasm for nuclear power.

Enthusiasm for nuclear power has been tempered by other realities. First, there are only three easily fissionable radionuclides (^{235}U, ^{239}Pu, and ^{233}U). Only ^{235}U occurs in nature in significant but limited quantities. Natural uranium consists of >99.3% ^{238}U and <0.7%

TABLE 2
Levels of Reactivity

Subcritical	Less than one fission is produced by neutrons induced from the previous generation of fissions. Energy output decreases.
Just Critical	Exactly one fission is produced by neutrons induced from the previous generation. Energy output is constant.
Supercritical	More than one fission is produced by neutrons induced by the previous generation of fissions. Energy output increases.

fissionable ^{235}U. In order to fuel a light water nuclear reactor the percent of fissionable ^{235}U must be increased to 2 to 5% usually 3%). Needless to say, some energy must be put into the mining and enrichment process. This energy must be subtracted from the energy ultimately produced to determine the net energy gain. When the percent of ^{235}U in uranium ore falls below a certain percentage, the energy required to mine and enrich it will exceed the energy which it will produce. Some estimate that the economically reasonable uranium reserves in the U.S. will be exhausted in the next century. The lack of an inexhaustible supply has generated interest in building reactors which will actually produce more fissionable materials (particularly ^{239}Pu) than they will consume. However, opposition to breeder reactors has been intense and the plans for a breeder reactor at Clinch River in the U.S. have been abandoned.

Fission of ^{235}U occurs spontaneously at only a very slow rate. The rate of fission and therefore the rate of energy production is greatly increased by bombarding the fissionable radionuclides with neutrons. Fission itself supplies the neutrons that are necessary to increase the rate of fission, therefore a rapid rate of energy production can be self-sustaining. On the average, fission of one ^{235}U nucleus produces 2.3 neutrons. If one of these neutrons (Table 2, Figure 2) causes fission of exactly one other ^{235}U nucleus, then constant energy production is achieved. Under this situation the nuclear reaction is said to be *just critical*. If less than one neutron causes fission of another ^{235}U nucleus, the nuclear reaction is not sustained, energy output decreases, and the reaction is said to be *subcritical*. When the neutrons from the fission of one ^{235}U cause fission of more than one ^{235}U nucleus, the energy output increases rapidly and the reaction is said to be *supercritical*.

Achieving this perfect balance of neutrons from one fission producing exactly one subsequent fission requires some ingenuity. Control rods which can be moved into and out of the reactor core can be used to absorb some of the excess neutrons. When the fuel is fresh, more neutrons will have to be absorbed than when the fuel is depleted. In addition, chemical neutron absorbers, also called poisons (e. g., boron), can be added to the water surrounding the fuel rods to provide some control over the percentage of neutrons which will cause additional fissions. Since an average 2.3 neutrons are produced with each fission of ^{235}U, 1.3 neutrons must be prevented from causing fission. In a normally operating reactor, one of the 2.3 neutrons will cause fission of another ^{235}U nucleus, approximately .65 neutrons will escape from the reactor vessel, and approximately .65 neutrons will be absorbed by the control rods or chemical poisons.

One subtlety about this process must be appreciated to understand how accidents can happen. The time between when a neutron is produced by one fission and when it interacts with another nucleus to cause another fission is very short, less than 10^{-4} s. If the ratio of fissions produced from one generation to the next is slightly in excess of one, the energy output increases rapidly due to the very short time between generations. For example, if the neutrons from one fission produced 1.001 fission, the power output of the next generation then would increase 2.7 times in one tenth of a sec and 21,917 times in one s (1.001^{1000} and $1.001^{10,000}$, respectively). Under these time constraints, control of a reactor could not be achieved by modulating these prompt neutrons. It would be impossible to move control

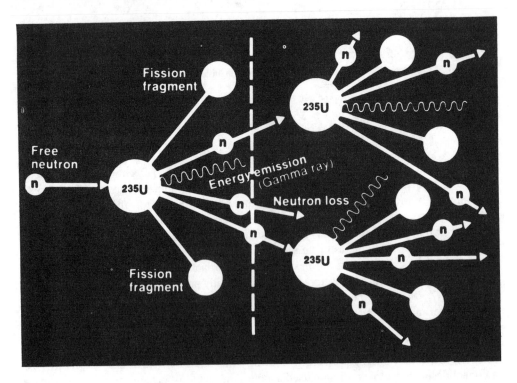

First Generation   Second Generation

FIGURE 2.   The fission process. First generation: A free neutron strikes a fissionable nucleus (^{235}U). The fission process results in 2 smaller nuclei (fission fragments) and an average of 2.3 neutrons (white circles labeled **n**). Second generation: In this example, 2 neutrons from the prior fission produce 2 more fissions. Under these circumstances energy output increases rapidly and the fission reaction is said to be supercritical.

rods in and out in such short time spans. Fortunately, about 0.5% of the neutrons in a uranium-fueled reactor are delayed neutrons. The time between when a delayed neutron is produced and when it causes a fission ranges from 0.2 to 56 s.[3] This much longer time constant allows for control of a nuclear reactor. The reactor is only allowed to be subcritical using prompt neutrons and criticality is achieved by the small addition of the delayed neutrons. In the accident at Chernobyl (described in detail in the next chapter), the reactor was allowed to go critical with prompt neutrons and therefore rapidly increased its energy output and exploded.

When neutrons are produced by fission they have very high energy. The chances of a neutron causing fission of another nucleus increases as the neutron loses energy and the density of the fissionable nuclei increases. Almost all reactors in the U.S. use ordinary (light) water as the moderator (the substance which absorbs the initial high energy of the neutron thereby increasing the chances of causing fission). The operating temperature and pressure of the reactor affect the density of the moderator and the density of the fissionable uranium. Therefore, changing pressure and temperature will also change the fission rate.

To prevent supercriticality accidents, nuclear reactors are designed with many redundant safety features which will automatically turn off the reactor when unexpected conditions (transients) are detected. Transients include abnormal temperatures, pressures, and flow rates. The automatic shutdown of a reactor, a scram, is said to be from the acronym *Safety Control Rod Ax Man*. The first research reactors were all rapidly shut down by cutting a rope which allowed control rods to drop into the reactor.[4] A literal interpretation of the word *scram*, "to go away quickly", seems just as appropriate.

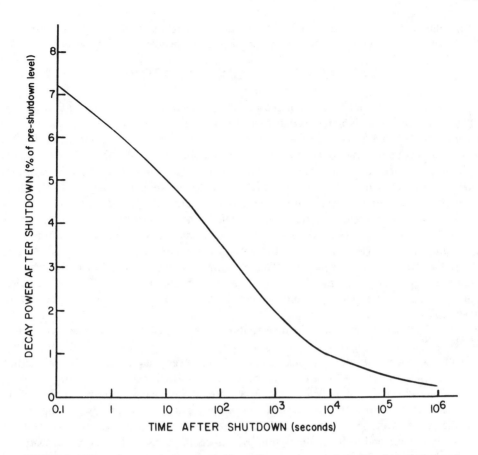

FIGURE 3.   Thermal power after reactor shutdown. Heat continues to be produced by the decay of
fission products after the reactor is shut down. The heat must be removed to prevent damage to the
reactor core. Failure to remove this heat resulted in extensive damage to the reactor core at Three Mile
Island.

10^2 s = 1.7 min
10^3 s = 0.7 d
10^4 s = 1.0 week
10^5 s = 2.3 months
10^6 s = 1.9 years

(From Nero, A. V., *A Guidebook to Nuclear Reactors,* University of California Press, Berkeley, 1979,
54. With permission. © 1979 The Regents of the University of California.)

Unfortunately, the energy produced by a nuclear reactor does not stop immediately once
the rate of fission is greatly reduced by the complete insertion of the control rods. Energy
output will continue at approximately 7% of the level that had been sustained (Figure 3).
The reactor must be continually cooled, even after a scram to remove this residual heat.
The damage to the reactor at Three Mile Island occurred *after* the nuclear reactor was made
subcritical. The core was extensively damaged because of failure to continue to cool the
reactor after shutdown had occurred.

Fresh, unused fuel rods are not very radioactive; however, highly radioactive byproducts
are produced by fission. The 7% continued energy production postshutdown comes from
the continued decay of large amounts of radioactive fission byproducts which accumulate
in the reactor. The decay heat of these fission products rapidly disappears initially, since
many of the fission products have very short half-lives. By 1 min after shutdown, the residual

energy output decreases to about 4% of the sustained operating level, by 1 h the output has decreased to 1.5%, and by the end of one day the output decreases to slightly less than 1%.

III. RADIONUCLIDE INVENTORY

Only a small amount (a few hundred curies of uranium) of the radionuclide inventory of an operating reactor is introduced as fuel. The total amount of radioactivity in a reactor (approximately 1000 MWe) that has been operating for 1 year is 15 billion Ci (Table 3). The additional radioactivity comes from three major sources. First, the nuclear fragments which are produced by fission are highly radioactive. The mass of the fission fragments tend to cluster around peaks in the vicinity of the atomic weights 95 and 140. The most important examples of the first group are krypton and strontium. The most important examples of the second group are iodine, xenon, and cesium. Another important fragment given off during fission is tritium. The second source for radioactivity is in nonfission reactions such as neutron capture. Neutron capture by heavy, more stable isotopes produces unstable radioactive elements as neutrons are added to them. Plutonium is produced in this manner. The third major source of radioactivity in the reactor is neutron activation of the fuel covering and structural materials. Radionuclides of cobalt, iron, nickel, chromium, and others are produced by activation.

The 15 billion-Ci inventory of radioactivity in an operating reactor is enormous. Some of the activity is in a gaseous form (xenon, krypton), making containment particularly difficult. Despite the difficulties, a normally operating power plant releases only a few curies of activity into the environment over the course of a year. Containment of the enormous amount of radioactivity in a nuclear reactor is accomplished using a four-part system. The first design feature to prevent the escape of radioactivity into the environment is to impregnate ceramic pellets with the radioactive fuel. The high melting point of the ceramic (2760°C) keeps the uranium and many of the fission byproducts in an insoluble solid state. Only the volatile byproducts (krypton, xenon, iodine) easily escape from the ceramic matrix in a normally operating power plant. The second barrier to the escape of radioactivity into the environment is the metal sleeves (fuel cladding) that the fuel pellets are placed in. This covering keeps most of the radioactivity within the fuel rods. Some of the radioactive gases do escape through tiny leaks in the fuel rod casings (Figure 4). The third level of containment is the reactor vessel itself. Any activity leaking from the fuel rods should be trapped in the sealed reactor vessel. The fourth level of containment is the containment building. This large structure is enclosing the reactor and can be closed off from the environment to trap any escaping radioactivity (Figure 5).

In addition to mechanical containment, two additional strategies are used to control the radionuclide inventory of a nuclear reactor. The first mechanism is filtration. Filtration systems chemically or physically separate radionuclides which have escaped into the plants liquid or gaseous waste stream. The second mechanism is holdup. Holdup prevents discharge of liquid or gaseous waste for long enough periods of time to allow substantial decay to occur. After a long enough period of time the waste stream can then be released into the environment.

When the reactor is shut down the radionuclide inventory decreases rapidly due to the decay of many short half-life isotopes. Once the reactor is shut down, the inventory rapidly decays to 5 billion Ci. One hundred fifty days after shutdown, the radionuclide inventory has decreased to 0.1 billion Ci.

IV. TYPES OF NUCLEAR POWER PLANTS

Fundamental differences in the design of nuclear reactors exist. Reactors which use

TABLE 3
Radioactivity in a 1000-MWe Light Water Reactor

Radionuclides	Half-life	Reactor inventory (10^6 Ci)	Health considerations; chemical considerations; and principal radiation
Tritium			
^{3}H	12.26 year	0.0723	Internal hazard; H_2O; β(0.019 MeV max)
Krypton			
83m	1.86 h	5.71	External irradiation; gaseous; β(0.67 MeV max for
85m	4.4 h	17.2	^{85}Kr)
85	10.76 year	1.16	
87	76 min	34.0	
88	2.8 h	49.0	
89	3.18 min	61.8	
90	33s	58.5	
Total		325	
Strontium			
89	52.7 d	71.6	Internal hazard to bone and lung; nonvolatile;
90	27.7 y	7.80	β(0.55 MeV max for ^{90}Sr)
Total		526	
Iodine			
129	1.7×10^7year	3.03×10^{-6}	Internal hazard to thyroid; highly volatile; β(0.8
131	8.05 d	71.9	MeV max for ^{131}I) and γ
132	2.26 h	103	
133	20.3 h	137	
134	52.2 min	156	
135	6.68 h	123	
136	83	54.0	
Total		1,017	
Xenon			
131m	11.8 d	0.582	External irradiation; gaseous; β(0.35 MeV max for
133m	2.26 d	3.29	^{133}Xe) and γ
133	5.27 d	137	
135m	15.6 min	36.8	
135	9.14 h	25.7	
137	3.9 min	132	
138	17.5 min	128	
139	43 s	107	
Total		680	
Cesium			
134	2.046 year	19.0	Internal hazard to muscle; volatile; β(1.176 MeV
137	30.0 year	9.92	max for ^{137}Cs) and γ
Total		595	
Zr, Nb, Mo, Tc, Ru, Rh, Pd, Ag, Cd, In, Sn, Sb		1,880	External and internal hazard; nonvolatile
Rare earths: La, Ce, Pr, Nd, Pm, Sm, Eu, Gd, Tb, Dy, Ho		4,140	External and internal hazard; nonvolatile
Total fission products		11,970	
Uranium			
237	6.75 d	108	External and internal hazard; nonvolatile; β(1.29
239	23.5 min	1,708	MeV max for ^{237}U) and γ
Total		1,816	

TABLE 3 (continued)
Radioactivity in a 1000-MWe Light Water Reactor

Radionuclides	Half-life	Reactor inventory (10^6 Ci)	Health considerations; chemical considerations; and principal radiation
Plutonium			
238	86.4 year	0.138	Internal hazard to bone, liver, lung, lymph; non-
239	24,390 year	0.0318	volatile; α(about 5 MeV for ^{238,239,240,242}Pu) and
240	6,580 year	0.0500	β(for ^{241}Pu)
241	13.2 year	12.4	
242	3.79×10^5 year	1.24×10^{-4}	
243	4.98 year	22.2	
Total		34.9	
Fissionable Pu (^{239}Pu + ^{241}Pu)			
Americium (241, 242m, 242, 243) and Curium (242, 243, 244)		1.14	Internal hazard; nonvolatile; α(5.5 MeV for ^{241}Am)
Total Actinides Th, Pa, U, Np, Pu, Am, Cm		3,614	
Activated Zircaloy cladding and Inconel spacers (Cr, Mn, Fe, Co, Ni, Zr, Nb, Sb)		12.9	Nonvolatile
Total fission products, actinides and cladding		15,600	

Modified from Nero, A. V., *A Guidebook to Nuclear Reactors,* University of California Press, Berkeley, 1979, 36. With permission.

naturally occurring water (light water) as the moderator and coolant are the most common reactors used to commercially produce electricity. Other types of reactors which are in common use include pressurized heavy water reactors, gas-cooled reactors and light water-cooled, graphite-moderated reactors. The pressurized heavy water reactor uses heavy water as the moderator and coolant. These reactors are used mostly in Canada. Gas-cooled reactors use helium as the coolant and graphite as the moderator. These reactors are found primarily in Great Britain. Light water-cooled and graphite-moderated reactors are used almost exclusively in the U.S.S.R. They have obtained great notoriety following the accident at Chernobyl.

Many of the basic principles of how a nuclear reactor works are the same for all types of power plants. Because of their widespread use, light water plants will be discussed in more detail. In addition, unique characteristics of water-cooled graphite-moderated reactors will be briefly discussed so that the accident at Chernobyl can be better understood. Two varieties of light water reactors have been installed at numerous sites. The first type is called a *boiling water reactor* and the second type is called a *pressurized water reactor*. Approximately one third of all operating commercial nuclear power stations in the U.S. are boiling water reactors.

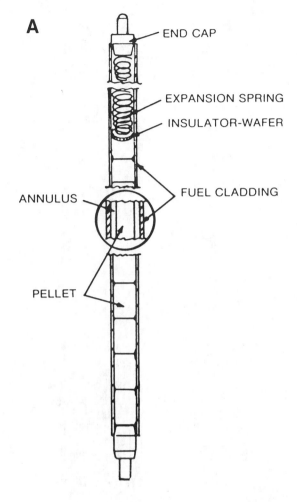

Fuel Rod

FIGURE 4. Fuel rod schematic. (A) Fuel rod: ceramic pellets measuring approximately 0.5 inches in diameter and 0.5—1.0 inch in length are stacked inside a tube to form a fuel rod. This design erects the first 2 barriers to prevent the accidental release of radionuclides into the environment. (From WASH-1250, reprinted in Nero, A. V., *A Guidebook to Nuclear Reactors*, University of California Press, Berkeley, 1979, 79.) (B) Fuel assembly: multiple fuel rods are inserted into a fuel assembly. Many fuel assemblies are in the reactor. (From WASH-1250, reprinted in Nero, A. V., *A Guidebook to Nuclear Reactors*, University of California Press, Berkeley, 1979, 77.)

All commercial boiling water reactors in the U.S. have been designed by General Electric. Steam is directly produced by the reactor itself and the steam from the reactor drives the turbines to generate electricity (Figure 6). Since the water used to generate the steam is directly in contact with the reactor, the steam is radioactive. The radioactivity is largely due to the formation of ^{16}N due to neutron activation of the oxygen in H_2O. Fortunately ^{16}N has a short half-life (7 s). Typically, the water flowing into the reactor has a temperature of 376°F and the water leaving the reactor has a temperature of 550°F. The pressure in the reactor is 7 MPa. The flow of coolant in a 1000-MW reactor is approximately 13,000 gal/s.

Reactors of different designs have different features. Boiling water reactors tend to have nonuniform power production since the water turns to steam as the coolant flows through

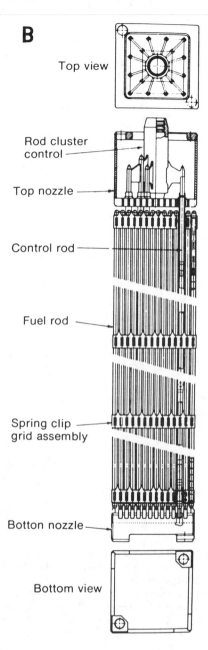

B

Top view

Rod cluster control

Top nozzle

Control rod

Fuel rod

Spring clip grid assembly

Botton nozzle

Bottom view

Fuel Assembly

the reactor. Because the water serves as a moderator which facilitates fission, less water and more steam means that the reactor produces less power at the top of the reactor than at the bottom. The power production can be made more uniform by a variety of design modifications. One intrinsic control system of light water-moderated reactors is that lack of water decreases the fission rate of the reactor due to the loss of its moderating effect.

Newer light water reactors tend to be pressurized water reactors. In the U.S. approximately half of the pressurized water reactors are made by Westinghouse, one quarter are made by Babcock and Wilcox, and one quarter are made by Combustion Engineering. The fundamental difference between pressurized water reactors and boiling water reactors is that

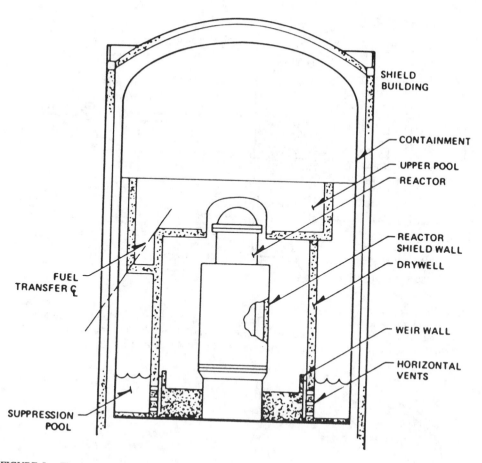

FIGURE 5. The reactor vessel and containment building for a boiling water reactor. In a normally operating power plant, the reactor vessel is sealed to prevent the escape of radioactivity. The containment building is also sealed should a release of activity occur. (From General Electric, reprinted in Nero, A. V., *A Guidebook to Nuclear Reactors,* University of California Press, Berkeley, 1979, 103. With permission.)

the water in a pressurized reactor is not turned directly into steam. Instead, the water flowing through the reactor (the primary coolant loop) flows through a steam generator (Figure 7). The water which is converted into steam in the steam generator (the secondary loop) never comes into contact with the water in the reactor, therefore, the steam produced is not radioactive. Coolant flow rates (primary loop) are similar to those in a boiling water reactor (17,000 gal/s), however, the pressure is higher (15.5 MPa) as is the temperature of the water entering (552°F) and exiting (615°F) the reactor vessel. This design is attractive since the radioactive water in the primary loop is confined to a smaller portion of the plant, thereby making the job of avoiding radiation exposure simpler. The average collective dose (man-rem per unit per year) is considerably less in pressurized reactors than in boiling reactors (Figure 8). Unfortunately, the price for this decrease in radiation hazard in the pressurized reactors is a more complex and slightly less efficient system. In particular, the maintenance and repair of steam generators has been a nontrivial task. To achieve acceptable heat transfer rates, the heated water of the primary loop flows through many small tubes in the steam generator (Figure 9). These small tubes heat the water in the secondary loop which surround the tubes. Rupture of these tubes with escape of the radioactive water in the primary loop into the secondary loop has been a difficult problem.

Almost one half of the reactors used to produce electricity in the U.S.S.R. are water-cooled, graphite-moderated reactors (Figure 10). In these reactors massive amounts of graph-

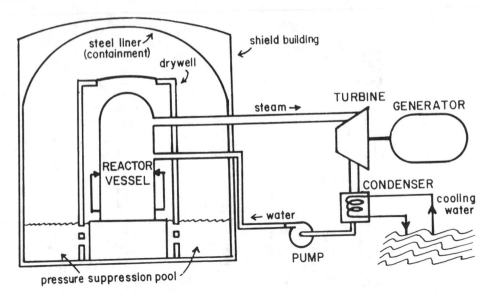

FIGURE 6.   The schematic of a boiling water reactor power plant. Steam is generated directly in the reactor vessel and flows to the turbine-generator system. The steam is then condensed and returns to the reactor vessel as feed water. (From Nero, A. V., *A Guidebook to Nuclear Reactors,* University of California Press, Berkeley, 1979, 96. With permission. © 1979 The Regents of the University of California.)

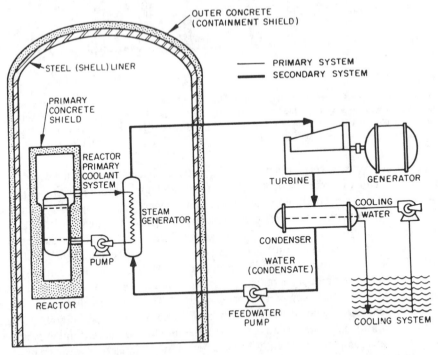

FIGURE 7.   Schematic of pressurized water reactor power plant. The primary loop contains steam which is produced by their reactor and flows to the steam generator. Water from the steam generator is then recycled as feed water to the reactor. The primary loop contains water which is radioactive. The secondary loop contains nonradioactive steam which is produced in the steam generator and flows to the turbine generator system. This water is then condensed and recycled as feed water to the steam generator. Ideally, the steam generator prevents mixing of the water from the primary loop and the secondary loop, therefore the water in the secondary loop is nonradioactive. (From ERDA-1541, reprinted in Nero, A. V., *A Guidebook to Nuclear Reactors,* University of California Press, Berkeley, 1979, 78.)

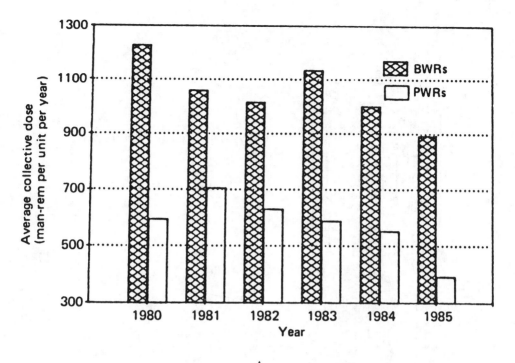

A

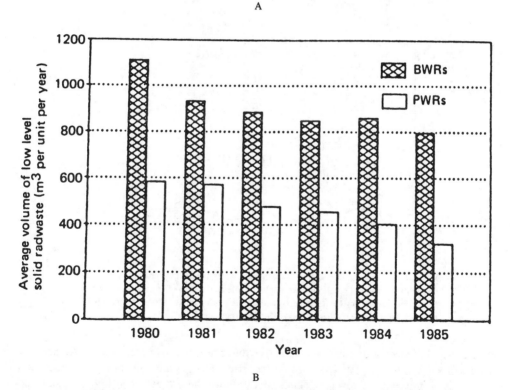

B

FIGURE 8. Collective dose and volume of radwaste for pressurized water reactors and boiling water reactors. (A) Because the radioactive water is less well confined in a boiling water reactor (BWRs) than a pressurized water reactor (PWRs), the collective dose to the worker is greater. (B) Boiling water reactors produce more rad waste than pressurized water reactors since the radioactivity is distributed over a larger volume. (From Nuclear Safety Review for 1985, International Atomic Energy Agency, Vienna, 1986, 5. With permission.)

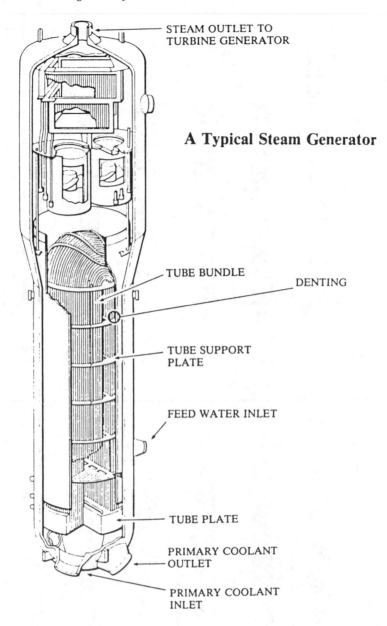

STEAM OUTLET TO
TURBINE GENERATOR

A Typical Steam Generator

TUBE BUNDLE

DENTING

TUBE SUPPORT
PLATE

FEED WATER INLET

TUBE PLATE

PRIMARY COOLANT
OUTLET

PRIMARY COOLANT
INLET

FIGURE 9.   A steam generator. Superheated water from the primary loop passes
through thousands of small tubes in a tube bundle in order to efficiently transfer the
heat from the primary to the secondary loop. Preventing leaks in these thousands of
tubes in the tube bundle has been a difficult maintenance problem.

ite are used because carbon is a less effective moderator than water. Since fewer neutrons
are absorbed by the graphite than would be absorbed by water, neutrons are used more
efficiently in this type of reactor. This system allows these reactors to operate using fuel
that contains only 2.0% of ^{235}U.

Two unique characteristics of graphite reactors contributed to the accident at Chernobyl.
First, the chance that a fission will occur increases when the temperature rises. The opposite
is true with light water reactors. The positive feedback of temperature on the rate of fissions
means that additional measures are required to prevent the reactor from going supercritical.

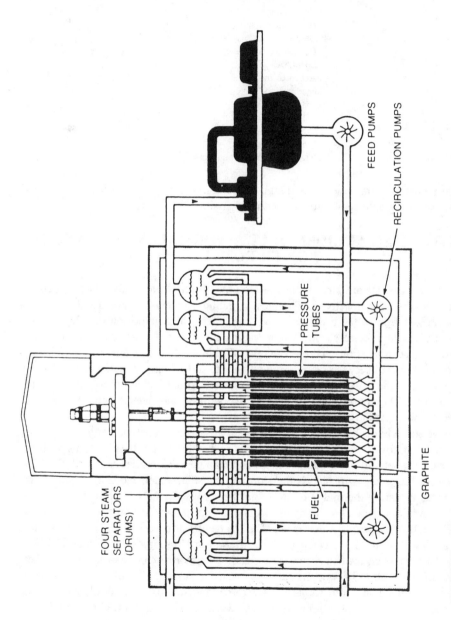

FIGURE 10. Schematic of a graphite moderated water cooled reactor. The large volume of graphite precludes a similar containment vessel as is used for a light water moderator reactor. (From Chernobyl: the Soviet Report, *Nucl. News*, 29, 1, 1986. With permission.)

TABLE 4
Types of Accidents

Major trauma only
    Burns
    Crush injuries
    Fractures from falls
    Electrocution
    Heat exhaustion
Exposure
    Opened reactor vessel
    Spent fuel
    Activated metal
Contamination
    External or Internal
        Primary loop
        Spent fuel pool
        Radwaste system
    Radioactive metal fragment

Second, the moderator, graphite, burns at high temperatures. The persistent fire at Chernobyl was due to burning graphite, not due to continued fission.

V. POTENTIAL ACCIDENTS AT A NORMALLY OPERATING POWER PLANT

Nuclear power plants are large industrial facilities. Many areas of the plant contain no significant amounts of radioactivity. The most common accidents are the accidents which one would expect from a facility with heavy equipment, high temperature, high voltage electricity, and high-pressure steam. Major trauma can occur due to steam burns, crush injuries, falls, heat exhaustion, and electrocution (Table 4). Major trauma due to falls and crush injuries are most likely to occur during outages for refueling and maintenance. During this time, the size of the work-force greatly increases in order to efficiently carry out refueling and maintenance. The combination of a larger work force and intense activity involving heavy objects increases the chances of an accident.

Extensive steam burns have resulted in the death of several nuclear power plant workers. Hospitals close to power plants must be prepared to handle severe burns. Burns with superheated steam appear different than the more common thermal injuries seen with fire. The intense heat of the steam will blanch the skin and cause an extensive third-degree burn. These atypical-appearing thermal burns must not be confused with local radiation injuries. Local radiation injuries have few if any immediate manifestations and are initially painless.

One example of an accident that resulted in the deaths of several workers due to burns occurred at Unit 2 of the Surry Nuclear Power Station in Virginia on December 9, 1986.[5] An 18-in. diameter main feedwater pipe to a steam generator ruptured, spraying 8 workers with steam and hot water. Six workers suffered extensive burns that resulted in four deaths. Two workers sustained only minor injuries. The three most seriously injured were evacuated from the site by helicopter. The remaining three workers were transported by ambulance. Radiation played no role in this accident. The walls of the pipe that ruptured had eroded from a nominal wall thickness of 0.50 in. to <.050 in.

Accidents involving radiation exposure/contamination *alone* occur but are almost never medical emergencies. Even patients who are exposed to potentially lethal doses require only supportive care initially. Death is most likely to occur 3 to 4 weeks after the accident. Earlier deaths are possible, but only when individuals are exposed to massive amounts of radiation for which there is no effective treatment. Patients who are only contaminated or who have minor injuries should be decontaminated first at the nuclear power plant. Any effort to make a hospital function as a decontamination center is misdirected. Hospitals have little expertise in decontamination. For these reasons, a radiation accident uncomplicated by major trauma is not best treated in a hospital emergency room. The main reason that a patient will be brought to an emergency room from a nuclear power plant is for treatment of major trauma, not for the treatment of radiation injury.

Accidental radiation exposure/contamination is more likely during outages. During refueling, the reactor vessel is opened. This increases the chances of radiation exposure/contamination by that route. In addition, areas and equipment in the plant which have become excessively contaminated during the normal operation of the plant are decontaminated or replaced during this time.

High exposures may occur when workers are close to an open, inadequately shielded reactor, spent fuel rods, or activated metal. One of the largest exposures which has occurred in a nuclear power plant in the U.S. occurred during a refueling and maintenance cycle at the Dresden Nuclear Power Station near Morris, Illinois, in March of 1981.[6] The opened reactor vessel was shielded with water and a large concrete radiation-shielding plug. Because of an inaccurate instrument, the water level in the reactor was thought to be higher than it really was. A contractor employee stood on an adjacent portion of the concrete shield as another portion was removed. The low water level provided inadequate shielding for the reactor and the worker was exposed to a whole-body radiation dose of 22 rem (0.22 Sv).

An exposure of a similar magnitude was reported by the Trojan Nuclear Plant in Columbia County, Oregon, in April 1978. Two radiation protection staff members were monitoring the plant for contamination during its refueling and maintenance cycle.[7] They were standing next to a fuel transfer tube when spent fuel rods were sent to the spent fuel pool. They thought that the tube they were standing next to was a ventilation shaft and that the fuel transfer tube was shielded with concrete. Their survey meters went off scale during the transfer of the spent fuel rods. It was estimated that their 22-s exposure resulted in whole-body doses of 27.3 and 17.1 rem (0.273 and 0.171 Sv).

Another potential source for an overexposure to radiation is activated metal. During fission, constant neutron bombardment of the initially nonradioactive metal in and composing the reactor vessel produces many radioactive nuclides. Metal removed from the reactor core can have dose rates of thousands of rads per minute at the surface. Some of the metal parts that are replaced during outages for refueling and maintenance are highly radioactive.

Radiation accidents which involve contamination require special precautions on the part of the attending hospital staff. Again it should be stressed that a patient should not be brought to a hospital emergency room for treatment of their contamination per se. The nuclear power plant personnel are much more skilled at decontamination than are the hospital staff. The reason that a patient would be brought to the emergency room would be for treatment of major trauma. In this setting, contamination with radioactivity is a nuisance and should not distract the medical staff from providing the appropriate medical treatment. In general, contamination with radioactive dirt should be treated the same way as is contamination with any hazardous waste. For example, the steps taken to care for a patient who is seriously injured and covered with sewage would be appropriate for taking care of the patient contaminated with radioactivity. Gowns and gloves would be worn to keep the attending personnel's clothes clean, and steps would be taken to prevent the room from becoming needlessly dirty.

Only a few principles need to be mastered in order to properly care for the radiation-contamination aspect of the accident. First it must be recognized that the paramedical and medical personnel are generally unfamiliar with radiation. This unfamiliarity is guaranteed to raise their level of anxiety during an accident involving radiation, and this distraction greatly increases the chances of making an error. In the past, patients have been grossly mistreated because of the medical staff's fear or lack of understanding of the significance of a radiation accident. Individuals have been refused admittance to emergency rooms and their radiation exposure has gone unappreciated for days.[8,9] To combat this unfamiliarity with radiation, it is very important to have radiation accident drills at least yearly and preferably several times a year. The Nuclear Regulatory Commission (NRC) requires yearly drills at hospitals which have been designated as support hospitals for nuclear power plants. These drills are invaluable since they give the medical staff a chance to think about their role in a radiation accident and a chance to ask questions about aspects which they do not understand. Radiation accidents occur infrequently, making drills essential. On the average, the support hospital for a nuclear power plant provides care for trauma twice a year. A radiation accident plan is now required for *all* hospitals by the Joint Commission of Accredited Hospitals.

Second, setting up procedures to facilitate communication between a nuclear power plant and the hospital is of utmost importance. Since medical personnel are unfamiliar with the jargon of the nuclear physicist and the nuclear physicist is unfamiliar with medical jargon, communication can be a complex task. Neither side wants to admit that they do not know what the other is saying. Drills are very helpful because they provide the opportunity to get the physicist and the health professional together so they can agree on terms that they will both understand. By far, communication is likely to be the weakest link during a radiation accident. Obtaining the initial information about an accident is greatly facilitated if a simple standard form is used to record the information (Figure 11) when a call from a power plant is received.[10] It is very important to record the name and phone number of the person reporting the accident so that additional information can be obtained as needed. Advanced notification of the arrival of the patient to the hospital is needed for the hospital to implement its radiation accident precautions.

The type of radiation accident determines whether or not precautions need to be undertaken (Table 4). Since the most common accident at a nuclear power plant will *not* involve radiation, no special precautions are needed. Nor are special precautions needed if an individual is only exposed to radiation. Individuals exposed to radiation (e.g., patients having a chest X-ray) are *not* radioactive.

Contaminated patients fall into three categories. Accident victims who have breathed in or swallowed radioactive materials are internally contaminated. Accident victims with radioactive dirt on their skin and clothes are externally contaminated. Finally, a patient may have a radioactive metallic fragment imbedded in a wound.

The contaminated patient requires special precautions. To the uninitiated, the precautions which are used to care for patients who are radioactive are often misunderstood. Areas of the hospital are roped off, the attending medical staff is gowned and gloved, floors are covered, etc. Since these precautions are unique to hospital personnel, it is not surprising that they regard radiation as uniquely hazardous. In fact, the special precautions serve only two main functions. First by wearing gloves and a mask the chances of ingesting radioactive material is decreased. It is important to prevent internal contamination, since it is much more difficult to remove unwanted radioactivity once it is inside the body. Second, the floor covering and the wearing of gowns simply make cleanup easier. Because Geiger counters are very sensitive instruments, cleanup following a radiation hazard accident is much more fastidious than cleanup following a biohazard, which cannot be so readily detected. Given the fact that cleanup will be so complete, it is simply made easier by the floor coverings, etc. Other than decreasing the chances of internal contamination, the precautions that are taken in caring for a contaminated accident victim do nothing to decrease the radiation dose to the attending medical staff. Fortunately, the radiation dose to which the attending medical staff and the accident victim are likely to be exposed from an accident at a normally operating nuclear power plant are not likely to be significant. The only exception would be a worker who is injured and has a highly radioactive metal fragment imbedded in a wound.

(To be used by Emergency Room Clerk to enter available data when a notification is received of the impending admission of a case involving radiation exposure or contamination.)

A. Person making notification:

Name _____ Date _____

Title _____ Affiliation _____

Address _____ Telephone _____

B. Patients to be admitted: Total number _____

Name (if available)	Injury but no radiation or contamination	Radiation Exposure	Internal Contamination	External Contamination	Contaminated wounds
1.					
2.					
3.					
4.					
5.					

C. Will patients be: surveyed for contamination? _____ Decontaminated _____

D. Nature of accident: Type radiation source _____

Other Details _____

_____

_____

E. Person in charge of radiation evalution: _____

F. Expected time of arrival (your hospital): _____

Notification taken by: _____

FIGURE 11.   Radiation incident report form. (From Shleien, B., *Preparedness and Response in Radiation Accidents*, HHS Publ. FDA 83-8211, August 1983, 246.)

The reasons why contamination with radiation is unlikely to be medically significant can be appreciated by considering the potential sources of contamination in a normally operating nuclear power plant. The fuel itself is very radioactive, but it is effectively controlled by the multilevel contaminant described earlier. Purification of the water which is in direct contact with the reactor also helps to maintain low levels of radioactivity. Typical radioactive contaminants of the water in the primary loop are listed in Table 5. The maximum permissible body burden (MPBB) is the maximum amount of a radioisotope to which an individual can be *chronically* exposed without exceeding the occupational exposure limits (5 rem [50 mSv]/year whole-body and major-organ dose). These levels of exposure have no direct measurable biological effect and are considered to be consistent with other risks

TABLE 5
**Major Radionuclides in One Liter of Primary Coolant From a
Pressurized Water Reactor**

	Coolant content μCi	MPBB μCi	Ml to exceed MPBB
^{3}H	400	1000	2,500
^{131}I	100	.07	7
^{134}Cs	.9	30	33,300
^{137}Cs	.9	30	33,300
^{54}Mn	9	20	2,222
^{60}Co	0.5	10	20,000

of employment. From examination of Table 5, it can be readily appreciated that the radiation risk of ingesting primary coolant is small. The major risk is from the ^{131}I. In the example that is given, the MPBB for ^{131}I would be exceeded by ingesting only 7 cc of primary coolant. Massive amounts of coolant would need to be ingested to exceed the MPBB for the other radionuclides.

The MPBB for ^{131}I is very low because radioiodine is highly concentrated in the thyroid gland. Compared to doses of ^{131}I that are *routinely* used to treat an overactive thyroid, the MPBB for ^{131}I is very small. To treat an overactive thyroid, 5 to 10 mCi (185 to 370 MBq) of ^{131}I are administered. The resulting radioactive dose will likely cause hypothyroidism that can be readily treated by administering exogenous thyroid hormone. Inconceivable amounts of primary coolant (50 l) would have to be ingested in order to give the 5 to 10 mCi (185 to 370 MBq) activity which is routinely administered to patients to treat an overactive thyroid.

Other possible sources of contamination in a normally operating nuclear power plant include the spent fuel pool and the water filtration and purification systems. The hazard of the water in the spent fuel pool is similar to the hazards of the activity in the primary coolant. Typical radionuclides found in the radwaste from the water filtration and purification systems and dry compressible waste are listed in Table 6.

The most serious accident in the U.S. involving trauma and contamination was an accident at Millstone at Waterford, Connecticut, in December 1977.[11] A hydrogen gas explosion occurred in the radioactive gas effluent stack. One worker was injured and contaminated when the metal door at the base of the stack was blown off by the blast. The highest dose rates measured at the surface of the individual's clothing was <200 mrem (2 mSv)/h. When the clothes were removed, the dose rates were lowered to 20 mrem (0.2 mSv)/h. The total exposure received by this individual was estimated to be 60 mrem (0.6 mSv) to the whole body and 323 mrem (3.23 mSv) to the skin. The exposure was primarily from the ^{138}Cs (a short half-lived decay product of noble gases; $T_{1/2}$ = 32.2 min). Medical injuries included a mild concussion and multiple skin abrasions. The contaminated areas of the patient required 5 washings. These washings were done over a period of 2 h and 20 min. The maximum dose to the attending medical personnel was 14 mrem. This dose is less than the radiation dose of a chest radiograph and is 1/50th of the radiation dose of many common diagnostic tests (upper gastrointestinal tract series, barium enema, CT scan). Hospital workers (i.e., radiology technologists) are routinely exposed to this level of radiation. For example, patients who are having diagnostic nuclear medicine studies are injected with small amounts of radiotracers to determine how well various organs are functioning. These patients are radioactive for several hours after they are injected. Typically a dose rate of 10 to 20 mrem (0.1 to 0.2 mSv)/h can be measured at a distance of 18 in from these patients. Medical personnel are accustomed to caring for these patients and do not express any undue concern about the risk of their own small radiation exposure.

At Chernobyl, enormous amounts of radioactivity were released from the reactor. The

TABLE 6
Typical Quantities of Radwaste Over a 6-Month Period at a Boiling Water Reactor

I. Spent Resins, Filter Sludges, Evaporator Bottoms, Diatomaceous Earth, Etc.

Nuclide	% of Total	Curies
^{60}Co	32.0	299.0
^{55}Fe	25.4	240.0
^{137}Cs	18.5	175.0
^{51}Cr	6.2	58.01
^{54}Mn	4.4	42.0
^{134}Cs	4.1	39.0
^{58}Co	3.6	34.0
^{89}Sr	2.4	23.0
^{90}Sr	1.5	14.0
^{59}Fe	0.9	8.1
^{65}Zn	0.4	4.0
^{103}Rv	0.4	3.5
^{140}Ba/La	0.3	2.6
^{131}I	0.2	2.1
Total	100	945

II. Dry Compressible Waste, Contaminated Equipment

Nuclide	% of Total	Curies
^{58}Co	46.0	7.0
^{60}Co	35.0	5.5
^{65}Zn	7.8	1.1
^{54}Mn	5.7	0.9
^{59}Fe	2.8	0.4
^{55}Fe	1.7	0.3
^{137}Cs	0.1	0.0
Total	100	15.0

firemen were externally and internally contaminated. Despite the severity of the accident, dose rates of only a few R/h were detected once the patients reached the hospital. The largest dose that any health care professional was exposed to at the hospital was a few rems (tenths of a Gy).

Since a patient from a nuclear power plant with internal contamination is very likely to be externally contaminated, patients with internal contamination will initially be treated the same as patients with external contamination. The only early clues to internal contamination will be that the activity does not readily decrease with washing and the circumstances of the accident. Early treatment of radioiodine ingestion is particularly important since treatment with stable iodine is very effective at decreasing the radiation dose. Treatment with stable iodine is discussed in detail later in this chapter.

The only event which could conceivably occur at a normally operating nuclear power

TABLE 7
Classification of Postulated Nuclear Power Plant Accidents

Class	Description	Examples
1	Trivial incidents	Small spills and leaks inside the containment
2	Small releases outside the containment	Small spills and leaks outside the containment
3	Radwaste system failures	Equipment leakage or malfunction, release from gas or liquid waste storage tank
4	Fission products to primary system (BWR)	Fuel cladding defects, off-design transients inducing fuel failures
5	Fission products to primary and secondary systems (PWR)	Fuel cladding defects and steam generator leaks, off-design transients, steam generator tube rupture
6	Refueling accidents	Fuel assembly drop, heavy object drop onto fuel in core
7	Spent-fuel handling accident	Fuel assembly drop in storage pool, heavy object drop onto fuel rack, fuel cask drop
8	Accident-initiation events considered in design-basis evaluation in the Safety Analysis Reports	Loss-of-coolant accidents (small and large), control rod ejection (PWR) or drop (BWR), steam line breaks (BWR), outside containment (PWR)
9	Hypothetical sequence of successive failures more severe than those postulated for establishing the design basis	

plant that may result in a significant radiation exposure to attending medical personnel would be an accident involving a metal fragment. As indicated previously, these fragments can be highly radioactive. The actual dose rate from the fragment, its size and location, its mechanical effect on the patient, and the patient's other injuries will affect the decision as to how rapidly the fragment should be removed. In general, rapid removal of the fragment, using long forceps to minimize the dose to the physician's hand, is desired. The fragment should temporarily be disposed of in a well-shielded container.

In summary, except for the rare instance of an embedded highly radioactive metal fragment, radiation contamination will play only a nuisance role in an accident at a normally operating nuclear power plant. Hospitals serving nuclear power plants must be prepared for major trauma which can and does occur at these large industrial facilities.

VI. POTENTIAL ACCIDENTS AT A MALFUNCTIONING NUCLEAR POWER PLANT

Because of the enormous radionuclide inventory of nuclear power plants, concern for the radiation aspects escalate greatly when there is a plant malfunction. Malfunctions can be trivial and have no effect on the overall operation and safety of the nuclear power plant, or they can be catastrophic and result in the release of enormous amounts of radioactivity. A listing of potential radiation accidents at nuclear power plants have been developed (Table 7).[12] Class 8 and 9 accidents have the potential for releasing large amounts of radioactivity into the environment.

Three Mile Island, Chernobyl, and Hollywood have combined to teach all of us about the dangers of Class 8 and 9 accidents. The dramatic Hollywood-style accident has been dubbed "the China Syndrome". In this accident the reactor goes supercritical. The increased output of power causes the reactor to explode. The explosion is due to extraordinary steam pressure as opposed to an actual nuclear explosion. (A nuclear explosion can only occur with uranium which has been enriched to greater than 90% ^{235}U. As mentioned before, reactor fuel contains about 3% ^{235}U.) The intense heat of the uncontrolled reaction will cause the fuel rod assemblies to melt. The carefully thought-out controllable geometry of the

TABLE 8
Possible Initiating Events for Major
Accidents at Nuclear Power Plants

Internal
   Loss of control of the reactor
      Human error
      Station blackout
      Fire
   Loss of coolant
External
      Earthquakes/tornadoes
      Terrorist
      Airplane crashes

reactor is lost and, under the worst possible conditions imaginable, a self-sustained intense, uncontrolled nuclear reaction results.

The molten fuel melts through the floor of the reactor vessel. When the intense heat from the uncontrolled reaction comes into contact with the earth's water, further steam explosions occur, spewing radioactive debris to the surface. According to the the Hollywood version, this out-of-control reactor disaster continues as the reactor burrows to the center of the earth. How it continues on to China has never been made clear.

Three Mile Island and Chernobyl have taught us that accidents at nuclear power plants can and will occur. Hopefully they have also taught us how to make nuclear power plants safer. From the beginning, attempts to identify the possible events that might initiate a major accident at a nuclear power plant have been made (Table 8). Once the possible initiating events are identified, efforts to avoid their occurrence are undertaken.

Prior to Three Mile Island, loss of control of the reactor due to human error was considered less likely than loss of control due to equipment failure. Since Three Mile Island, it has been recognized that avoiding human error is an extremely important factor in maintaining the safe operation of a nuclear power plant. At Three Mile Island, the plant operators became confused by the bewildering sequence of events. Through a series of blunders, safety systems which had automatically been invoked and would have prevented damage to the reactor core were mistakenly turned off. Three Mile Island taught us that operators need more training and that the presentation of the important complex data at the time of an accident has to be simplified.

Despite these lessons about human error, a second, more devastating accident occurred at Chernobyl. The primary cause of this accident again was human error. Numerous safety systems were turned off to conduct a test prior to routine shutdown of the reactor. In this case, the operators apparently did not know that they were operating the reactor in a very unsafe manner.

Equipment failures that should be considered as possible initiating events for major accident include station blackout, fire, and a loss of coolant accident (LOCA). A station blackout occurs when all the electrical power to the nuclear power plant is lost. Total loss of electricity would mean loss of control of the reactor. Although the control rods for the reactor can be inserted by gravity, electricity is needed for pumps to provide the necessary coolant to remove the residual heat from the reactor following shutdown. To deal with this eventuality, nuclear power plants have redundant diesel-powered emergency generators on site. There have been several instances of station blackout that have required use of these backup generators.

Fire also has the potential to cause loss of control of the reactor. An often-cited accident in Brown's Ferry, Alabama, occurred when a fire threatened to burn through the electrical wires which connected the reactor control center with the reactor. Had the fire burned through the wiring, all of the redundant safety systems would have become inoperative. Because of this accident, reactors are now equipped with duplicate, spatially separate wiring for critical system components.

A LOCA is thought to be the most likely cause of a major nuclear accident. If there is a complete break in one of the large pipes of the primary loop of a light water reactor, enormous quantities of coolant can be lost in a very short period of time. To prevent disastrous consequences of a major loss of coolant, three things must be assured. First, the reactor must be immediately scrammed by fully inserting the control rods. Second, enough water from a secondary source must be available to keep the reactor covered. Third, a mechanism to continue to pump coolant through the reactor must exist.

In the case of a LOCA, the reactor should be automatically scrammed because of the transients (abnormal pressure, temperature, and flow) that a major LOCA would cause. Because it is very important to shut off the reactor quickly, there is great concern when there is an "Anticipated Transient Without Scram" (ATWS). ATWS are considered to be a very serious malfunction and they are carefully investigated by the nuclear industry and the regulatory bodies. The potentially serious consequences of an ATWS can be readily avoided by manually scramming the reactor. A prompt manual scram requires a very vigilant well-trained reactor operator.

In order to keep the reactor covered with coolant during a LOCA, large quantities of water are always available to be added into the primary loop by the emergency core cooling (ECC) system. This system has to work not only at the normal operating temperatures and pressures of the reactor, but also at the extraordinarily high temperatures and pressures that may occur during an accident. High-speed injections of large amounts of water into a super-heated, high-pressure system create many technical problems that must be overcome.

The ECC not only provides the water to keep the reactor cooled but the capability to circulate the water to provide continued cooling of the reactor to remove the residual decay heat once it has been shut down. The break in the primary loop must be isolated and alternative routing of the coolant must be provided.

Less severe LOCAs can occur when one or more tubes in the primary loop of the steam generator ruptures. The most publicized accident of this type occurred on January 25, 1982, at the Robert E. Ginna nuclear power plant in upstate New York.[13] Rupture of a tube in the steam generator resulted in the loss of 700 gal/min of primary coolant into the secondary loop. The ECC is designed to cope with water losses of a much greater magnitude.

The major problem after an initiating event occurs is quickly understanding what went wrong and how to fix it. An abnormal reading in the reactor control center may be due to a true event or a malfunction of the monitoring equipment. The emergency systems are used infrequently; therefore, they must be constantly tested to be certain that they will work when needed. In addition, operators need to be well trained in using systems which they hope they will never have to use.

In addition to equipment failures, other external events must be considered as potential initiating events for a major accident at a nuclear power plant. External events include tornadoes, hurricanes, explosions (from terrorist activities or during a war), and airplane crashes. Several nuclear power plants have been built where there is the potential for severe earthquakes (Figure 12). These plants have been specially designed to withstand severe earthquakes. The containment building itself serves two purposes. First, it serves as the final barrier to prevent the escape of radioactivity. Second, it serves as a barrier to protect the reactor from external forces (weather, explosions, and airplane crashes). The containment building is made of steel liner surrounded by reinforced concrete that is several feet thick (Figure 13). Security at nuclear power plants is tight to prevent the plant from being sabotaged from within.

When all is said and done, accidents in both normally functioning plants and malfunc-

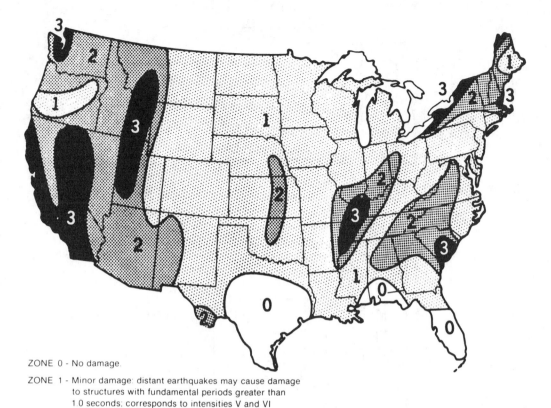

ZONE 0 - No damage.

ZONE 1 - Minor damage: distant earthquakes may cause damage
to structures with fundamental periods greater than
1.0 seconds; corresponds to intensities V and VI
of the M.M.° Scale.

ZONE 2 - Moderate damage: corresponds to intensity VII of the M.M.° Scale.

ZONE 3 - Major damage: corresponds to intensity VIII and higher of the M.M.° Scale.

FIGURE 12.   Seismic risk map of the United States. (From United States Earthquake, 1968, U.S. Coast, Geodetic Survey, U.S. Department of Commerce, 1960.)

tioning plants occur, despite all of the steps that are taken to prevent them. A small increase in the risk of death accompanies most human activities (Table 9). In the U.S., there have been no deaths directly attributed to radiation exposure from a commercial nuclear power plant. The deaths which have occured are largely due to thermal burns. This sort of death (steam burns) is just as likely to occur at a conventional fossil fuel-burning power plant as a nuclear power plant. Despite Chernobyl and Three Mile Island, many still believe that there are fewer deaths per KW of electricity produced by nuclear power than by fossil fuel-burning plants. Death from fossil fuel-burning plants may be due to mining, air pollution, and ultimately the greenhouse effect.

The types of injuries for which health professionals should prepare at a malfunctioning nuclear power plant are generally the same as one would expect at a normally functioning plant (burns, crush injuries, fractures, and electrocution). At Three Mile Island, there were no acute injuries, despite the fact that 70% of the core was damaged. Damage to the core greatly increases the chances of significant radiation exposure and contamination. At Three Mile Island, a large amount of the radionuclide inventory was released from the core and distributed throughout the entire primary loop. A considerable amount of activity was released into the containment building. Some areas of the plant had exposure rates of over 1,000 R/h. Relatively small amounts of activity were released into the environment; therefore, physical damage to the public was negligible.

The emergency action levels that have been agreed to by the NRC and the Federal

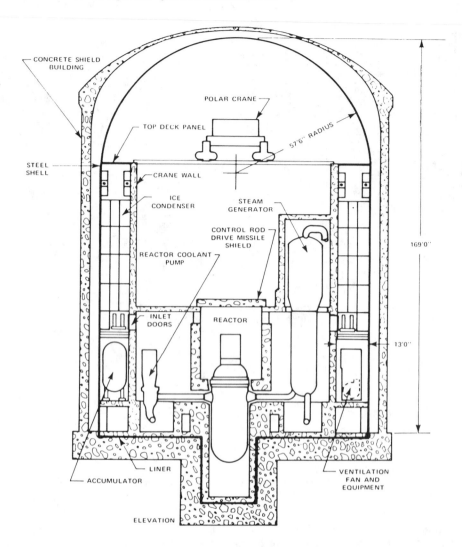

FIGURE 13. Containment building. The containment building is composed of a concrete shell which is several feet thick in places with an inner steel shell. In addition, the reactor vessel itself is enclosed in concrete. This is a design by Westinghouse Electric Corp. (From Westinghouse, reprinted in Nero, A. V., *A Guidebook to Nuclear Reactors*, University of California Press, Berkeley, 1979, 87. With permission.)

Energy Management Agency provide a readily available indication of the level of concern for potential hazard to the public in the event of an accident at a nuclear power plant (Table 10). The Environmental Protection Agency (EPA) protective action guides (PAGs) (Table 11) consider the maximum projected whole-body and thyroid exposures.[14] Calculating the projected maximum doses to the public, given the uncertainty and confusion that acutely accompanies an accident, is very difficult, therefore, the threshold for escalating the emergency action level is low. Declaration of an emergency action level automatically invokes a complex chain of events. Detailed description of the appropriate response has been published elsewhere.[15]

Prior to Chernobyl, it was assumed that there would be a time lag from the time that an accident occurred at a nuclear power plant to the time that there was a release of significant amounts of radioactivity. In the reactor safety study[16] it was assumed that 2 to 30 h would be required before significant melting of the core would occur following a major malfunction.

TABLE 9
Everyday Risks

Activity	Deaths/year (Estimate)	Activity	Deaths/year (Estimate)
1. Smoking	150,000	13. Bicycles	1,000
2. Alcoholic beverages	100,000	14. Hunting	400
3. Motor vehicles	50,000	15. Home appliances	200
4. Handguns	17,000	16. Fire fighting	195
5. Electric power	14,000	17. Police work	160
6. Motorcycles	3,000	18. Contraceptives	150
7. Swimming	3,000	19. Commercial aviation	150
8. Surgery	2,800	20. Nuclear power	100
9. X-rays	2,300	21. Mountain climbing	30
10. Railroads	1,950	22. Power mowers	24
11. General aviation	1,300	23. School football	23
12. Large construction	1,000	24. Skiing	18

Adapted from Mettler, F. A. and Moseley, R. D., *Medical Effects of Ionizing Radiation*, Grune & Stratton, Orlando, FL, 1985, 253.

TABLE 10
Emergency Action Levels of Nuclear Power Facilities

Emergency action class	Level of plant function	Potential releases of radioactivity	Immediate Action
Unusual event	Potential degradation of level of plant safety	No release	Bring operating staff to readiness—provide systematic handling of information and decision-making
Alert	Actual or potential substantial degradation of level of plant safety	Small fraction of EPA PAGs[a]	Assure emergency personnel are ready to respond. Provide offsite authorities with current status
Site area emergency	Actual or likely major failures in plant function	Releases not expected to exceed EPA PAGs	Fully mobilize emergency personnel in nearsite environs. Dispatch onsite and offsite monitoring and communications teams
General emergency	Actual or imminent substantial core degradation or melt	Releases reasonably expected to exceed EPA PAGs offsite	Sheltering until assessment whether or not evacuation indicated and feasible

[a] EPA PAGs: Environmental Protection Agency's Protective Action Guidelines (see Table 11).

Emergency planners would have a few hours to warn and potentially evacuate the public. In Chernobyl, the initial event was a supercritical excursion that blew the reactor apart with a massive steam explosion. Enormous amounts of radioactivity were released immediately. Controversy exists as to whether or not the immediate release of radioactivity could occur with light water reactors such as those used in the U.S.[17] Unlike Chernobyl's graphite-moderated reactor, light water reactors have a containment building that is designed to withstand a sizable reactor explosion. Light water reactors also have a safety feature that is

TABLE 11
EPA Protective Action Guidelines

Population at risk	Projected whole-body gamma dose (rem)	Projected thyroid dose (rem)
General population	1—5[a]	5—25[a]
Emergency workers	25	125
Lifesaving activities	75	—[b]

[a] When ranges are shown, the lowest value should be used if there are no major local constraints in providing protection at that level, especially to sensitive populations. Local constraints may make lower values impractical to use, but in no case should the higher value be exceeded in determining the need for protective action.

[b] No specific upper limit is given for thyroid exposure since, in the extreme case, complete thyroid loss might be an acceptable penalty for a life saved. However, this should not be necessary if respirators and/or thyroid protection for rescue personnel are available as the result of adequate planning.

intrinsic to their design. Whereas graphite reactors increase the rate of fission as the temperature rises (positive feedback), light water reactors decrease their fission rate as the temperature rises (negative feedback). For this reason, it is thought that a light water reactor cannot explode and release large amounts of radioactivity without any warning. If there were a major accident that had the potential for releasing large amounts of radioactivity, the hospital's role would change little from its role in a radiation accident of lesser magnitude. The hospital's major concern will still be the treatment of major life-threatening trauma. The radiation aspect of the accident requires no complicated acute intervention. Risk to the hospital staff from radiation may increase, but hospital workers will always have a tremendous advantage over rescuers who are working on-site.

During a major accident, health care may be complicated by at least three factors. First, the designated support hospital may be evacuated if it is located within the evacuation zone (usually a ten-mile radius around the plant). Second, a major accident may result in a large number of casualties. Nearly 250 individuals required hospitalization following the Chernobyl accident. Obviously an accident that involves this many injuries requires rapid stabilization and triaging of patients to other medical centers. Third, the public will naturally turn to hospitals for advice regarding their radiation exposure and possible contamination. Some mechanism to rapidly refer these patients to other facilities must be established. The hospital must use their scant resources to care for the seriously injured. If decontamination on a large scale is necessary, it is best performed by nonhospital personnel at some other public facility (schools, etc.).

The public's concern about the safety of nuclear reactors is largely due to the very small possibility of a very large accident involving the massive release of radioactivity. Rasmussen has suggested that a nuclear accident leading to 3,300 early fatalities and some 45,000 cancers over a 40-year period following the release has a probability of occurence of 1 in a billion per reactor per year.[16] In order to put this probability into perspective, the probability of 3,000 deaths due to a large airplane crashing into a full sports stadium is estimated to be 1/10,000 per year in the U.S. These numbers lead to the conclusion that it is 1000 times more likely that an airplane crash will cause acute deaths of the same magnitude as the worst imaginable reactor accident.

The release of any amount of radioactivity by a nuclear power plant is of great concern to the public. Malfunctions of nuclear reactors resulting in releases of radioactivity have occurred in the past and will undoubtedly occur in the future. The potential health consequences of the release of radioactivity vary for each radionuclide. The health consequences are affected by the physical half-life of the radionuclide, its decay scheme, its chemical and physical form, and its behavior in biological systems.

TABLE 12
Accident Releases of ^{131}I to the Environment from Nuclear Facilities

Accident	Year	Amount of ^{131}I (Ci)	Maximum offsite dose to thyroid (rems)
Windscale	1957	20,000	16
SL-1	1961	80	.035
Hanford	1963	60	.03
Savannah River	1964	153	1.2
Three Mile Island	1979	20	0.005
Chernobyl	1986	7,300,000	250

Krypton and xenon are noble gases. The primary health concern following release of these gases into the environment is external exposure. Neither gas is very soluble, so internal contamination from absorption through the lungs is minimal. Multiple krypton radionuclides are produced (Table 2). All krypton radionuclides have half-lives of 3 h or less, except for ^{85}Kr, which has a half-life of 10.76 years. Xenon's radionuclides also are short-lived ($T_{1/2}$ <12 d). The short half-life of the noble gases and the enormous dilutional effect of the atmosphere make contamination of environment with the noble gases a short-term biological concern.

Iodine is also highly volatile and is likely to be released along with the noble gases. Iodine has received a great deal of attention for several reasons. First, it is present in reactors in great quantities. Second, its volatility makes release into environment during an accident likely. Third, iodine is concentrated in our food chain (especially milk) and in our bodies, resulting in a potentially large dose to the thyroid. Fourth, effective treatment for internal contamination exists. It is difficult to put the enormous quantities of radioiodine in a reactor into perspective. ^{131}I is used in the treatment of thyroid cancer and other thyroid diseases. A dose of 100 mCi (3700 MBq) of ^{131}I will deliver a dose of 50,000 to 100,000 rem (500 to 1000 Sv) to the thyroid gland, resulting in complete destruction of the normal gland. Despite the enormous dose to the thyroid, the dose to the rest of the body is only 50 rem (0.5 Sv). The approximately 70,000 Ci of ^{131}I in an operating 1000 MW reactor is enough ^{131}I for 70 million 100-mCi (3700 MBq) ablative doses of ^{131}I. These 70,000 Ci of ^{131}I are only a fraction of the radioiodine inventory (since ^{129}I through ^{136}I are also present). These facts have created healthy concerns over the potential effects of accidental iodine releases. Fortunately a number of other factors help to decrease the potential disastrous effects of an accidental radioiodine release. First, the amount of radioiodine which has been released in previous accidents is less than what would have been predicted. There is now evidence that iodine combines with other substances (e.g., cesium) at the high temperature of a malfunctioning reactor, making the iodine considerably less volatile. The percentage of the radioiodine inventory released at Three Mile Island was very small (Table 12). In the Chernobyl accident, only 20% of the radioiodines were released, despite the fact that 100% of the noble gases were released.[17] In addition, it is important to remember that only a fraction of the radioiodine released will end up in humans. Human contamination will be from inhalation and the ingestion of contaminated food and water.

The Food and Drug Administration (FDA) protective action level for iodine contamination is 25 rem (0.25 Sv) to the thyroid gland. It has been recommended that governments intervene in any situation that would potentially result in this exposure to the general population. No meaningful analysis of the cost/benefit ratio of this recommendation has been performed for small and large releases of radioiodine. It is likely that the cost/benefit ratio of this recommendation varies with the circumstances surrounding the iodine release. In any case, the 25 rem (0.25 Sv) protective action level is quite conservative. The American

Thyroid Association suggests that a level of 100 rem (1 Sv) be used as the threshold for initiating intervention. The dose to the thyroid gland from a routine diagnostic ^{131}I thyroid scan (100 μCi administered to the patient by mouth) is 80 to 100 rem (0.8 to 1.0 Sv). Use of ^{131}I for diagnostic scans is now discouraged because other radioiodines (^{123}I) have better physical characteristics and deliver one tenth the radiation dose.

Long-term followup studies in patients who have had diagnostic ^{131}I scans have not revealed an increased incidence of thyroid cancer.[18] Increased incidences of thyroid cancer have been noted in patients who have received external radiation therapy to the head and neck. It has been estimated that 400 to 500 rad (4 to 5 Gy) of radiation is necessary to be carcinogenic in the thyroid. Because of its distribution in the thyroid and its mechanism of decay, it has been estimated by some that ^{131}I is 1/30 as carcinogenic as X-rays.[19] Cancer induction following exposure to radioiodine has been reported in the Marshall Islanders, who were accidentally caught in nuclear fallout following a test explosion in the Bikini Atolls.[20] It has been estimated that the islanders received 28 to 580 rad (0.28 to 5.8 Gy) to their thyroids from ^{131}I and 5 to 9 times more of a dose was received from the short half-life iodine radionuclides, giving a total dose of 280 to 5,000 rads (2.8 to 50 Gy) to their thyroid. In addition, the islanders were exposed to an average of 150 rad (1.5 Gy) of external radiation. These values compare to the 5000 to 10,000 rad (50 to 100 Gy) dose to the thyroid, which is commonly administered for *treatment* of hyperthyroidism with [131]I. The most recent evaluation of the 251 islanders who were exposed shows that 2 developed thyroid atrophy, 46 (18%) developed thyroid nodules, and 8 (3%) developed thyroid cancer. The expected number of benign thyroid nodules would be 6.3% and the expected number of thyroid cancer would be 0.7%. No thyroid atrophy would be expected to occur spontaneously.

The carcinogenic effect of the radioiodine ingestion by the Marshall Islanders is in conflict with long-term followup studies in patients *treated* with ^{131}I for hyperthyroidism.[18] The differences may be due to some synergistic effects of the short half-life of radioiodine and the external radiation. Fortunately, thyroid cancer, benign nodules, and hypothyroidism induced by radioiodine can be treated quite effectively. These abnormalities take many years to develop (10 to 20 years minimum).

A number of different protective actions are possible when the environment is acutely contaminated by radioiodine. First, the population can be kept inside buildings with their windows closed. Second, the population can be evacuated. Third, stable iodine can be given to prevent uptake of radioiodine by the thyroid gland. Fourth, food and water can be carefully monitored to prevent ingestion of contaminated materials. Which actions should be taken and when they should be taken are controversial.[21-24]

In the setting of an acute accident, decision-making can become more difficult. If a brief release of radioactivity has occurred, the dose to the population may be minimized if they are kept indoors with windows closed as the cloud of radioactivity passes over. Evacuating the population at this point may increase their exposure, since it will require that they go outdoors. If necessary, evacuation could occur after the radioactive plume has passed. The difficulty with this approach is that future events may be unpredictable during an accident at a nuclear reactor. If the releases continue, evacuation of the population may be the wisest action.

The role which administration of stable iodine should play is unclear. If exposure to radioiodine is prevented by evacuation and screening the food supply, stable iodine may not be needed. The logistics of administering stable iodine in a severely contaminated environment may be insurmountable. The wisdom of distributing stable iodine in a controlled setting where contamination is minimal and food and water supplies can be monitored can be questioned. Fortunately, small quantities of radioiodine can be easily detected in food; therefore, screening the food supply is possible. The economic implications of screening food supplies can be lessened, since contaminated food can be redirected to processes which require time. For example, it may be possible to salvage milk contaminated with ^{131}I by using it to make cheese. The 8-d half-life of ^{131}I means that much less radioiodine will be in the cheese after several weeks of processing and curing. The decision to administer stable iodine is often a political one. Distribution of iodine is sometimes undertaken to allay the public's great anxiety regarding radiation. During the Chernobyl accident, the psychological and political benefits of stable iodine distribution outside the U.S.S.R. were often more apparent than were the medical benefits.

Tritium is another radionuclide of potential concern. By far, the most common chemical form of tritium in a nuclear reactor is water. The potential biological hazard due to tritium is minimal due to several factors. First, the amount of tritium in a nuclear reactor is, comparatively speaking, small. Second, since water is present in such great quantities on earth and in living organisms the dilution factors are great. Finally the *biological* half-life of tritium in an organism is short (10 to 12 d); therefore, the radiation dose due to internal contamination rapidly decreases if further ingestion is prevented.

[137]Cs is the radionuclide that is likely to be of greatest long-term biological importance in a catastrophic accident that results in a massive release of fission products. Cesium gains its biological importance from its biological and physical properties. Biologically it is a potassium analog. When ingested, it is rapidly and nearly completely absorbed. Once absorbed, its biological half-life in the body is relatively long, about 100 d. Like potassium, cesium is widely distributed in the body, especially in the muscles. Physically, cesium is volatile, so significant amounts of activity are likely to be released into the environment in a catastrophic reactor accident. The physical half-life of ^{137}Cs is the longest of all the cesium radionuclides (30 years); therefore, it will remain a concern for many decades. Of all the radionuclides in the reactor, cesium is most likely to be responsible for the greatest whole-body dose to the population. In some ecosystems (e.g., Lapland), cesium is concentrated by plants (e.g., lichen) and animals (e.g., reindeer), resulting in a human dose that is several orders of magnitude higher than would otherwise be expected. Since ^{137}Cs is a high-energy gamma emitter, a significant amount of the population dose is from external irradiation.

[90]Sr is the last of the radionuclides in a nuclear power plant that is likely to have significant long-term biological sequelae when released into the environment in large quantities. Since strontium is nonvolatile it is much less likely to escape from a reactor. Approximately 25 to 30% of inhaled or ingested strontium is absorbed. Since it is a calcium analog, half of the absorbed strontium (10% of the ingested strontium) accumulates in bone. Once in bone, strontium remains there with a biological half-life of several years. The accumulation in bone results in a potentially high dose to the bone and bone marrow. Production of bone tumors and leukemias are the primary concern. Since strontium is a beta emitter, it is primarily an internal hazard.

The remaining radionuclides in the enormous inventory of a nuclear reactor are unlikely to play a significant role in the biological consequences of a nuclear reactor accident. Their biological impotence is due to three possible factors. First, radionuclides with short physical half-lives (<1 d) are of less significance since they rapidly disappear from the environment. Second, radionuclides that are nonvolatile are less likely to be released in significant quantities. Third, many radionuclides are in a chemical form which is poorly soluble and/or they do not enter into biological systems.

V. SUMMARY

In summary, with almost 300 nuclear power plants operating worldwide, the safety of nuclear power will soon be better known. The consequences of the two widely publicized major reactor accidents at Three Mile Island and Chernobyl will be discussed in the next chapter. Over the next decade we will learn whether or not the lessons learned from these accidents have made nuclear power safer. In the meantime, we must be well prepared to take care of patients injured in accidents at normally operating and at malfunctioning power plants. It would be tragic if lack of preparation and /or fear of radiation resulted in mistreatment of patients. It is hoped the information presented in this chapter will help health care professionals better care for patients of radiation accidents that occur at nuclear power plants.

REFERENCES

1. World list of nuclear power plants, *Nuclear News,* 30, 61, 1987.
2. Nuclear Safety Review for 1985, International Atomic Energy Agency, Vienna, 1986.
3. **Nero, A. V.,** *A Guidebook to Nuclear Reactors,* University of California Press, Berkeley, 1979, 260.
4. **Ford, D.,** *Cult of the Atom,* Simon and Schuster, 1981, 28.
5. Report to Congress of Abnormal Occurrences, NUREG-0090 Vol 9, No. 4, 1987, 7.
6. Faulty reading leads to 21-rem exposure, *Nuclear News,* April 1981.
7. Report to Congress of Abnormal Occurrences, NUREG-0090, Vol 1, No. 2, 1978, 3.
8. **Barlotta, F. M.,** The New Jersey Radiation Accidents of 1974 and 1977, in *The Medical Basis of Radiation Accident Preparedness,* Hubner, K. F. and Fry, S. A., Eds., Elsevier/North Holland, New York, 1980, 151.
9. **Parmentier, N. C., Nenot, J. C., and Jammet, H. J.,** A Dosimetric Study of the Belgian (1965) and Italian (1975) Accidents, in *The Medical Basis of Radiation Accident Preparedness,* Hubner, K. F. and Fry, S. A., Eds., Elsevier/North Holland, New York, 1980, 105.
10. **Shleien, B.,** Preparedness and Response in Radiation Accidents, HHS Publ. FDA 83-8211, August 1983, 246.
11. NRC Licensee Event Report from Millstone Nuclear Power Station, December 27, 1977.
12. **Glasstone, S. and Jordan, W. H.,** *Nuclear Power and Its Environmental Effects,* American Nuclear Society, La Grange Park, IL, 1980.
13. Generator Tube Rupture at R.E. Ginna Nuclear Power Plant, NUREG-0909, 1982, Nuclear Regulatory Commission, April 1982.
14. Manual of Protective Action Guides and Protective Actions for Nuclear Events, EPA 520/1-75-001, U.S. Environmental Protection Agency, Washington, D.C., September 1975 (Revised June 1980).
15. **Shleien, B.,** Preparedness and Response in Radiation Accidents, HHS Publ. FDA 83-8211, Health and Human Services, Washington, D. C., August 1983, 135.
16. Reactor Safety Study, Rasmussen rep., WASH 1400 (NUREG - 75-014), U.S. Nuclear Regulatory Commission, Washington, D.C., October 1975.
17. Report on the Accident at the Chernobyl Nuclear Power Station, NUREG 1250, Nuclear Regulatory Commission, Washington, D.C., 1987.
18. **Holm, L. E., Dahlquist, I., Israelsson, A.,** et al., Malignant thyroid tumors after iodine-131 therapy. A retrospective study, *N. Engl. J. Med.,* 303, 188, 1980.
19. **Maxon, H. R., Thomas, S. R., Saenger, E. L.,** et al., Ionizing irradiation and the induction of clinically significant diseases of the human thyroid gland, *Am. J. Med.,* 63, 967, 1977.
20. **Lessard, E.,** et al., Thyroid absorbed dose for people at Rongelop, Utirik and Sifo on March 1, 1954, Brookhaven National Lab, BNL 51882, UC48, March 1985.
21. **Becker, D. V.,** Physiological basis for the use of potassium iodide as a thyroid blocking agent: logistical issues in its distribution, *Bull. N.Y. Acad. Med.,* 59, 1003, 1983.
22. **Shleien, B.,** Recommendations of the use of potassium iodide as a thyroid-blocking agent in radiation accidents: an FDA update, *Bull. N.Y. Acad. Med.,* 59, 1009, 1983.
23. **Yalow, R. S.,** Risks in mass distribution of potassium iodide, *Bull. N.Y. Acad. Med.,* 59, 1020, 1983.
24. **Robbins, J.,** Implications for using potassium iodide to protect the thyroid from low level internal irradiation, *Bull. N.Y. Acad. Med.,* 59, 1028, 1983.

Chapter 17

THE THREE MILE ISLAND AND CHERNOBYL REACTOR ACCIDENTS

Henry D. Royal

TABLE OF CONTENTS

I. THREE MILE ISLAND

A. HOW THE ACCIDENT HAPPENED

The accident at Three Mile Island occurred at 4 a.m. on March 28, 1979.[1-5]At that time, the Three Mile Island reactor unit II was operating at 97% of its maximum power. Three problems which contributed to the accident began days to hours before 4 a.m. First, there had been a persistent slow leak of reactor coolant from the pressurizer. The pressurizer (Figure 1, Containment Building) is a large vessel filled with steam and water. Pressure in the reactor vessel can be more easily regulated with this cushion of compressible steam. The leaking coolant emptied into the reactor coolant drain tank. Because the leak was small, the operators had no difficulty maintaining normal water levels in the pressurizer and normal pressure in the reactor. They had calculated that the leak was below the limits specified by the Nuclear Regulatory Commission (NRC) that would have required that they take immediate remedial action. In reality, the leak actually exceeded the NRC limits, although the exact size of the leak played no significant role in the accident.

The leak of reactor coolant was thought to be occurring either through the electromatic relief valve or through the pressurizer safety valves. These valves are designed to relieve any abnormally high pressure that develops in the reactor. They automatically open when a preset high pressure is exceeded in the reactor coolant system. The electromatic relief valve was designed to open at a lower pressure than do the safety valves. The leakage ultimately contributed to misleading the reactor operators to believing that there was not a serious leak of coolant.

The second problem which may have contributed to the accident was that the block valves on the pipes which carried auxiliary feed water to the steam generator (Figure 1, Turbine Building) had inadvertently been left closed when it was serviced two days prior to the accident. The third problem, which the reactor operators were busily attempting to repair, occurred 11 hours prior to the accident. In the process of transfer of resins from the demineralizer (Figure 1, Turbine Building) to the resin regeneration tank (not shown in the figure), a blockage in the transfer line developed. During the process of trying to clear this blockage, water backed into the condensate pumps. This caused the condensate pumps to fail and the accident at Three Mile Island began in earnest.

Without the condensate pump, the water, returning from the turbine back to the steam generator via the main feed water pump, was no longer cooled by the condenser and thus the temperature increased. Within one second of the condensate flow stoppage, the main feed water pumps to the steam generator stopped as designed. Almost simultaneously the main turbine tripped. For the time being no water was flowing through the secondary loop of the reactor. The secondary loop is the main way that the heat generated from the reactor is normally removed from the reactor. The plant is designed to be able to continue to remove heat via the secondary loop by initiating flow through the auxiliary feed water to the steam generator. This water is already cooled since it comes from the condensate storage tank. At Three Mile Island the three auxiliary feed water pumps started up by design and by 14 s after the loss of the main feed water they had reached full pressure. Unfortunately, because the valve between the auxiliary feed water pumps and the steam generator (see above) had been left closed, this means of providing heat removal was inoperative. After 8 min of not providing any heat removal from the reactor, the operators discovered that the auxiliary feed water valves were in the wrong position and they opened these valves. Part of the delay in recognizing that the auxiliary feed water valves were closed has been blamed on the fact that routine maintenance tags were hanging on the control panel blocking the auxiliary feed water valve position indicators. The significance of the 8-min delay in providing feed water to the secondary loop is controversial.

The lack of heat removal by the secondary loop caused the temperature and pressure of

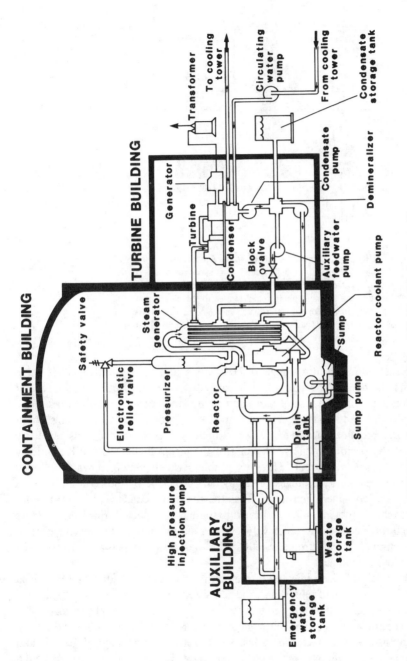

FIGURE 1.   Schematic of the Three Mile Island Nuclear Power Plant.

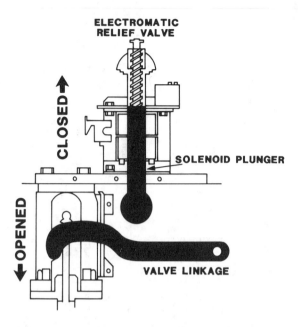

FIGURE 2.   Schematic of the electromatic release valve. Loss of coolant from the Three Mile Island reactor occurred because the valve in valve linkage remained in the open position, despite the fact that the solenoid plunger had moved to the closed position. The light in the control room which indicated that the valve had closed as expected showed the position of the solenoid plunger rather than directly detecting the position of the valve linkage.

the reactor to increase which in turn triggered the opening of the electromatic relief valve some 3 to 6 s after the condensate pump had failed. At 8 s into the accident, the reactor scrammed, due to the fact that the reactor pressure had increased beyond preset limits. With the control rods fully inserted into the reactor, the nuclear reaction ended within one second. Heat was continually produced however, at approximately 7% of the previous level, by continued decay of the fission products. Opening of the electromatic relief valve quickly brought the pressures back to normal. The only problem which remained was continued heat removal from the reactor to dissipate the decay heat produced by the fission products.

Initially things seemed under control. At 13 s after the initial condensate pump failure, the pressure in the reactor coolant system returned to normal as expected, due to the release of pressure through the electromatic relief valve. When the pressure in the reactor coolant system returned to normal, the electromatic relief valve was designed to automatically close preventing further loss of coolant.

Closure of the relief valve is indicated in the control room by an indicator light. That light indicated that the valve had closed as expected when the reactor returned to normal pressure. Because the indicator light showed that the valve was closed, the operators assumed that there was no significant loss of coolant from the reactor. It took a long time to dissuade the operators from this belief. In fact, the indicator light sensed the position of the solenoid switch which operated the valve but not the position of the valve itself (Figure 2). Although the indicator light indicated that the valve was closed, the valve was stuck in an open position and loss of coolant was continuing at a rapid rate. If the operators had recognized that the valve was stuck in its open position they could have manually closed the valve and totally prevented subsequent damage to the reactor core.

There were other clues that could have tipped off the operators that the relief valve had not closed. For example, instruments in the control room monitored the temperature of the pipes leading from the stuck open valve to the drain tank. An abnormally high temperature would indicate that hot coolant was still escaping from the reactor. The operators did check the temperature in these pipes; however, they thought that the high temperature was due to the continued slight valve leakage of which they were aware before the accident. An additional method for monitoring flow to the drain tank was a pressure indicator of the drain tank. Unfortunately this indicator was on a panel behind the approximately 7-ft-high primary control panel on which all critical instruments were placed. The operators did not check this pressure indicator.

As the reactor coolant pressure dropped, due to the open electromatic relief valve, the high pressure injection emergency pumps that add water to the primary coolant system were automatically tripped at 4.5 min into the accident. The operators believed that a loss of coolant accident was not possible since they thought the relief valve had closed and the water level in the pressurizer was high. For these reasons, they manually turned off the emergency core cooling system. The operators believed that the high water level in the pressurizer meant that there was plenty of coolant in the reactor. In fact, the high water level indicated that steam and then water was escaping through the still open electromatic relief valve.

At approximately 3 min into the accident, the relief valve on the reactor coolant drain tank lifted and reactor coolant began to accumulate in the reactor sump pump area. The sump pump began to pump 140 gal/min of minimally radioactive coolant to the waste storage tank in the auxiliary building. This tank had a ruptured pressure relief disk and therefore the radioactive coolant spilled to the floor of the auxiliary building. By 10 min into the accident, a second reactor building sump pump started, increasing the rate of flow to the auxiliary building to 280 gal/min. The second sump pump was automatically turned on because the level of the escaping coolant in the sump area exceeded 4.4 ft.

At this point, the operators continued to be very confused. A cacophony of alarms were sounding throughout the control room involving numerous plant systems. The operators were unable to tell which alarms were real and which were false or what were causes and what were effects. The operators had chosen to believe that the electromatic relief valve had closed as the control panel indicated and that the high water level in the pressurizer confirmed that a loss of coolant accident was not happening.

By 16 min into the accident, the temperature rose sufficiently so that steam voids were forming throughout the system. Additional alarms began to sound as the reactor coolant pumps began to malfunction when they were required to pump steam instead of water. At 18 min into the accident, the reactor building exhaust showed ten-fold increase in the reading of radioactive emissions. These readings were also not located on the front panel, therefore they were obscured from the operators' view. At this point, the primary coolant that was leaking into the reactor and auxiliary buildings was not highly radioactive, since damage to the fuel rods and fuel pellets had not yet occurred.

By 32 min after the beginning of the accident, the core temperature went off scale, although the reactor pressure, reactor coolant temperature, and pressurizer level all remained stable. At 50 min into the accident, the operators called an on-call duty officer and the operating engineer to the site. They were still unsure of what had gone wrong. At 1 h and 11 min into the accident, the temperature in the reactor building had increased so that reactor building cooling was automatically turned on.

Because of the steam voids which were occurring through the system, the reactor coolant flow had been steadily decreasing. The operators were worried that if they continued to operate the pumps with little coolant passing through them that they could ruin a pump seal and induce a large loss of coolant accident. Alarms indicating excessive vibration of the reactor coolant pumps induced them to turn off one set of reactor pumps. At 1 h and 41 min into the accident, severe vibrations due to steam voids continued to occur in the two remaining reactor coolant pumps. The operators decided to trip these two pumps in order to avoid seal failure. The operators believed that natural circulation would adequately cool the reactor if no loss of coolant accident had occurred. In fact, the temperature and pressure of the reactor were well outside the pressure/temperature conditions for establishing natural circulation. At this point, the damage to the reactor had become irreversible.

Two hours after the start of the accident, a conference call was established between the control room operators and officials of the Three Mile Island plant. These officials included the station superintendent, the vice president of generation, and the Babcock and Wilcox site representative. The conferees discussed various possibilities including the fact that the electromatic relief valve might have been open; however, it was reported to be shut. Conferees decided to restart the reactor coolant pumps and all report to the control room. The conference call lasted 38 minutes. At 2 h and 18 min after the accident, the electromatic relief valve was finally noted to be stuck open and it was manually closed.

By 2 h and 38 min after the accident began, radiation monitors revealed a 100-fold increase in the radiation levels in the primary coolant. This rise in radiation levels indicated some damage had occurred to the fuel rods. A reactor coolant pump was restarted 2 h and 54 min the accident. The pump ran for 19 min before it was again shut off because of vibrations. The reactor pressures began increasing dramatically because the electromatic relief valve had been closed

At 2 h and 58 min into the accident, radiation levels of 600 R/h were noted in the primary coolant line and a "site emergency" was declared. The radiation levels rapidly increased. There were 50 to 60 people in the control room attempting to resolve the crisis. At 3 h and 38 min into the accident a "general emergency" was declared. By 4 h and 20 min after the accident, radiation monitors in the containment building recorded 600 R/h. This radiation level rapidly increased to 1000 R/h at 4 h and 40 min into the accident. By 5 h after the initiation of the accident the radiation levels reached 6000 R/h. Despite these very high levels of radiation in the containment building, there was no significant leakage of activity; therefore, off-site evacuation was not considered.

By 6 h after the accident, the airborne radiation levels in the unit 2 control room required the evacuation of all but the essential personnel. Communication in the unit 2 control room was hampered by the use of respirators. Even at this point, with all the consultants, it was thought that the core was still covered with coolant. They were reluctant to start the reactor coolant pumps for fear of a vibration-induced pump seal failure and subsequent loss of coolant. At 7.5 h after the start of the accident, the electromatic relief valve was reopened in an attempt to depressurize the reactor so that coolant flow could be reestablished. Depressurization of the reactor caused more steam formation but allowed for some heat removal via the relief valve.

At 9 h and 50 min after the beginning of the accident, a hydrogen explosion occurred within the containment. Under normal circumstances, hydrogen in the primary loop is beneficial to prevent oxidation; however, under the conditions of the accident hydrogen accumulated in the containment. There was also fear that a hydrogen bubble had formed inside the reactor and that there might be an explosion in the reactor vessel itself. Whether or not there ever was a hydrogen bubble in the reactor remains controversial. The utility insists that even if hydrogen had been present in the reactor vessel that it would not have exploded because there was not sufficient oxygen in the reactor vessel to support an explosion.

Since depressurization of the reactor increased the steam voids, it was not possible to use the reactor coolant pumps. At 13.5 h after the accident it was decided to repressurize the reactor to collapse the existing steam voids so that cooling with the reactor pumps could be attempted. At 15 h and 45 min after the accident the reactor coolant pumps were restarted. Coolant flow to the damaged reactor was finally reestablished and cooldown proceeded relatively uneventfully.

TABLE 1
Release of Radionuclides into the Environment

Radionuclide	TMI[3]	Chernobyl[22]	Atmospheric Testing[7]
^{133}Xe	10	45	—
^{85}Kr	.043	.5	4.3
^{131}I	.00002	7.3	19,000
^{89}Sr	0	2.2	2,432
^{90}Sr	0	.22	16
^{106}Ru	0	1.6	324
^{137}Cs	0	1	25.9
^{144}Ce	0	2.4	810
^{140}Ba	0	4.3	19,000
^{95}Zr	0	3.8	5,395

Note: Table entries are in MCi.

The poor performance of the operators during the Three Mile Island accident is difficult to comprehend in a vacuum. It is clear that their training was inadequate. Providing proper training for a reactor operator is complicated by the fact that very few decisions need to be made during the normal operation of a reactor. It is only when an unusual sequence of events combines to cause unexpected reactor behavior that the operator has to make important decisions. Because this rarely happens, operators have not, in the past, been well trained to meet these emergencies.

In their previous training it had been stressed that the pressurizer should never be allowed to become completely filled with water. A "solid" pressurizer made it much more difficult to maintain a steady pressure in the reactor. When the reactor is operating normally the water level in the pressurizer is a good indicator of the amount of coolant in the primary loop. To avoid a solid pressurizer, they had been taught to cut back on the water added to the reactor coolant system. The high water levels in the pressurizer misled the operators to believe that the primary loop was filled with coolant, when in fact the primary loop was filled with superheated radioactive steam. Their decisions to countermand the automatic safety systems directly resulted in the accident.

B. HEALTH CONSEQUENCES

For the first few days of the Three Mile Island accident there was a great deal of concern regarding the potential health consequences of the accident. Because of lack of administrative preplanning, the decision-making process was not well defined. In addition, accurate information necessary to make a rational decision was not always available.

In the weeks following the accident, a careful assessment of the health impact of the accident was performed.[6] The actual physical harm to the public was judged to be minimal. Only noble gases and a small amount of iodine escaped from containment (Table 1).[7] The noble gases were primarily ^{133}Xe ($T_{1/2}$-5.3 d) and ^{135}Xe ($T_{1/2}$-9.2 h). Ten MCi (3.7×10^{17} Bq) of the estimated 140 MCi (5.2×10^{18} Bq) of ^{133}Xe in the core escaped. Only 10 KCi (3.7×10^{14} Bq) of the estimated 70 MCi (2.6×10^{15} Bq) of ^{131}I in the reactor's core was released to the environment.

The best estimate of the collective dose to the population within a 50-mi radius of the plant was 3300 person rem (33 person Sv) (Table 2). The population within the 50-mi radius was 2 million. The average dose to an individual in this population was <2 mrem (20 μSv). This is comparable to the radiation dose received when flying from New York to Los Angeles round trip. It was estimated that there would be 325,000 naturally occurring cancers in this population and that one additional radiation-induced cancer might occur. The estimates of collective population varied from 1600 person rem to 5300 person rem (16 to 53 person

TABLE 2
Estimated Dose to the Population

	Size affected (Radius in kilometers)	Population	Dose (Person rem)	Average dose (rem)
TMI	80	2×10^6	3300^a	.002
Chernobyl	30	1.35×10^5	1.6×10^{6a}	12
	Worldwide	3×10^9	6×10^7	0.02
Atmospheric testing	Worldwide	3×10^9	3×10^{9a}	1.0
Airplane travel	Worldwide	3×10^9	2.0×10^{5b}	.006
Background radiation	Worldwide	3×10^9	4.5×10^{8c}	.150

[a] Cumulative committed dose
[b] Per year in 1978[7]
[c] Per year

TABLE 3
Collective Dose to Population 0—50 Miles from Three Mile Island Nuclear Station March 28 Through April 3, 1979

Radius (mile)	Collective dose person rem	Total population	Average individual exposure (mR)
0—1	51.2	658	77.8
1—2	66.7	2,017	33.1
2—3	482.2	7,579	63.3
3—4	352.2	9,676	36.4
4—5	76.4	8,891	8.6
5—10	810.0	137,474	5.9
10—20	137.4	577,288	0.24
20—30	27.3	433,001	0.063
30—40	1.9	237,857	0.0069
40—50	0.3	713,210	0.00048
TOTAL	2,005.7	2,165,651	0.92
	(2,000)		(0.9)

From Rogovin, M. and Frampton, G. T., NUREG/CR 1250, U.S. Nuclear Regulatory Commission, Washington, D.C., 1979.

Sv). The Department of Energy estimated a collective dose to the population to be approximately 2000 person rem (20 person Sv) and provided a detailed dose estimate based on the distance from the plant (Table 3, Figure 3, Figure 4).

The closest populated area to the plant was 0.5 mi east northeast of the plant. The maximum dose to an individual in this area assuming no shelter during the entire period of the accident was 83 mrem (0.83 mSv). An individual was identified who was on Hill Island, 1.1 miles north-northwest of the plant, during part of the period of higher exposure. The best estimate of the exposure of this individual during the 10-h period is 37 mrem (0.37 mSv). The highest radiation dose measured by an on-site monitor outside the containment building was 1020 mrem (10.2 mSv). All of these dose estimates are likely to be overestimates because they are skin doses and they do not account for any dose reduction due to being indoors or due to leaving the area.

Despite the fact that the physical health effects of the accident at Three Mile Island were trivial, there appears to have been a measurable psychological impact of this accident.[8,9] Prior to the accident at Three Mile Island, the psychological impact of accidents at nuclear power plants were not considered.

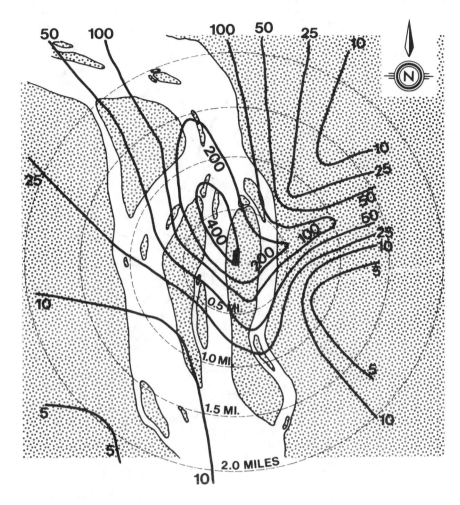

FIGURE 3. Isodose curves (mrems) for the cumulative dose within 2 mi of Three Mile Island due to release of radioactivity from the period of March 28 through April 3, 1979. They are based on Department of Energy aerial radiation surveys.[6]

C. THE CLEANUP

The accident at Three Mile Island created an enormous and unique highly radioactive mess that needed to be cleaned up. The recovery effort following the accident at Three Mile Island was divided into four areas. First, the reactor had to be stabilized. Second, the containment building had to be decontaminated so that maintenance of instrumentation and equipment that kept the reactor in a stable state could be undertaken. Third, the damage to the interior of the reactor vessel needed to be assessed. Fourth, the reactor needed to be disassembled and defueled. Final decommissioning of the plant would be delayed.

For the first month following the accident, all the efforts were directed towards controlling the reactor and preventing releases of radioactivity. Fortunately, the reactor remained well enough instrumented to permit engineers to monitor its condition. The containment building, however, was completely inaccessible because it held large amounts of radioactive water and gas. The auxiliary building was also heavily contaminated. It was estimated that there were 1900 m³ of contaminated water in the reactor building and 1500 m³ of water in the auxiliary building.

Because of the hydrogen explosion, the physical condition in the containment building was unclear. Radiation levels as high of 10,000 R/h had been measured in the containment

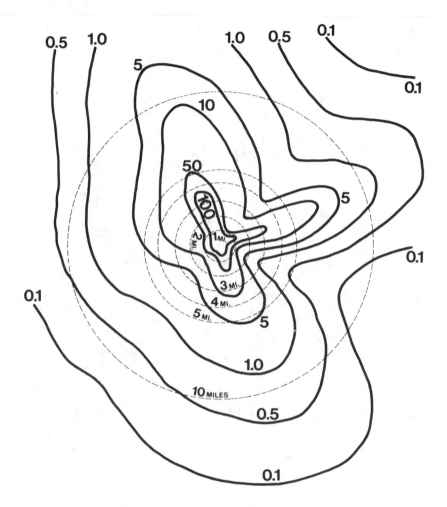

FIGURE 4.   Isodose curves (mrems) for the cumulative dose within 10 mi of Three Mile Island due to release of radioactivity from the period of March 28 through April 3, 1979. They are based on Department of Energy aerial radiation surveys.[6]

building at the time of the accident. In order to prevent leakage of radioactive gas and water from the containment building, the pressure within the containment building was initially held at lower than atmospheric pressure.

The job of the recovery team was further complicated by the fact that the cleanup efforts had to undergo intense public scrutiny.[10,11] All significant procedures for recovery had to be reviewed and approved by the NRC. Approximately 800 to 900 procedures ranging from a one- to 100-page proposals were inspected each year by the NRC staff.

An example of the public relations problems faced by the recovery team was the venting of the 43,000 Ci (1.6 × 10^{15} Bq) of ^{85}Kr gas which was largely responsible for the atmospheric radiation dose in the containment building. Very early on the recovery team decided that the simplest and most reasonable way to eliminate the ^{85}Kr from containment was to release it into the atmosphere in controlled amounts. The public was very skeptical of this solution. After much public debate the krypton was finally vented in July, 1980 (over 1 year after the accident). The maximum total radiation exposure at any point off-site during the entire period of venting was 0.02 mrem (0.2 μSv).[12]

After the krypton was vented it was possible to enter the containment for a brief period of time to visually assess the damage. On July 20, 1980, two engineers entered the Three

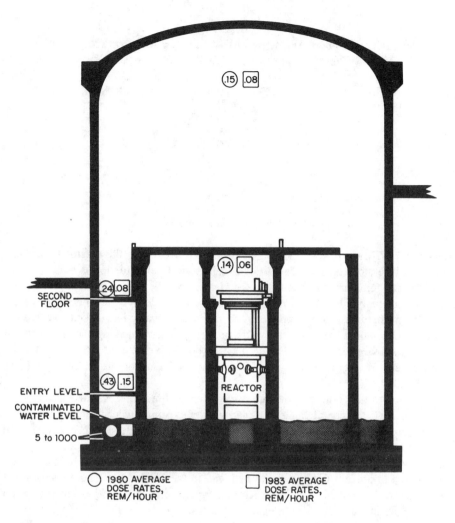

FIGURE 5. Schematic of the containment building at Three Mile Island indicating the radiation doses in various parts of the plant in 1980 and 1983.

Mile Island reactor building for a 20-min inspection. During their inspection they measured radiation doses up to 40 R/h (Figure 5).[13] The initial estimates of the radiation dose to the workforce involved in cleanup was between 2000 to 8000 person rem (20 to 80 person Sv); however, as time went on the radiation dose to the workforce has been revised upward to 46,000 person rem (460 person Sv). The radiation dose to the workforce cleaning up following the accident will be greater than 10 times the collective radiation dose to which the public was exposed to.

In order to decontaminate the large amount of highly radioactive water, Metropolitan Edison installed an ion exchange system — EPICOR II — several months after the accident (Table 4). It was submerged in the spent fuel pool to provide adequate shielding. Plans for disposing of this tritium-tainted water are under consideration.[14]

Assessment of the damage to the interior of the reactor was begun between July and August of 1982. At this time, the first television inspection of the inside of the reactor was completed. A large void in the reactor occupying at least 9.3 m³ of the 34 m³ core was detected (Figure 6). This void was formed when between 35 and 45% of the fuel rods and the uranium fuel pellets melted. For this to happen, temperatures in the reactor had to exceed 2800°C. At least 70% of the core was damaged. Figuring out how to remove the congealed mass of highly radioactive fuel posed no simple task.[15,16]

TABLE 4

Radioactivity of Spilled Water at TMI-2 Before and After Processing with EPICOR II System Compared with the Federal Law 10 CFR 20 Levels

Radionuclide	Before processing, nCi/l	After processing, nCi/l	10 CFR 20, nCi/l
^{137}Cs	45,900,000	4.40	20
^{134}Cs	8,300,000	6.60	9
^{89}Sr	1,200,000	0.10	3
^{90}Sr	3,100,000	0.29	0.3
Tritium	440,000	440,000.00	300
Gross beta and gamma emissions	67,000,000	6.30	None

Note: 1 nCi = 3.7 × 10^4 Bq. CFR = Code of Federal Regulations.

By late 1987 over 70% of the fuel had been removed from the reactor to the national engineering laboratory outside Idaho Falls, Idaho, and final defueling is expected in 1990 (Figure 7). The remaining problem with the cleanup will be decontaminating the basement of the containment building. Half of the projected radiation dose to the workforce is expected to come from this phase of the project. The radioactive water has leaked into the porous concrete blocks which make up the walls of the basement, making cleanup particularly difficult. This final phase of the cleanup may not be completed until robotics technology is available, perhaps not until the year 2000. The total cost of the cleanup will exceed $1,000,000,000.

In addition to the enormous cleanup effort, Three Mile Island resulted in an enormous effort by the NRC to generate an action plan to alter existing nuclear reactors in an attempt to make them safer.[17-20] The regulations included more than 130 items. Many items dealt with human factors. For example, better training was required for reactor operators. In addition, two senior reactor operators were required per shift. A number of hardware changes were required to prevent failures which had lead to the Three Mile Island accident. Much more extensive and explicit requirements for emergency plans for accidents at nuclear power plants were formulated. A major step after the accident was centralization of emergency planning within a single agency, the Federal Emergency Management Agency (FEMA).

II. CHERNOBYL

A. HOW THE ACCIDENT HAPPENED

The worst accident in the history of nuclear power occurred at the Chernobyl Nuclear Power station in the Ukraine on April 27, 1986 (Figures 8 and 9).[21-27] This accident released enormous amounts of activity into the environment and shocked the nuclear power industry with the realization that an accident considered to be most unlikely to occur had become a reality. The accident at Chernobyl has initiated an international effort to understand what happened, how similar accidents could be prevented in the future, and what the long-term effects of the accident will be. The International Atomic Energy Agency (IAEA) and the Soviet Union had a preliminary post-accident review in Vienna from August 25th through August 29th, 1986.[20] Sixty-two countries and 21 international organizations were represented.

Just as with Three Mile Island, it is very instructive to carefully review the events that lead up to the Chernobyl catastrophe. The sequence of events appear to be highly improbable, even in retrospect. The post-accident management by the Soviet government was remarkable.

The Chernobyl Nuclear Power Station was one of 15 RBMK-type reactors (Figure 10) operating in the Soviet Union. Four of these units were operating at the Chernobyl site. Two additional units were under construction at the site.

Hypothesized Core Damage Configuration
(226 Minutes)

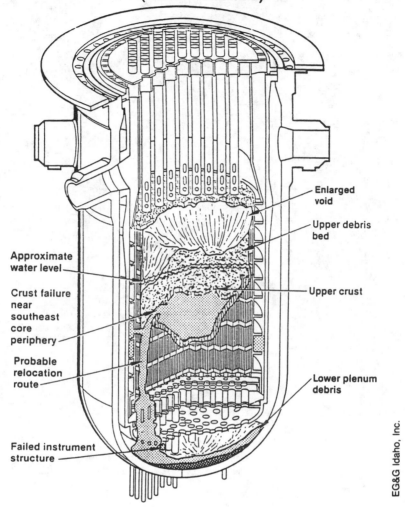

FIGURE 6.   Schematic of the damage to the reactor core at Three Mile Island. The 9.3-m³
void which was created when the fuel rods melted and actually flowed to the bottom of the
reactor vessel is shown. The fact that the reactor vessel was not breached and that the molten
mass of fissionable fuel resolidified remains incompletely understood. (From Booth, W.,
Science, 238, 1342, 1987. With permission.)

The accident occurred as the operators were attempting to test whether or not the inertia
of the rotor of a turbogenerator was sufficient to supply temporary electricity to the power
plant in the event of a station blackout. This electricity would only be needed during the
few seconds between the loss of electrical power from the grid and the start up of standby
emergency diesel generators. A test of this sort had been conducted earlier in 1982 and in
1984; however, the results were unsatisfactory because the voltage had fallen off much more
rapidly than the inertial energy of the turbine rotor. A new voltage regulation system had
been installed in an attempt to overcome this problem. The test was to be done in conjunction
with a routine shutdown of the reactor for maintenance since the test was to be performed
at low power. The next planned maintenance period was more than 1 year away so there
was some urgency to complete the test.

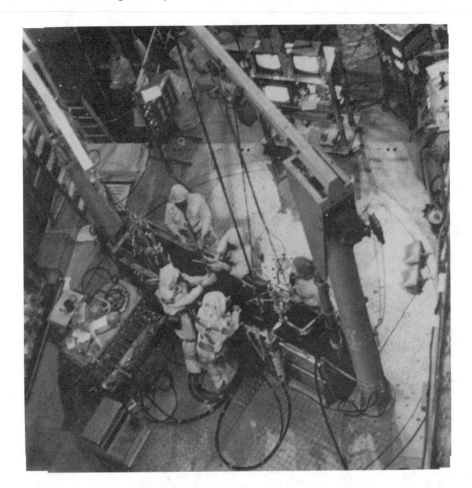

FIGURE 7. Working in the pot. Over 200,000 lb. of the approximately 300,000 lb. of core debris has been removed from the reactor vessel of Three Mile Island by men using long-handled tools to chop, pry, and remove chunks of the resolidified mass. (From Booth, W., *Science,* 238, 1344, 1987. With permission.)

At 1 a.m. on April 25th, the output of the reactor was decreased from 100% (3200 MW) to half of that in a period of 5 min (Figure 11). At 2 p.m., the emergency core coolant system (ECCS) was isolated from the reactor. This isolation was done in order to prevent the ECCS from automatically tripping when the turbogenerator was isolated from the reactor. The start of the test was then unexpectedly postponed at the request of a local electricity dispatcher who wanted the plant to remain at 50% power in order to meet the electrical demand. For the next 9 h the reactor continued to produce electricity to meet this demand. During this time, the ECCS remained disconnected from the reactor. Although this factor played no part in the accident, it is remarkable that the reactor would have been operated for so long without the ECCS in operation.

At 11:10 p.m., preparations were resumed to begin the turbogenerator test. For technical reasons the optimal power output to conduct the tests was 700 to 1000 MW. Since the automatic control system that operated the control rods was not designed to operate the reactor at this level, most of the automatic control system was turned off and the control rods were operated manually. When manual reduction of the power output of the reactor was attempted, there was an overshoot in the power reduction and the level fell to below 30 MW.

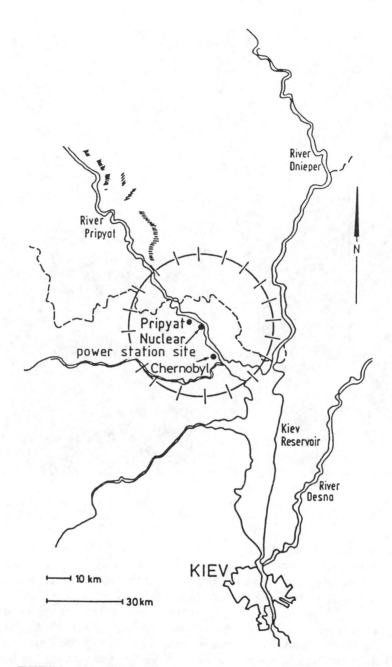

FIGURE 8.   Map of the Chernobyl Nuclear Power Station site. (From Summary Report on the Post Accident Review Meeting on the Chernobyl Accident, Saf. Ser. 75-INSAG-1, International Atomic Energy Agency, Vienna, 1986.)

By 1 a.m. on April 26th, the operators were able to raise the power back to 200 MW. Bringing the reactor back to this level was difficult due to a xenon poison buildup that occurred during the excursion to lower power. Xenon in the fuel was absorbing neutrons, making it difficult to increase the rate of fission. In order to compensate for the xenon buildup, the operators had to pull far too many control rods out of the reactor. This resulted in a situation in which the reactivity worth of the remaining control rods was equivalent to 6 or 8 fully inserted rods. The reactor was not designed to be operated below 30 rod equivalents without special authorization, and below 15 rod equivalents continued operation

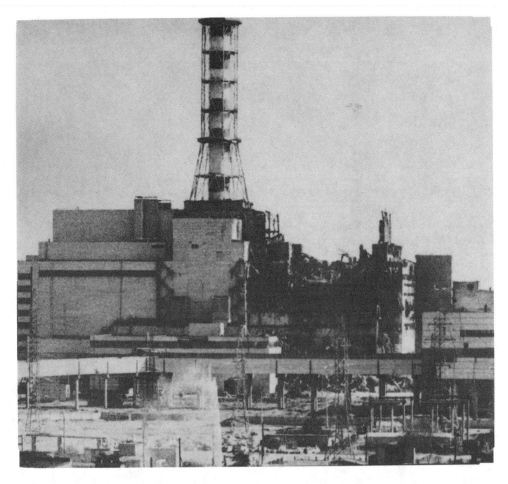

FIGURE 9.   Aerial photograph of the Chernobyl Nuclear Power Plant shortly after the accident. (From *Nucl. News,* 29(13), 59, 1986. With permission.)

of the reactor was forbidden. At this point, the reactor was in a very dangerous state. Not only do the control rods of this type of reactor move more slowly than control rods of other types of reactors, they actually can increase the reactivity of the reactor when they are initially reinserted. If the reactivity of the reactor increased, it would be difficult to control.

Having already been delayed, the operators were very intent on getting the reactor up to an acceptable power level for the test. Because of this they ignored the touchy state the reactor was in and they decided to continue on. In addition to the fact that too many control rods had been withdrawn, the reactor was also unstable for other reasons. The reactor was at a power that was considerably lower than had been planned, and therefore had considerably less hydraulic resistance of the core. This produced an increase in coolant flow which subsequently resulted in increased turbulence. The consequence of this increased flow was the creation of coolant conditions in which a small temperature increase could cause extensive flashing to steam. While all of this was occurring, the steam pressure and water level in the steam separation drums also dropped below emergency levels. The operators blocked the resulting signals to the low levels to the emergency protection systems in a continuing attempt to keep the reactor running long enough for the test to be started. At 1:19 a.m., the feed water supply to the reactor was increased in an attempt to restore the water level in the steam separation drums. This resulted in a decrease in coolant temperature and a decrease in steam production which caused negative reactivity. To compensate, the automatic control

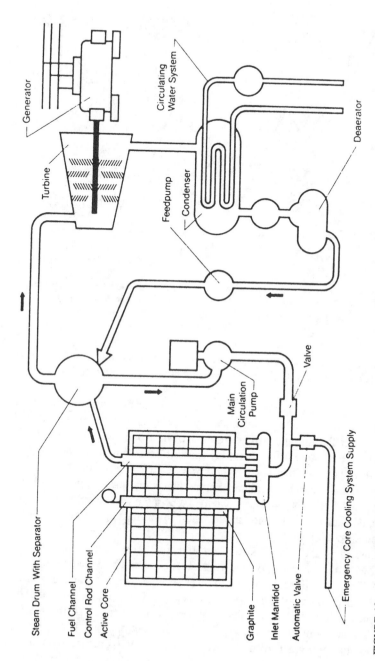

FIGURE 10. Schematic of the RMBK-1000 graphite-moderated, water-cooled nuclear power plant. (From Report on the Accident at the Chernobyl Nuclear Power Station, NUREG 1250, Superintendent of Documents, U.S. Government Printing Office, Washington, D.C., 1987.)

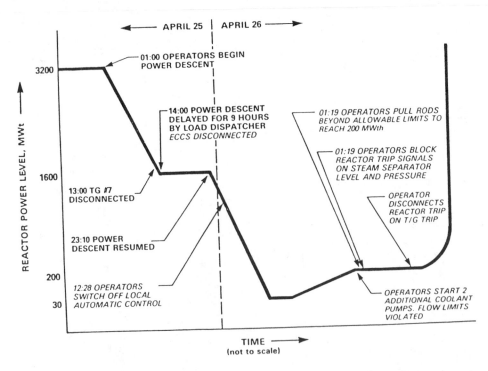

FIGURE 11.   Graph of the major events leading to the Chernobyl accident. The reactor power during the time leading up to the accident is plotted. The time axis is not to scale. (From Report on the Accident at the Chernobyl Nuclear Power Station, NUREG 1250, Superintendent of Documents, U.S. Government Printing Office, Washington, D.C., 1987.)

rods were fully withdrawn plus the operators attempted to further withdraw manual rods as well. The operators overcompensated and the automatic control rods began to move back in.

At 1:22 a.m. the reactor parameters had stabilized and the decision was made to start the actual turbine test. In case they wanted to repeat the test again the operators blocked the emergency protection signals from the turbine stop valve which they were about to close so that it would not scram the reactor. Just before they shut off the steam to the turbine they reduced the feed water flow back to initial levels which were required for the test conditions. This resulted in an increase in the coolant temperature that subsequently increased the reactivity of the reactor. At 1:22:30 the operators obtained a printout from the fast reactivity evaluation program which indicated that they should shut down the reactor immediately. They delayed long enough to start the test.

At 1:23:04 the turbine stop valve was closed. Shortly thereafter the reactor power began to rise sharply. The RBMK reactor has a positive void coefficient so that when the coolant flashed to steam further increases in reactivity and power resulted which further increased the temperature and steam production. The operators desperately attempted to manually scram the reactor seconds before the uncontrollable supercritical excursion of the reactor occurred. A few seconds later a number of shocks were felt in the control room. The operators saw that the control rods had not reached their lower stops and therefore deactivated the rods to let them fall by gravity.

At about 1:24 a.m. observers outside the plant reported 2 explosions, one after another. A summary of the violations of the operating procedures at the Chernobyl IV nuclear power plant are presented in Table 5. If any one of the first five violations had not been committed, the accident probably would not have happened.[22]

TABLE 5
Operator Violations of Procedures[22]

Violations	Consequences
1. Power level below that specified by procedures	Large positive void reactivity coefficient Reactor difficult to control Overall power coefficient positive
2. Control rods mispositioned	Unauthorized (and probably unanalyzed) configuration Emergency protective system ineffective
3. Operated all eight main circulation pumps, with coolant flow exceeding authorized levels	Reduced voiding but coolant temperature near saturation
4. Blocked reactor scram signal from loss of both turbine generators	Lost automatic scram protection at start of test
5. Blocked reactor scrams on water level and steam pressure in the drum separator	Lost reactor protection system based on thermal parameters
6. Turned off the emergency core cooling system	Lost possibility of reducing severity of accident

The accident was the result of a prompt critical reactivity excursion and subsequent steam explosion. The explosion literally blew the top off the reactor. The complacency with which this test was conducted was due to the fact that the test was really perceived as a mechanical/electrical test rather than a test of the nuclear reactor itself. An electrical engineer, not a nuclear physicist, was in charge. The reactor, operating at low power, was regarded as being safer than one operating at high power.

B. ACUTE HEALTH CONSEQUENCES
At the time of the explosion there were 444 workers on site. Two hundred and sixty-eight of the individuals were construction workers and 176 were staff members. There were three medical technicians on duty. During the first half hour following the accident, 29 patients were admitted to the medical station at the power plant. At this time, medical teams from Pripyat were requested. In order to avoid extensive contamination of the medical station, all patients were stripped of water-soaked contaminated clothing and given necessary first aid prior to entering the medical station. At 6:40 a.m. a specialty team from Moscow lead by Dr. Guskova was notified of the accident. This team arrived at noon, approximately $10 \frac{1}{2}$ h after the accident.

There were two immediate deaths. One worker was killed during the collapse of part of the building. A second individual died $5 \frac{1}{2}$ h after the accident from extensive thermal burns.

The number of people on site grew as hundreds of additional personnel were called in for rescue, plant control, and firefighting operations. The initial assessment of radiation dose was difficult. Many of the plant's radiation monitors had been destroyed in the explosion. Dosimetry for individuals was unavailable because the dosimeters were either off-scale, contaminated, or lost in the confusion.

Triaging patients for acute radiation syndrome was based on a rapid medical evaluation. Vomiting was regarded as a reliable indicator of a potentially lethal radiation exposure. The time to onset of vomiting could be used qualitatively to determine the approximate dose (Table 6). Although nausea and vomiting may be due to other causes, the absence of nausea and vomiting for the first 6 h following the accident reliably excluded patients with high enough radiation exposure to cause the acute radiation syndrome that would potentially be fatal.

In addition to using the patient's symptoms and the initial fall of the lymphocyte count to estimate whole-body dose, cytogenetic studies were also carried out. Cytogenetic studies

TABLE 6
Characteristics of Patients with Acute Radiation Syndrome

Dose range (RAD)	Onset of nausea and vomiting (h)	Number of patients	Number of deaths	Time until death (d)
80—200	2	31	0	—
200—400	1—2	43	1	96
400—600	0.5—1	21	7	16—48
600—1600	0.5	20	20	10—91
	TOTAL	115	28	

From United Nations Scientific Committee on Effects of Atomic Radiation, Sources, Effects and Risks of Ionizing Radiation (appendix), Report to the General Assembly, United Nations, New York, 1988.

are very laborious and results cannot be obtained earlier than 48 to 55 h after the withdrawal of blood for lymphocyte culture.

The radiation exposure of the patients in Chernobyl was a complicated radiation injury. The core of the reactor had been vaporized in the intense fire which followed the explosion. Since many of the fission products are medium- to high-energy beta emitters, workers and emergency personnel on site were exposed to extensive beta radiation to the skin. The protective clothing which the firefighters wore was made of a porous canvas material that allowed highly contaminated water to seep through and come into contact with the skin. Ultimately this exposure caused extensive beta burns to the skin and resulted in many of the deaths (Table 6).

Although accurate dosimetry in the reactor building was not available, it is estimated that the exposure rate was a few hundreds rads per hour. These survivable exposure rates existed because much of the radioactivity was being carried away by the radioactive plume which formed following the explosion and the subsequent fire. In addition, the sides of the reactor were intact, so some shielding of the reactor core was still present. Of the nearly 1000 individuals who were screened, 115 patients were hospitalized with acute radiation syndrome.

Ultimately 28 of the 115 patients died of radiation injuries. One additional patient died shortly after the accident of thermal burns and one died immediately from trauma at the site. There were no deaths in patients who were estimated to receive under 200 rem (2 Sv) whole-body dose. Only one of these patients suffered from any significant skin burns (Table 6). One of the 43 patients who were estimated to have between 200 and 400 rem (2 to 4 Sv) died. Only 10 of these patients had significant skin burns. Seven of the 21 patients who had an estimated whole body dose between 400 and 600 rem (4 to 6 Sv) died. Their deaths occurred between 16 and 48 d after the accident. Six of the seven people that died in this group had suffered from severe beta burns to the skin. Twenty patients were estimated to have between 600 to 1600 rem (6 to 16 Sv). Eight of these patients had beta burns to 60 to 100% of their body and two of these patients also had high levels of internal contamination.

Nineteen of the 22 patients with more than 600 rem (6 Sv) of radiation received a bone marrow or fetal liver transplant.[28] Seventeen of 19 of these transplant recipients died. Two other victims who did not receive transplants also died. The death in this group occurred from 14 to 91 d after the accident. The two transplant recipients who lived rejected the transplant and regenerated their own marrow. The experience with bone marrow transplants in this group of patients suggests that the role of bone marrow transplantation will be quite limited.

The combination of beta "burns" to the skin and whole-body radiation is a particularly lethal one. The beta burn begins to manifest itself 14 d after the injury at the time when the suppression of the hemopoietic system is just becoming a problem. At the time when the patient is least able to cope with infection, the beta burn to the skin provides an enormous portal for entry of infection. Many of the deaths were due to sepsis.

Severe skin burns developed in 56 persons. These burns were very difficult to treat and proved to be a major complicating factor. It is thought that many of these burns could have been prevented and thus many lives saved had the rescue personnel worn clothing that was better suited for preventing extensive contamination of the skin with medium- to high-energy beta radiation.

Eight of the medical attendants who were working on site developed the acute radiation syndrome. One of the medical workers on site, a young physician, later died. The radiation exposure to medical workers off-site was much less. Some of the medical personnel at Hospital #6 in Moscow received 4 to 5 rem (40 to 50 mSv) to whole body and 35 to 40 rem (0.35 to 0.40 Sv) to the hand during the first 2 weeks following the accident. Prior to the Chernobyl accident, plans called for decontamination of patients at the scene of the accident or at the regional hospitals. The magnitude of the accident at Chernobyl along with the thermal injuries to the skin made complete decontamination prior to transfer to definitive care hospitals impossible.

Although personnel at the site were exposed to radioactive aerosols containing fission and activation products, the levels of internal contamination were far below those that significantly contributed to the development of the acute radiation syndrome. Only two subjects with extensive thermal burns of the skin had high levels of internal contamination but even this was not clinically significant. There was no significant contribution to the total radiation dose from neutrons. ^{24}Na activity in these patients was negligible.

Viral infections of the herpes type were very prominent in the accident victims. These infections were effectively treated with an antiviral drug (acyclovir). Use of fresh unpooled platelets was also quite helpful in treating the patients' thrombocytopenia.

C. POPULATION DOSE

One hundred and thirty-five thousand people living within 30 km of the site were eventually evacuated and evaluated for radiation exposure. The population of Pripyat was not evacuated immediately following the accident. Although the delay in the evacuation of the population of Pripyat was portrayed by some as a callous action on the part of the Russian officials, this delay was very well thought out. The initial indication following the accident was that the greatest bulk of the radioactivity had been released acutely. By keeping the population of Pripyat indoors while the released activity was rapidly diluted in the atmosphere, their radiation dose would be decreased. In addition, the only evacuation route from Pripyat would have brought the population closer to the disabled power plant and would thus potentially expose the population to a higher radiation dose. The third problem with an immediate evacuation was that the evacuation had to be well-coordinated, otherwise the radiation exposure of the population would increase. Eventually some 1500 buses were used to evacuate the population. Evacuation was finally undertaken when the persistent fire at the power plant caused continued release of radioactivity.

The evacuation of Pripyat started on the morning of April 27th. Roads had been treated with a special polymer to prevent resuspension of radioactive dust by the buses. The evacuation of the 45,000 people from Pripyat was executed in less than 3 h. The success with which the population of Pripyat was evacuated is indicated by the fact that the average per capita dose for the 45,000 evacuees was calculated to be 3.3 rem (33 mSv). The comparable unsheltered dose from the time of accident to the evacuation was estimated to be 10 to 15 rem (100 to 150 mSv). The average individual exposure for the 135,000 evacuees within 30 km was estimated to be 12 rem (120 mSv). At the time that the decision was made to evacuate Pripyat the radiation exposure rate was 1 rem (10 mSv) per hour. The evacuees showered and were given new clothing when they arrived at the reception centers to which the evacuation buses took them. Their old clothing was destroyed.

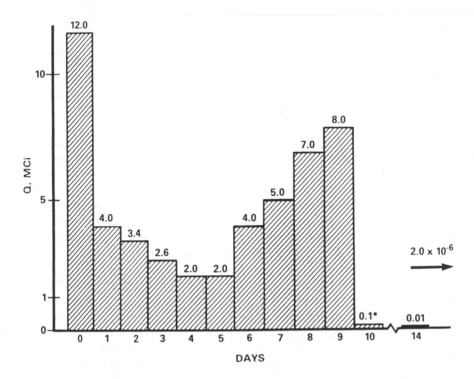

FIGURE 12.   Bar graph of the amount of radionuclides released into the atmosphere in the days following the accident at Chernobyl. (From Report on the Accident at the Chernobyl Nuclear Power Station, NUREG 1250, Superintendent of Documents, U.S. Government Printing Office, Washington, D.C., 1987.)

The release of radioactivity from the reactor exceeded previous releases of radionuclides in reactor accidents by several orders of magnitude (Table 2). The release continued over a 10-d period of time as the Russians struggled to extinguish the graphite fire (Figure 12). The release rate decreased from day 1 through day 5 due to the bombardment of the open reactor with 5000 tons of materials (boron carbide—40 tons, dolomite—800 tons, clay/sand—1800 tons, and lead—2400 tons). The increased release of radioactivity from day 6 through day 9 was thought to be due to heatup of the fuel by the residual decay heat and possible carbidization of the uranium dioxide, making it easier for fission products to escape. The Soviets attribute the rapid falloff of radioactive release on day 10 to the introduction of cold nitrogen into the reactor vault and the formation of less volatile compounds of fission products as a result of their interaction with the material deposited.

It was estimated that 0.3 to 0.5% of the core was deposited on site, 1.5 to 2% of the core was deposited within a 20-km radius, and 1 to 1.5% of the core was deposited beyond 20 km. It has been estimated that the maximum dose received off site was approximately 30 to 40 rem (300 to 400 mSv).

The maximum collective external dose delivered to the 135,000 evacuees in the 30 km area around the plant was estimated to be 1.6×10^6 person rem (1.6×10^4 person Sv), or an average of 12 rem (120 mSv) per person. On the basis of that collective dose and assuming a cancer risk factor of about $2^{-5} \times 10^{-4}$/person rem, approximately 300 to 700 excess fatal cancers in the evacuee population would be attributed to the accident. Measuring these excess cancers will be difficult since in the course of normal events about 12% of the evacuees will normally die of cancer (approximately 16,000).

The inhabitants of the 30-km zone were given potassium iodide to minimize the uptake of radioiodine.[29] Extensive monitoring, particularly in children (100,000 were measured in

TABLE 7
Estimates of Additional Cancer Deaths to Result From Chernobyl

No. of deaths (%)	Estimator[a]
5100 (0.5)	Beninson (International Commission on Radiologic Protection)
10000 (0.10)	Rosen (International Atomic Energy Agency)
40000 (0.42)	Legasov (Soviet Atomic Energy Agency)
100000 (1.05)	Cochran (Natural Resources Defense Council)

Note: Total number of deaths expected in the next 70 years from all other causes: 9,500,000.

[a] Name of individual cited in report by Norman and Dickson;[30] the organization each represented is indicated in the parentheses.

Modified from Adelstein, S. J., *JAMA*, 258, 655, 1987.

all) was undertaken. From the monitoring, it was estimated that most absorbed doses to the thyroid gland from inhaled or ingested radioiodines was less than 30 rem (300 mSv). Several hundred children may have received a thyroid dose as high as 250 rem (2.5 Sv). The risk of hypothyroidism appears to be negligible below a dose of approximately 1000 rem (10 Sv). If one assumes that the collective thyroid dose was about 4×10^6 person rem (4×10^4 person Sv), the number of excess thyroid cancers due to the Chernobyl accident would be approximately 100 to 250; 10% of these would be expected to be fatal. In addition, a somewhat larger number of benign thyroid nodules might occur. This excess incidence of thyroid cancers and benign nodules may be detectable since background incidence rates are expected to be low.

Another concern in the evacuated population is the possibility of radiation-induced birth defects, particularly mental retardation. The data based on the atomic bomb survivors at Hiroshima and Nagasaki suggest that the risk of mental retardation is about 4×10^{-3}/rem if the fetus is exposed during the critical period (8 to 15 weeks postconception) of gestation. Since a population of 135,000 people would be expected to include about 300 women during this critical period of pregnancy, the number of babies born with retardation due to the radiation exposure can be calculated. If one assumes the average individual dose to the evacuated population was 12 rem (120 mSv), one would estimate that 15 children may be retarded as the result of the exposure. An excess of this magnitude may be detectable since fewer than 3% of all children in developed countries suffer from mental retardation. Despite careful monitoring of the pregnant women no excess in children who are mentally retarded has been noted.

Estimates of the long-term consequences of the accident at Chernobyl and on the health of the very large population of people who have been exposed to small amounts of radiation have varied greatly[30-33] (Table 7). Generally, these estimates assume a nonthreshhold model for radiation carcinogenesis. If the body's repair mechanisms are able to repair the damage of low levels of radiation, the deaths from low levels are only theoretical. The increase in radiation exposure to populations greater than 1000 km from the plant are similar to the difference in exposure due to natural differences in background levels of radiation.

REFERENCES

1. **Rubinstein, E.,** The accident that shouldn't have happened, *IEEE Spectrum,* 16(11), 33, 1979.
2. **Mason, J. F.,** The technical blow by blow, *IEEE Spectrum,* 16(11), 33, 1979.
3. **Rogovin, M. and Frampton, G. T.,** Three Mile Island. A report to the commissioners and to the public, NUREG/CR 1250, U.S. Nuclear Regulatory Commission, Washington, D.C., 1979.
4. **Collins, D. M.,** Health Physics Lessons Learned in Reactor Accidents, U.S. Nuclear Regulatory Commission, Superintendent of Documents, U.S. Government Printing Office, Washington, D.C.
5. **Kemeny, J. G., Babbitt, B., Haggerty, P. E., et al.,** Report of the President's Commission on the accident at Three Mile Island. The need for change: the legacy of TMI, Superintendent of Documents, U.S. Government Printing Office, Washington, D. C., 1979.
6. Ad Hoc Population — Dose Assessment Group, Population dose and health impact of the accident at the Three Mile Island Nuclear Station, May 10, 1979, Superintendent of Documents, U.S. Government Printing Office, Washington, D. C.
7. **Annex, E.,** Exposures resulting from nuclear explosions, in, *Ionizing Radiation: Sources and Biological Effects,* UNSCEAR, United Nations, New York, 1982.
8. **Dohrenwend, B. P., Dohrenwend, B. S., Warheit, G. J., et al.,** Stress in the Community: a report to the President's Commission on the accident at Three Mile Island, *Ann. N.Y. Acad. Sci., U.S.A.,* 365, 159, 1981.
9. **Dohrenwend, B. P.,** Psychological implications of nuclear accident. The case of Three Mile Island, *Bull. N.Y. Acad. Med.,* 59, 1060, 1983.
10. Pragmatic Environmental Impact Statement Related to Decontamination In and Disposal of Radioactive Waste Resulting from March 28, 1979, Accident at TMI Nuclear Station, Unit 2, NUREG 063 Nuclear Regulatory Commission, Superintendent of Documents, U.S. Government Printing Office, Washington, D.C., 1983.
11. NRC Plan for Cleanup at Three Mile Island, Unit 2, NUREG 0698, Nuclear Regulatory Commission, Superintendent of Documents, U.S. Government Printing Office, Washington, D.C.
12. Krypton-85 in the atmosphere—with specific reference to the public health significance of the proposed controlled release at Three Mile Island, NCRP Commentary Number 1, National Council on Radiation Protection and Measurements, Washington, D.C., 1980.
13. **Devine, J. C.,** A Progress Report: cleaning up TMI, *IEEE Spectrum,* 18(3), 44, 1981.
14. Guidelines for the release of waste water for nuclear facilities with special reference to the public health significance of the proposed release of treated waste waters at Three Mile Island, NCRP Commentary No. 4, National Council on Radiation Protection and Measurements, Washington, D.C., 1987.
15. **Adam, J. A.,** A slow comeback, *IEEE Spectrum,* 21(4), 27, 1984.
16. **Booth, W.,** Postmortem on Three mile Island, *Science,* 238, 1342, 1987.
17. **Eisenhut, D. G.,** NRC as referee, *IEEE Spectrum,* 21(4), 33, 1984.
18. **Fischetti, M. A.,** Band-aids and better, *IEEE Spectrum,* 21(4), 39, 1984.
19. Clarification of TMI Action Plan Requirements, NUREG 0737 Nuclear Regulatory Commission, Superintendent of Documents, U.S. Government Printing Office, Washington, D.C.
20. NRC Action Plan Developed as a Result of the TMI Accident, NUREG 0660 Nuclear Regulatory Commission, Superintendent of Documents, U.S. Government Printing Office, Washington, D.C.
21. Summary Report on the Post Accident Review Meeting on The Chernobyl Accident, Safety Ser. 75-INSAG-1, International Atomic Energy Agency, Vienna, 1986.
22. Report on the accident at the Chernobyl Nuclear Power Station, 1987, NUREG 1250, Superintendent of Documents, U.S. Government Printing Office, Washington, D.C.
23. Implications of the accident at Chernobyl for safety regulation of commercial nuclear power plants in the United States, August 1987., NUREG 1251, U.S. Nuclear Regulatory Commission, Washington, D.C.
24. **Norman, C.,** Chernobyl: errors and design flaws, *Science,* 233, 1029, 1986.
25. Chernobyl: the Soviet Report, *Nucl. News,* 29(13), 59, 1986.
26. The Chernobyl Accident, *Nucl. News,* 29, (8), 87, 1986.
27. **Fischetti, M. A.,** The puzzle of Chernobyl, *IEEE Spectrum,* 23(7), 34, 1986.
28. **Gale, R. P.,** Immediate medical consequences of nuclear accidents. Lessons from Chernobyl, *JAMA,* 258, 625, 1987.
29. **Becker, D. V.,** Reactor Accidents: public health strategies and their medical implications, *JAMA,* 258, 649, 1987.
30. **Adelstein, S. J.,** Uncertainty and relative risks of radiation exposure, *JAMA,* 258, 655, 1987.
31. **Norman, C. and Dickson, D.,** The aftermath of Chernobyl, *Science,* 233, 1141, 1986.
32. **Fry, F. A.,** The Chernobyl reactor accident: the impact on the United Kingdom (1987 Mayneord Lecture), *Br. J. Radiol.,* 60, 1147, 1987.
33. **Clarke, R. H.,** Reactor accidents in perspective, *Br. J. Radiol.,* 60, 1189, 1987.

Chapter 18

INSTRUMENTATION AND PHYSICAL DOSE ASSESSMENT IN RADIATION ACCIDENTS

Charles A. Kelsey and Fred A. Mettler

TABLE OF CONTENTS

I. INTRODUCTION

In the management of a radiation accident patient, a hospital must have instrumentation available to locate and assess the amount of radioactive contamination as well as to assess absorbed radiation dose to both the patient and the medical staff. The purpose of this chapter is to describe (1) basic types and characteristics of radiation monitoring instruments, (2) methods for assessing personal absorbed dose, and (3) how to use physical methods to assess absorbed dose to the patient.

One of the most important steps in coping with a radiation accident should be taken before any accident occurs. This step is the assembly and periodic testing of a radiation instrumentation kit. Such a kit should contain instrumentation for real-time detection of various types of radiation that might be expected, as well as being able to assess both high and low levels of radiation exposure. The kit should also contain devices such as film badges that can be used to estimate individual absorbed doses. It is important that any kit be tested and inventoried at least every 6 months.

II. RADIATION DETECTION INSTRUMENTS

Radiation detection instruments generally measure either alpha particles or beta/gamma radiation. Only a very sophisticated and expensive piece of equipment can measure alpha as well as more penetrating radiation types. The extremely short range of alpha particles usually requires a special alpha detector, and such meters are very delicate since the detector portion must have a window thin enough to permit passage of alpha particles. High activity alpha emitters are found almost exclusively in defense facilities or in very large research facilities and, in general, it is not necessary for most hospitals to have an alpha detection capability. Some of the difficulties related to alpha detection equipment have been outlined in Chapter 4. As was pointed out in that chapter, most weapons-grade plutonium contains sufficient other radionuclides such that one may choose to detect low energy X-rays rather than the alpha particles themselves.

Beta- and gamma-emitting radionuclides are in common use throughout industry and medicine and accidental contamination with such radionuclides is a real possibility. Thus, a hospital should maintain an instrument for detection of these radiations. Various types of radiation detection instruments are shown in Table 1.

A. IONIZATION CHAMBER SURVEY METERS

Ionization survey meters contain an air-filled chamber for detection purposes. These ionization meters can operate over a wide range of radiation levels. Thus, if high exposure levels are suspected, an ionization chamber should be initially utilized. The range of such meters is on the order of mR to thousands of rads per hour. Unfortunately, such ionization chambers often have a relatively slow (several seconds) response time, and this means that the detector probe must be moved slowly over suspected areas. The ionization survey meter shown in Figure 1 has a thin mylar end window protected by a plastic endcap. The endcap must be removed only when searching for beta contamination. If the window is torn or punctured, the detector cannot be used and must be returned to the supplier for repair.

B. GEIGER-MUELLER (GM) COUNTERS

Geiger counters are the instruments of choice for radiation surveys when one is attempting to localize areas of contamination or detect very small amounts of radiation. The detector, or probe, on the Geiger counter contains a pressurized gas in a sealed tube. Geiger counters are relatively fast in responding and relatively inexpensive. Most Geiger survey probes have a protective cover over a thin entrance window so that the machine can be used to detect

TABLE 1
Radiation Survey and Monitoring Instruments

Instrument Type	Type of radiation detected	Typical use	Minimum X-ray Energy Detected	Typical dose rate or dose range	Advantages	Disadvantages
Ionization chamber survey meter	X, gamma, beta	Survey	20 keV	5 mR/h—500 R/h	Response independent of photon energy	Slow response, low sensitivity
Pencil dosimeter	X, gamma	Personnel monitoring	50 keV	200 mR—200 R	Small, inexpensive, instant reading of integrated dose	May discharge if dropped
Film	X, gamma, beta	Personnel monitoring	20 keV	>10 mR	Measures integrated dose, gives permanent record	Must be processed under controlled conditions. Heat and vapor can produce false readings
TLD	X, gamma	Personnel monitoring	20 keV	>10 mR	Measures integrated dose, gives permanent record	Must be processed before reading is available
Geiger-Mueller counter	X, gamma, beta	Survey	20 keV	0.5—20 mR/h	Rapid response, rugged instrument	Very energy dependent
Scintillation counter	X, gamma, beta	Survey	20 keV	0.05—20 mR/hr	Very sensitive reading response	Fragile, expensive

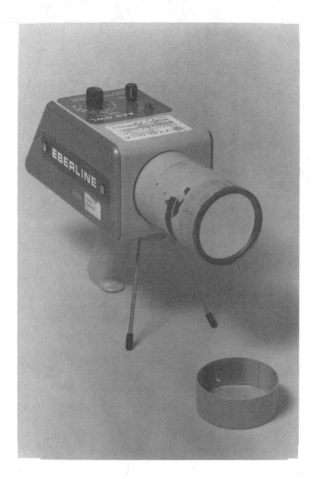

FIGURE 1.   Ionization survey meter.

poorly penetrating radiation (such as beta) when the shield is moved into the open position. Figure 2 shows a Geiger counter with the probe having its protective shield partially rotated to expose the thin window underneath. Both the instruments shown in Figure 2 and 3 are civil defense-type instruments. The instrument shown in Figure 2 is a low-range instrument with a maximum exposure range of 50 mR/h. The instrument shown in Figure 3 has a maximum rate of 500 mR/h, but since it does not have a probe or thin window, it has no beta sensitivity.

The first application of such monitoring or survey instruments is to determine whether or not the patient is contaminated. This is accomplished by performing a radiation survey of the patient. The detector is slowly scanned over areas of suspected or possible contamination (Figure 4).

Prior to performing a survey, it is important to ascertain whether or not each instrument is functional. With instruments which operate on batteries, this is usually done by initially turning the selector switch to the "BAT" or "BATT" position. If the batteries are adequate, the indicator needle on the meter will go near the top end of the scale face. After this is done, one turns the selector switch to the X 1 position. This will allow the survey instrument to begin detecting. If the instrument has an audible output or makes a clicking sound, background radiation should be identified. For many Geiger-type meters, background radiation is about 60 clicks/min. Often it is useful to have a very tiny radioactive "check" source taped on the side of the instrument case. The probe should be placed next to this

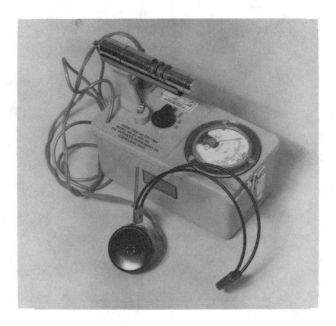

A

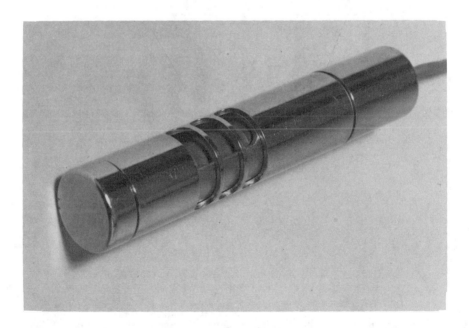

B

FIGURE 2.   (A). Model CDV-700 low-range Geiger counter. (B). Geiger counter probe with thin window partially open.

tiny source and the needle should show a response. Once this is done, one can begin surveying for contamination. Any indications of radiation levels higher than natural background radiation are potential areas of contamination and, in general, areas which register more than twice the background level are considered contaminated.

Contamination usually refers to the presence of unsealed and unwanted radionuclides;

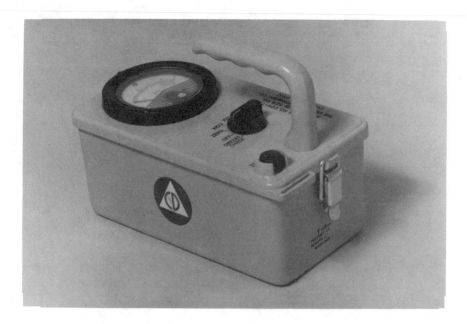

FIGURE 3.   Model 715R high-range Geiger counter.

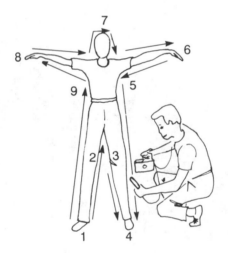

FIGURE 4.   Survey of an individual. The same survey pattern is
repeated on the back of the individual.

however, survey meters are also capable of detecting continuous radiation emitted from
other sources, such as an encapsulated radioactive source used perhaps for industrial radiography. If a radiation field is present, it is difficult to assess the possibility or presence
of contamination on a patient until the patient is removed from the radiation field. This is
because the survey meters are essentially unable to distinguish between radiation from a
source and radiation emanating from radioactive contamination. Use of the audio portion of
the meter has both advantages and disadvantages. If the audio portion is turned off, one
must simultaneously watch both the position of the probe with respect to the patient and the
meter. Under these circumstances, it is easy to touch the probe to a contaminated area and
contaminate the probe itself. To avoid contaminating the probe, it should be covered with

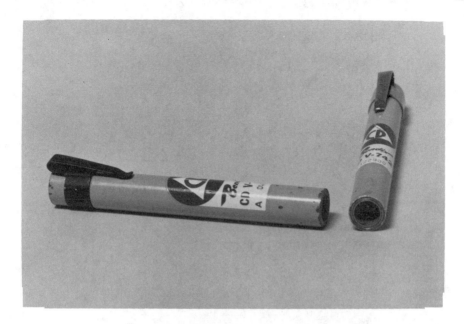

FIGURE 5. Personnel or "pencil" dosimeters.

a plastic food storage bag or a surgical glove. The main disadvantage of the use of the audio portion is that in situations in which the patient is already apprehensive about radiation, even a small amount of contamination will result in a significant audio output. This may significantly increase the patient's apprehension and concern out of proportion to the actual hazard.

C. SCINTILLATION DETECTORS

Scintillation detectors are much more expensive than either ionization chambers or Geiger-type counters. They are also very sensitive to physical shock. However, these disadvantages are overcome by a considerably improved efficiency. These detectors utilize a dense crystal. Interaction of ionizing radiation with the crystal results in a scintillation, or light flash, which is recorded by a photomultiplier tube. The major advantage of such a detector over the other types of detectors is that it is possible to assess the energy of the incident radiation since the intensity of the light flash is proportional to the amount of energy. Another advantage of such a detector is that once the energies of the incident radiation are identified, one can identify the radionuclide involved.

III. PERSONNEL DOSIMETERS

The purpose of personnel dosimeters is to provide an estimate of individual absorbed dose. Hospital personnel are already familiar with at least one form of these devices, i.e., film badges. There are two basic types of personnel dosimeters, the pencil or pocket dosimeter and the thermoluminescent dosimeter (TLD) or film badge.

A. PENCIL OR POCKET DOSIMETERS

These devices are approximately 1.5 cm in diameter, about 15 cm long (Figure 5) and have a clip to attach the dosimeter to the user's clothing. The dosimeter is basically an air-filled ionization chamber. The dosimeter must be charged prior to use (Figure 6A). This is performed by pushing down on the dosimeter while the distal end is inserted into a charging device. When this is done, the scale at the end of the device is illuminated and, by turning

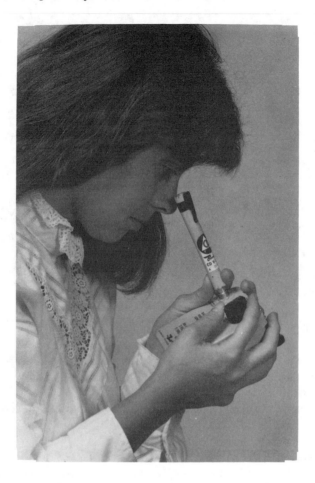

A

FIGURE 6.   (A). Pencil dosimeter being charged using the charging unit. The dosimeter must be pushed down to engage the charging unit contacts. (B). Reading the pencil dosimeter by looking toward a light.

a knob on the charger, the scale indicator can be positioned to the zero mark. This charges the unit and, as ionization occurs, the charge within the unit is reduced and the indicator line moves up the scale. Reading the dosimeter requires no special instrumentation and can be done immediately. Reading is accomplished by looking through the dosimeter at a bright light as illustrated in Figure 6B. An example of the image that one might see at the end of a dosimeter is shown in Figure 7.

Pencil ionization dosimeters are easy to use and do provide an instant measure of the accumulated exposure to that portion of the individual. Thus, while caring for a patient who is contaminated, one is able to occasionally look at the dosimeter to obtain an estimate of one's own absorbed dose. Unfortunately, the pencil dosimeters do not provide a permanent record and, thus, it is important to record this information. Another disadvantage is that these dosimeters are very sensitive to shock and they may go offscale by being dropped on the floor or bumped against a hard surface. Pocket dosimeters can be purchased in a varied range of sensitivities, for example from 0 to 100 mR or 0 to 10 R. Overall, the accuracy of the devices is not as great as TLDs or film badges.

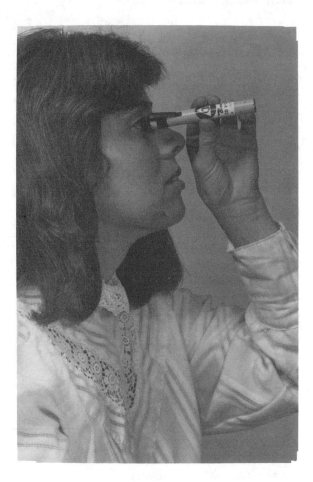

FIGURE 6B.

B. THERMOLUMINESCENT DOSIMETERS

These devices are very similar in appearance to a standard film badge. Both TLDs and film badges suffer from the disadvantage of not providing an instantaneous readout and the absorbed dose to an individual is only ascertained after the fact. TLDs contain crystalline or powdered material which, when heated, gives off light in proportion to the amount of radiation absorbed. These materials are very sensitive to radiation and yet they are very stable. TLDs are able to store the information without being read for days or months. They are also reusable, since after heating or annealing, they are again ready to accumulate information. TLDs are able to record absorbed doses accurately in the range of 10 to 1,000,000 mR. Unfortunately, the TLD is unable to provide information concerning the energy of the incident radiation. Another disadvantage is that only one reading of the crystalline material is possible, and if a mistake is made while processing, it is not possible to retrieve the information.

C. FILM BADGES

In contrast to a TLD, the film badge is able to provide a permanent record. Film badges are not as sensitive to radiation as TLDs; however, they are able (through placement of shielding outside the film) to give some estimate of the incident radiation energy as well as the absorbed dose. There are technical problems which have limited the use of film badges in some accident situations, such as stapling the film badge to a piece of paper prior to

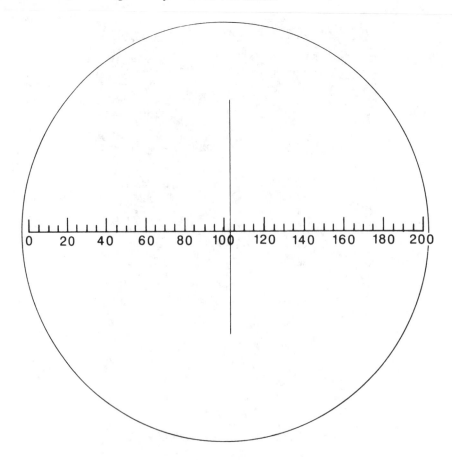

FIGURE 7.   Example of pencil dosimeter scale reading of 103 mR.

processing and allowing light to leak onto the film through the staple hole. Additionally, leaving a film badge in an area which is hot (in excess of 130°F.) also will cause the emulsion to be darkened when processing occurs. Film badges tend to be somewhat less inexpensive than TLDs. Both TLDs and film badges must be replaced periodically as they will record accumulated natural background radiation prior to, during, and after an accident, thus a TLD or film badge which has been in storage for 6 months will already have a baseline reading of between 50 and 150 mR.

It is important during management of a radioactively contaminated patient to have the film badge or TLD in a protected environment. If contamination from the patient were to get on the film badge, it would continue to expose the film badge or TLD even after it was taken off and thus give an erroneously high reading. In most radiation accident management situations, it is prudent to wear both a pocket or pencil dosimeter and either a TLD or film badge. This allows one to have an instantaneous and accessible estimate of radiation dose (from the pencil dosimeter) as well as a slightly more accurate method (TLD or film badge) that can be processed after the accident.

There is always a great discussion as to the proper placement of personnel dosimeters. Generally, they are worn either on the collar or at the belt level. Presently there are no regulations which require placement in a certain anatomical location. Most of these devices also have a serial number which should ultimately be placed on a dosimeter log and recorded with the wearer's name and social security number. The reading of the pen dosimeter should also be recorded on the same sheet of paper and an example of a dosimeter log is provided in Appendix 1, Section 6.

IV. PHYSICAL ASSESSMENT OF ABSORBED DOSE

At absorbed doses in excess of 25 rad (0.25 Gy) to the whole body and in excess of 100 rad (1.0 Gy) to the extremities, ultimate patient management depends on biological dosimetry and tissue response. In such instances, film badges and TLDs are only of supporting value. With lower absorbed doses, however, there are few if any biological findings and in these circumstances, personnel dosimeters, accident reconstruction, and history are the most important factors in dose assessment. The methods of biological assessment have been discussed earlier in Chapters 5, 6, and 8.

A. USE OF PERSONNEL DOSIMETERS

Some of the limitations of these devices have been discussed earlier in this chapter. Of course, their use for dose estimation purposes is only helpful in an accidental situation where an occupationally exposed person who was already wearing such a dosimeter was involved in the accident. In over half the accidents which are evaluated each year, no dosimeters have been worn. Another limitation is that dosimeters only will measure the dose to the single point on the body where the dosimeter was worn. Several graphic examples have been given in other chapters which indicate that in accidental situations there may be extreme dose gradients over very short distances and thus a film badge or TLD worn on the waist may not accurately reflect midline body dose or maximal dose to the patient, both of which are much more clinically relevant. Another difficulty with personnel dosimeters is the limitation imposed by the beam direction and possible shielding of the dosimeter by the body. For example, if a personnel dosimeter has a reading of 20 rad (0.2 Gy), this will not be clinically significant if, in fact, it was an entrance dose. If, however, this represents the exit dose from the patient and the radiation was not very penetrating, then the entrance dose on the opposite side of the patient from the film badge could have been hundreds of rads (Gy). As has been pointed out in Chapter 2, probably the most common type of serious radiation accident involves handling of an unsuspected but highly intense radioactive source. In these circumstances, the fingers of the hand may have absorbed doses in excess of 10,000 rad (100 Gy), but due to the inverse-square law and rapid dropoff of radiation exposure with distance, a film badge worn on the belt may only have recorded 50 rad (0.5 Gy). One could easily imagine similar problems with dosimeter interpretation when a radioactive source was inadvertently placed in a pocket and the dosimeter was worn on the collar. Although there are significant limitations to use of data from such dosimeters, they do at least provide a single data point in time and space which is better than nothing.

B. HISTORY

The importance of early, detailed, and accurate recording of the accident history cannot be overemphasized. The following will present at least a partial list of data that should be obtained in order to have a useful history:

- Name of patient
- Employer
- Company
- Physical injuries and treatment
- Skin surface contamination, including location, dose rate, and decontamination procedures utilized, if applicable.
- Internal contamination, including radionuclide chemistry, particle size, and suspected route of contamination (other useful information in this regard would include nasal counts, wound counts, whole-body counts, and bioassay samples already collected.)
- Evaluation of exposure to penetrating radiation, including precise location and position of patient relative to the radiation source at the time of exposure

- Exact time and duration of exposure
- Was dosimeter worn? Where? What type?
- Where is the current location of the dosimeter?
- Symptoms such as nausea, vomiting, anorexia or diarrhea and the exact time of occurrence of each
- Have blood counts or cytogenetic samples been obtained for biologic dosimetry purposes?
- Home phone number of individual as well as contact at work
- Were any other individuals present during the accidental exposure and if so who were they and where are they?
- Has source of exposure been terminated or does a possibility for continuing exposure of other persons still exist?

Such a history will quickly identify whether you are dealing with a significant radiation accident, an incident, or essentially a nonaccident or imaginary event.

C. ACCIDENT RECONSTRUCTION

Often the history will be sufficient to give a fairly reasonable dose estimate, provided the nature of the radiation source is accurately identified. In circumstances in which there has been a very steep gradient of exposure or in which several people are involved and there may be shielding, reconstruction of the accident situation may be useful. In such circumstances, a phantom of soft tissue equivalent which has a skeleton within it can be utilized. Such Rando-type phantoms are made with horizontal sections, each being about 1 cm thick. There are holes in which TLDs can be placed while the accident is reconstructed. If the source of exposure is then activated again, one may determine with a reasonable degree of accuracy what the dose distribution was within the body. Such reconstruction may be useful to determine prognosis and therapy of the patient. As one example, it is often difficult for clinicians to determine the best spot to look for surviving bone marrow and phantom reconstructions can give dose estimates to the bone marrow in different portions of the skeleton.

V. RADIATION ACCIDENTS, INCIDENTS, AND NONACCIDENTS

Significant accidents have had their criteria listed in Chapter 2. Generally, these represent whole-body absorbed doses under 25 rad (0.25 Gy) and doses to extremeties under several hundred rad (several Grays). At absorbed-dose levels less than these, biological damage is minimal and biological changes are difficult, if not impossible, to detect. We prefer to classify exposures from this range down to acute exposures in the range of 1 rad (10 mGy) as radiation *incidents*. In this dose range there would be no detectable nonstochastic effects, although there may be a slightly increased risk for stochastic effects such as cancer.

Events in which acute doses approach the range of the natural background that one might receive in a year or lower (<200 mrad or 2 mGy) essentially represent *nonaccidents*. Unfortunately, the potentially exposed person may not see it this way and future legal problems are certainly a possibility. Thus, even in situations where absorbed dose is likely to be non-existent or negligible, it is still useful to document incidents and nonaccidents in a file. Such files should contain at least some elements of the history, allegations, and how the conclusion was reached that the exposure was negligible. It is also important to meet with the individual, discuss the event, and reassure him or her. Of course, every radiation safety officer has at least one story of the amount of time and effort taken to deal with an individual who is convinced that he or she is a victim of alien death rays, a malfunctioning television set, or microwave oven which is influencing his or her personality and vital energies. There is no easy solution to such problems other than reassurance, although in most cases this is of little avail and the person will leave unhappy and attempt to seek another source of consultation.

At this point, it may be useful to give several examples of how physicians would handle specific incidents or nonaccident events that occur in hospital settings. Useful tables and information for all such situations can be found in References 1 to 3.

A. EXAMPLE 1

A pregnant hospital visitor mistakenly arrives on a patient transport elevator. In the same elevator is a radiation therapy patient being returned to the floor after having had a ^{137}Cs implant performed. The pregnant visitor is concerned about the radiation exposure and asks whether she should have an abortion. An estimate of the dose to the fetus can be made with a few simple calculations. Measurement of the patient reveals that the highest radiation level 1 m from the patient was <50 mR/h. The elevator ride could only have taken a few minutes. Thus the surface dose to the visitor was about 3 mrem (30 μSv). The fetus was shielded inside the mother and the fetal dose, therefore, is probably in the range of 1 to 2 mrem (10 to 20 μSv). The patient can then be reassured and told than no fetal abnormalities have been identified in humans at dose levels of <10 rem (100 mSv) to the fetus. The patient can also be told that the amount of radiation received is approximately the same amount of cosmic radiation that the fetus would get if the mother flew in a jet from New York to Los Angeles.

B. EXAMPLE 2

A 26-year-old mother was asked to hold her 2-year-old son while a skull series was obtained. Six weeks later the radiology department was notified that the mother was pregnant at the time she held her son and did not remember being given a lead apron to wear. The technologist who performed the examination cannot remember anything about that specific examination. An estimate of the radiation dose to the fetus can be made on the basis of determining whether the mother held the son's skull directly over her abdomen or was sitting next to the table. In the worse case, where the mother was in the direct X-ray beam, the surface exposure to the mother's abdomen was probably in the range of 200 mrad (2m Gy). Attenuation by the mother's overlying soft tissues in this case would be a factor of 4. Thus fetal exposure is in the range of 50 mrad (0.5 mGy). One could explain to the mother in this instance that this is about the same amount of additional radiation as if the mother had spent half of her pregnancy in Denver or Salt Lake City as compared to some city at sea level.

C. EXAMPLE 3

A patient in the hospital has been injected with 20 mCi (740 MBq) of ^{99}Tc phosphate for a bone scan. Four hours later a nurse spills the urine collection bag on the floor of the patient's room. The nurse estimated that she was in the room for approximately 20 min while cleaning up the spill, without realizing the urine was likely to contain radioactivity. Approximately half of the injected dose is expected to be eliminated in the urine in the first several hours. Thus, if 10 mCi (370 MBq) of technetium were spread on the floor and the physical decay was calculated, the exposure level to the waist of a person standing in the middle of such a spill would be approximately 30 mR/h. Assuming the nurse had bent over to clean up the spill, the dose may be slightly higher than this per hour though if she had only spent 20 min in the area, it is unlikely that she has received a whole-body dose of >20 mrad (0.2 mGy).

D. EXAMPLE 4

A nurse in the recovery room has had her film badge report returned and the reading was an absorbed dose of 50 rad (0.5 Gy). Obviously, such a dose, if true, is a significant radiation accident and had this represented an exit dose on the patient, whole-body midline dose could easily exceed 100 rad (1 Gy). Thus, one should immediately contact the nurse and find out whether or not there has been a history of nausea, vomiting, or anorexia. A complete blood count (CBC) with a differential should also be performed to evaluate the absolute lymphocyte count. Assuming both of these yield negative results, one may assume that the midline body dose did not exceed 50 rad (0.5 Gy). Unfortunately, one would like to be sure the dose was not even this high and cytogenetic analysis could be performed. Cytogenetic evaluation for dicentrics is usually capable of determining if the individual received an absorbed whole-body dose in excess of 10 rad (0.1 Gy). The cytogenetic examination takes approximately 1 week of a technologist's time to perform. While waiting for these results one can evaluate the environment of the nurse to determine whether there may be an unsuspected radioactive source. This can be done with a survey meter in the working environment, and if the nurse had taken the personnel dosimeter home, it would be also prudent to survey the nurse's automobile and home. One could also call the film badge company to find out whether there had been an error or some unusual occurrence in processing that particular film badge or batch of badges.

E. EXAMPLE 5

A thyroid cancer patient has just received a therapeutic dose of 100 mCi (3700 MBq) of ^{131}I. A few minutes later the patient vomits and a significant amount of the material contaminates a nurse standing nearby. If one third of the material is on the nurse's clothing, then a reasonable representative dose rate to the skin is 40 mrad (0.4 mGy)/h/cm². This dose rate would be a 50/50 mixture of gamma and beta components. We assume that there is a 20-min delay before the nurse can change clothes and the whole-body dose is in the range of 200 mrad (2 mGy). The important aspect of such an accident in dose evaluation is to determine how long the material remained on the nurse, since iodine can be absorbed through the skin and rapidly concentrated by the thyroid. If only 1% of the 30 mCi (1100 MBq) on the nurse was absorbed through the skin, the absorbed dose to the thyroid of the nurse is about 300 rad (3 Gy). Use of blocking agents has been discussed in Chapter 10 and, in this particular instance, administration of a supersaturated solution of iodide or a potassium iodide tablet would have been very important to block radioiodine uptake by the thyroid.

VI. SUMMARY

In summary, there is a wide variety of survey instruments which can be utilized both in accident management and in estimation of absorbed dose. Personnel dosimeters also may be used, but have some limitations which must be recognized. In cases in which there has been a significant radiation accident, use of biological indicators should take precedence over physical assessment of dosimetry. Accident reconstruction can be useful in patient management to give an idea of the absorbed dose distribution throughout the body. Physical dosimetry becomes particularly important in estimation of lower absorbed doses where no biological damage is evident. Probably the most important aspect of dose estimation is in obtaining an accurate and detailed history.

REFERENCES

1. **Shleien, B. and Terpilak, M.,** *The Health Physics and Radiological Health Handbook,* Nuclear Lectern Associates, Olney, MD, 1984.
2. **Kereiakes, J. G. and Rosenstein, M.,** *Handbook of Radiation Doses in Nuclear Medicine and Diagnostic X-ray,* CRC Press, Boca Raton, FL, 1980.
3. **Glaze, S., Schneiders, N., and Bushong, S. C.,** A computer assisted procedure for estimating patient exposure and fetal dose in radiological examinations, *Radiology,* 145, 187, 1982.

Chapter 19

JUDICIAL AUTOPSY OF RADIATION ACCIDENTS

Phillip M. Kannan

TABLE OF CONTENTS

I. INTRODUCTION — SCIENCE OUTSIDE THE LABORATORY

If a radiation accident leads to litigation, science and law will be focused on the events and relied on to resolve the dispute. The interaction of these two disciplines will be very complex; it certainly goes beyond a separatist's view that science will provide the substance, and law the procedure for adjudicating the issues. In analyzing the relationship of science and law, one must keep in mind that throughout its history, science has been influenced by many social, nonscientific forces. On some occasions, science could not avoid the interference; on others, it chose not to avoid it. An example of the first type of intervention taken from the science of astronomy and one of the second type taken from medicine will be discussed briefly to illustrate how complex the interaction between science and social forces can be.

Nicholas Copernicus postulated the heliocentric system of the universe which was contrary to the accepted interpretation of the Scriptures. Because of the "strong opposition and violent hostility that would be aroused by the propagation of his theory", he refused to publish it until the year of his death in 1543. And hostility there was. Vaucouleurs described it as follows:

"The battle aroused by the new system . . . lasted for more than three centuries during which, as Bigourdon pointed out, *'Science very frequently played only the smallest part.'* "

"Feeling that they were losing the battle on the factual front, the defenders of the traditional teachings . . . turned to the temporal power of the Church . . . and after long and tortuous debate, they managed to have Copernicus' book placed on the Index in 1616 . . ."[1]

A recent, in fact continuing, example[2] of science choosing to be influenced by a social force involves efforts of the American Psychiatric Association to include three new psychiatric disorders in its official diagnostic manual. The disorders are premenstrual syndrome, self-defeating personality, and sadistic personality. The opposition to including these disorders did not come from the psychiatric community, but from feminist groups, and it was not based on scientific arguments. The opponents argued that diagnoses of either of the personality disorders could provide a defense to prosecution for wife-beating and child abuse, and the other disease would stigmatize women with menstrual problems. As of this date, a compromise has been reached. The conditions will be included in an appendix of the manual. The meaning of this is unclear since never before has a "disease" been in an appendix. It cannot represent a solution since it solves neither the psychiatrists' nor the feminists' problem.

In the U.S., courts have been pressed into the service of making scientific decisions and at times have rejected the consensus which represented the judgment of an entire branch of science. One such incidence of this occurred in *Helling* vs. *Carey*.[3]

Ms. Helling first consulted Dr. Carey in 1959 for myopia; he prescribed contact lenses. He saw her several times in 1967 and 1968 for what he concluded were problems related to the lenses. In October 1968 (when Ms. Helling was 32), for the first time he tested her eye pressure and field of vision and found she had primary open-angle glaucoma. She had no peripheral vision and greatly reduced central vision. In the lawsuit filed by Ms. Helling against Dr. Carey, the medical experts for both Dr. Carey and Ms. Helling all testified that the standards for the profession did not require routine pressure tests for glaucoma for patients under 40 years of age. The Supreme Court of Washington, made up of lawyers not physicians, disagreed with the profession of ophthalmology. It stated:

"The precaution of giving this test to detect the incidence of glaucoma to patients under 40 years of age is so imperative that irrespective of its disregard by the standards of the ophthalmology profession, it is the duty of the courts to say what is required to protect patients under 40 from the damaging results of glaucoma."[4]

As this case shows, standards of a profession can be disregarded by a court. However, such decisions are very rare; compliance with professional or industry standards is a strong defense. This is an important fact in radiation litigation because the radiation industry is so heavily regulated. The role of standards is discussed later in this chapter.

The intervention of courts in science is not an infrequent event. David L. Bazelon, Senior Circuit Judge, U.S. Court of Appeals for the District of Columbia Circuit, Washington, D.C. stated "The caseload of our court today predominately involves challenges to federal administrative action relating to the frontiers of technology."[5] At the same time Judge Bazelon points out that courts are being called upon to resolve scientific questions, he acknowledges the technical inadequacy of judges to do so. He asks, "What judge knows enough to understand issues on the frontiers of nuclear physics, toxicology, and other specialities informing health and safety regulations?"[6]

The answer is there are none; they must be educated in each case. However, there are few lawyers with sufficient scientific background to prepare and present a case involving such issues in a way that will facilitate the courts' efforts to understand and properly resolve the issues, and there are few scientists who understand the judicial process well enough to aid the court.

Each deficiency reduces the probability that a scientifically valid result will be reached. While there is no quantitative way to estimate how these deficiencies combine — additively, multiplicatively, or more likely exponentially — it is clear that the worst case occurs when all three are present in the same case. These deficiencies are discussed below.

The litigation which almost always follows radiation accidents in the U.S. presents the opportunity for the conjunction of these three. Such cases involve unfamiliar forces, measured in unfamiliar units, with uncertain effects over extended time. Moreover, the injury which is alleged to have resulted from radation exposure is likely to have many nonradiation causes.

To see that the last stage of a radiation accident is almost always litigation, consider the case of William Jack Eppes vs. Duke Power Company.[7] Mr. Eppes, an employee of Duke Power Company, worked on one occasion for 2 h and 25 min in a radiation control area. During this time, he wore protective clothing consisting of a paper suit which was taped at the wrists and ankles, rubber shoes, and a helmet with an air line attached. He wore a badge-dosimeter on his chest. He testified that he removed his helmet and face mask for approximately 4 to 5 min. His badge-dosimeter had a reading of zero.

Mr. Eppes developed multiple myeloma and filed a claim with the South Carolina Workers' Compensation Commission alleging that this 2 h and 25 min of exposure and other unspecified radiation during his 11 years of employment with Duke Power Company caused the disease. Although there was mention of this other possible exposure, the adjudication in fact involved only the 2 h and 25 min of exposure. The Commission found that the external dose was 8 mrem and the internal dose was 10 mrem. Thus, there was an 800-page record, a voluminous exhibit file, and a 73-page decision in a battle over 8 and 10 mrems.

The court which tries the case filed after a radiation accident will be called upon to make a decision based on uncertainty. That is an inherent property of all trials. It results from the fact that a trial is an attempt to recreate the past through the testimony of witnesses and documents. However, memories are inexact, imperfect, subject to bias, incomplete, and documents require interpreters who will introduce their bias, understandings, and limitations. This uncertainty of facts gives rise to a risk that an incorrect decision will be made by the judge.

II. REDUCING RISK OF INCORRECT DECISION IN RADIATION LITIGATION

One way to reduce the risk of an incorrect decision is to reduce the uncertainty faced by the judge. This conclusion has certain implications for a physician who may be called upon to treat a radiation-accident victim. The first is that such a physician wants a record of his treatment of the victim. Written procedures regarding treatment of such victims which specify what the physician planned to do may be the basis of what was actually done. Often they help sharpen memories by providing a framework. The usual procedure of patient care often generates an important part of a written record of the treatment. Requests for services from support groups such as pathology laboratories and the reports generated are vital parts of the record. Instructions to staff, orders to the hospital pharmacy, every scrap of paper that is pertinent must be collected and saved.

An important part of the standard procedure is obtaining the written consent for the proposed treatment from the patient. To withstand legal challenge, this must be "informed consent". Generally, this must include a disclosure of the significant risks associated with the proposed treatment and alternatives to it. This includes those risks which the physician knows or should know that a reasonable person in the patient's position would consider significant in making a choice among the treatment alternatives.[8]

There are often documents other than the hospital and physician records which are of critical importance in litigations arising from a radiation accident. These are documents from the accident site. These include periodic reports filed with the Environmental Protection Agency, the Nuclear Regulatory Commission, and various state agencies, and appraisals and audits conducted by or for such agencies. Such reports may indicate such things as what radioactive material is present, at what levels, and what safety record and accident history the facility has. Service records and manufacturer's specifications for any equipment involved in the accident may prove useful. There may be accident reports resulting from internal investigations or an investigation by a regulatory agency of the state or federal government.

Any document of the type described in the above paragraphs should be obtained and preserved. They will be useful in reconstructing the accident for the court at trial. Since they are likely to have been prepared not with a view to litigation, they are often open and frank.

All documents should be carefully reviewed, summarized, indexed, and securely stored. All documents, including all copies, should be in one place. Access to these should be controlled by one person. This is an effort to ensure that when they are needed to reconstruct the past in preparation for trial and at trial, the documents will be available and accessible.

III. EXPLAINING SCIENCE TO JUDGES OR JURIES

A second way to reduce the risk of an incorrect decision in radiation litigation is to have the science involved in the case explained in court by experts in such a way that the judge or jury can understand it. Explaining science to laymen in such a way that it will be comprehended is not an impossible task. In commenting on his book *The Making of the Atomic Bomb*, Richard Rhodes stated, "Niels Bohr once said he could explain all of physics without using a mathematical formula."[9]

This is the sort of explanation the judge or jury will need. That science can be made comprehensible to judges is clear to anyone who reads Judge Kelly's decision in Johnston vs. The U.S.;[10] this decision reads like a primer in radiation. The judge's education resulted from the "teachings from superb witnesses". To be a superb witness, technical knowledge is necessary, but not sufficient. The scientist-witness must understand the context, that is, the trial, in which his testimony will be given. The importance of context to meaning is not unique to judicial proceedings. Consider the following statement regarding Greek history: "Until recently, the story of the Bactrian Greeks has been relegated to Indian history, where it has no meaning, but now, fragmentary evidence has been sorted and arranged, so that we have, not four, but five Hellenistic dynasties."[11]

The scientist-witness must "sort and arrange" his evidence to meet the needs of the court. In order to do that, however, the scientist-witness must understand the basic workings of the judicial process. He must know the context into which his testimony will fit; otherwise, it will have the same fate in the trial that the Kingdom of Bactria suffered in Indian history.

Giving the scientist-witness the background necessary to understand the context means explaining to him the judicial process starting with the document which initiates it. He must understand the trial strategy and the role his testimony will play in it. Not only will this aid the scientist-witness, but as the following discussion shows, it will also help his attorney prepare and present his case.

The judicial process is begun when a person called the plaintiff files with the court a document called a complaint. The rules for federal courts, which have served as a model for states, describe the complaint as "a short and plain statement of the claim showing that the pleader is entitled to relief and a demand for judgment for the relief to which he deems himself entitled."[12]

The rules under which radiation accidents will be litigated typically call for a period, called the discovery period, during which each party can obtain information and documents from the other. For each party, the purposes of discovery are (1) to find out what it does not know, (2) to find out what the other party knows, (3) to pin down the other party's version, and (4) to marshal and focus evidence.

The federal rules[13] enable each party to serve written questions, called interrogatories, on the other which must be answered under oath, provided they are reasonably calculated to lead to the discovery of admissible evidence. The scientist-witness has a very important role to play regarding interrogatories. First, he should advise his attorney of the information to seek through interrogatories. For example, if the plaintiff is alleging that he has cancer of the lungs which resulted from exposure to radiation from an accident in the defendant's facility, the scientist-witness would be aware of the possible "host" factors in radiation carcinogenesis and would help his attorney prepare questions to develop the information needed to evaluate these possible factors.[14]

Second, he should assist his attorney in the preparation of answers to the interrogatories served by the other side. Both of these activities give the scientist-witness important information which will assist him in understanding the factual context in which his testimony will be placed.

In the discovery period, each party will be able to obtain all documents which are reasonably associated with the action.[15] The scientist-witness can assist his attorney in this endeavor. In the example given above, the scientist-witness will know of medical procedures which involve radiation to the patient. He will know to suggest types of documents which usually result from such medical procedures. Moreover, he will be able to identify other possible causes of the cancer and assist his attorney in preparing specific requests for documents which may be relevant to those causes. For example, if stomach cancer is the disease, the physician can suggest that, since hiatal hernia can cause this disease, the attorney should inquire as to whether or not the claimant had such a condition and if so, request all pertinent documents. The scientist-witness will also be able to identify regulatory reports which contain relevant data. The data which the document production phase of discovery process reveals will add to the scientist-witness' understanding of the theories being developed by each party and will enhance his ability to put his testimony in context to be more useful to the judge later at the trial.

The third method of discovery which most judicial proceedings include is the taking of depositions.[16] This is the answering under oath of questions posed by the other party's attorney. The questioning will take place outside the courtroom (no judge will be present), and it will be transcribed verbatim. A deposition properly taken will reveal all that the witness knows about the case and will freeze his version. If, later at a trial, the witness deviates from the version given at a deposition, he will be confronted and questioned about "changing his story". Thus, it is very important to be well prepared for a deposition. The witness should know what to expect in it and have the testimony he intends to give later in court well under control.

IV. WHO IS THE TEACHER AND WHAT SHOULD BE TAUGHT?

At the beginning of litigation which results from a radiation accident, it is clear who the teacher is. It is the scientist-witness. He must teach his attorney the fundamental scientific concepts which are operative in the case. The lawyer probably does not know what ionizing radiation is. He probably does not understand the concept of radiation dose, dose response, and the many other scientific concepts involved. The discovery process is a good time for the scientist to educate the lawyer. He should receive a course in the basic concepts of radiation which are relevant to the litigation. This is not an effort to make the lawyer a health physicist or physician. It is not necessary that he know and understand the equation:

$$\overline{Z}^2 = \zeta D + D^2$$

where Z is the microdosimetric quantity specific energy, D the absorbed dose, and ζ is the ratio of the second and first moments of the frequency distribution of specific energies produced by single events.[17]

Neither the lawyer nor the judge needs this information and certainly neither needs to be able to derive it or to understand how it is derived. The scientist must give sufficient detail to explain his version in a technically valid way, but not so much that it becomes incomprehensible to a layman. A scientist who cannot teach an introductory course in his field because he has difficulty bringing the level down to what is consistent with the background of the the students will have problems striking the proper balance between information that illuminates an issue and detail which obscures it.

At the same time that the attorney is a student learning from the scientist, he is a teacher from whom the scientist learns about the judicial process and learns how to be a deponent and how to be a witness. Neither of these skills is innate; they must be learned. The lawyer-teacher faces the same dilemma regarding what to teach as did the scientist-teacher. The intricacies of the hearsay rule are of no use to the scientist. However, a solid understanding of leading questions can be of great use. The scientist, who is familiar with the notion of approximation and estimation, will quickly understand that it is better for him to give his answer in his own words rather than allowing someone else to choose words which may only be an approximation to the answer he wishes to give. His words will provide a more exact response and are preferable.

Two legal concepts which the lawyer should explain carefully to his medical expert witness are "preponderance of evidence" and "reasonable degree of medical certainty".

In a radiation case, the jury, if there is one, is the trier of fact; if there is no jury, the judge will be the trier of fact. In either event, the trier of fact must resolve the disputed factual issues. In almost all the cases the standard applied by the trier of fact is proof by a preponderance of the evidence. This amounts to proof which leads the trier of fact to find that the existence of the contested fact is more probable than its nonexistence.[18] Put in other words, it is synonymous with the term "greater weight of the evidence".[19]

This is the test most likely to be applied in litigation resulting from a radiation accident. However, there are radiation cases which apply a different standard called the substantial factor test. The first case to do so was Allen vs. The U.S.[20] This test was stated as follows:

"Where a defendant who negligently creates a radiological hazard which puts an identifiable population group at increased risk, and a member of that group at risk develops a biological condition which is consistent with having been caused by the hazard to which he has been negligently subjected, such consistency having been demonstrated by substantial, appropriate, persuasive, and connecting factors, a fact finder *may* reasonably conclude that the hazard caused the condition absent persuasive proof to the contrary offered by the defendant."[21]

If applied, this test in effect changes the requirement from plaintiff having to provide causation to plaintiff only having to prove that he has a condition "consistent with having been caused" by the negligent conduct of the defendant. The quantum of proof necessary for this is "substantial, appropriate, persuasive, connecting". Clearly, this test is less demanding than the "preponderance of the evidence" standard.

There is no short definition for "reasonable degree of medical certainty". This standard applies to the physician who is called to testify and accepted by the judge as an expert witness. After relevant facts have been made available to him, the physician will be asked if he has an opinion to a reasonable degree of medical certainty whether or not those facts caused the injury. If he says that he does, he will be allowed to give that opinion. The purpose of imposing the reasonable degree of medical certainty standard is to prevent the giving of testimony that is merely speculative or conjectural. Testimony given in terms of "distinct possibility" or "might have been" will not be accepted to prove a causal connection. It will be called speculative and rejected by the courts.[22]

The requirement of a reasonable degree of medical certainty ensures that the physician will apply the standards of his profession rather than his individual view. The question is whether or not a reasonable practitioner of the profession in his practice of it could form an opinion based on these facts. If he concludes that giving an opinion is consistent with those standards, he will be allowed to give it. One court phrased this requirement as follows:

"Physicians must understand that it is the intent of our law that if the plaintiff's medical expert cannot form an opinion with sufficient certainty so as to make a medical judgment, there is nothing on the record with which a jury can make a decision with sufficient certainty so as to make a legal judgment."[23]

There is no fixed probability associated with this standard. In fact, one court has held it was erroneous to assign a probability to it. The first time the case was tried, a physician certified as a medical expert (this concept is discussed below) testified that there was a 90% probability that the automobile accident from which the litigation resulted caused plaintiff's hernia. The court of appeals for Missouri held that this was not substantial evidence of causal connection between the hernia and the accident.[24] When the case was retried, the same physician testified that within reasonable medical certainty he was of the opinion that the hernia was caused by the accident. This was accepted by the trial court and upheld by the court of appeals.[25] A radiation case holding that statistical evidence showing a greater than 50% probability that radiation caused the injury does not satisfy the reasonable degree of medical certainty standard is discussed below.[26]

Ultimately, the judge is the student and the trial presents the opportunity for each party to teach him in litigation what resulted from a radiation accident. Each party will rely on documents and witnesses to persuade him to see the events as it does. This will be done by presenting witnesses who testify about facts. They are necessary in this type of litigation because they reconstruct the event. However, facts are not enough to decide the issues presented in such cases; opinions are also needed.

The court will have rules which determine what qualifications a witness must have before he can give opinions as part of his testimony. The Federal Rules of Evidence which apply to all trials in federal court, and serve as a model for other courts, state:

"If scientific, technical, or other specialized knowledge will assist the trier of fact to understand the evidence or to determine a fact in issue, a witness qualified as an expert by knowledge, skill, experience, training, or education, may testify thereto in the form of an opinion or otherwise."[27]

A witness qualified to give opinion testimony is called an expert witness.

The structure of an expert's opinion testimony should resemble that of Euclid as he developed geometry or Peano as he developed the real numbers. The assumptions should be clearly identified and each conclusion and opinion should be supported by what has been developed previously. Careful preparation, coordination, and understanding by the expert and his lawyer are essential for this type of expert testimony. If properly done, it minimizes the risk that cross-examination will be effective.

An expert witness, of course, is permitted to give his opinion only in the field in which he has been recognized as an expert by the court. In radiation litigation, the two fields in which such testimony will always be called for are dose estimation and causation. Generally, dose estimations require one trained in radiation physics or health physics or, if cell damage is used to estimate dose, in cytogenetics. Opinions on causation are usually only given by physicians with some knowledge, skill, or experience in radiation effects. However, state workers' compensation laws may qualify experts in other fields to give opinions regarding causation; for example, in Krumback vs. Dow Chemical,[28] a Colorado statute required a claimant to show causation by "reasonable probability". The appeals court of Colorado held that as a matter of law, a health physicist was qualified to give an opinion regarding causation. Absent legislation to the contrary, causation should only be proved by medical testimony. In fact, when the health physicist who was allowed to give an opinion on causation in Krumback testified in a later court case, the judge characterized his report on causation by saying it is "not a medical opinion but is statistical sophistry".[29]

It is important to note that in the federal rule quoted above, expert testimony is not limited to giving opinions. The expert witness may also give an exposition of scientific or other principles relevant to the case. This is of great significance in radiation cases because it is an effective way to educate the judge or jury, if there is one, regarding the basic science involved in the case.

Part of learning to be a witness is learning how to respond to cross-examination. The general idea is to have cross-examinations resemble a cat-and-cat, rather than a cat-and-mouse, game. Some of the basic rules usually given to a witness are:

1. He is to listen to the question and if he understands it, to respond truthfully to it in his own words.
2. He is not to answer questions he does not understand.
3. He is not to argue with the lawyer cross-examining him.
4. He is not to lose his temper.
5. He is not to speculate or guess.

Developing an opinion in the manner of Euclid's model suggested above makes it easier to comply with these and similar rules on cross-examination. More important, however, such testimony will be easy for the judge to follow. If he learns from it, it will have served its purpose.

V. RADIATION STANDARDS AND STATISTICAL EVIDENCE

Radiation safety standards are often involved in radiation litigation. It is important that their meaning be explained to the court. If the dose to the plaintiff exceeds an applicable standard, the plaintiff may attempt to have the trier of fact infer that violation of the standard is proof that the plaintiff's injury was caused by the radiation. The theory and history of these standards make it clear that such an inference would not necessarily be correct. Referring to the standards, the judge in Johnston vs. U.S. stated:

"These standards have ranged from 72 rem/year down to 5 rem/year, but the reductions have not been made because there was any evidence of harm at the higher levels. The reductions were made because hospitals and industry could and were operating at these much lower doses already so there was no good reason to have standards set way above common practices."[30]

If the dose is below the applicable standard, defendant should be able to successfully argue that no harm resulted.[31] Referring to the 5 rem/year standard, Judge Foley found:

"The standards were established after thorough scientific review by the world's leading experts and are continually reviewed. Compliance with the standards is proof of a reasonable standard of conduct."[32]

When a court does reject compliance with professional or industrial standards as a defense, it is weighing the cost of meeting a higher standard against the potential benefit that would result from the new standard. Judge Learned Hand[33] suggested as a formula for this approach comparing the product of the probability of injury times the gravity of the resulting injury with the burden of adequate precautions. When a court balances such broad interests, it is, in effect, acting like a legislature and is being guided by "considerations of expediency and public policy".[34]

That the court in Helling vs. Carey (discussed above) engaged in this legislative type process is shown in the following quote from a concurring opinion:

"Where its (glaucoma's) presence can be detected by a simple, well-known, harmless test, where the results of the test are definitive, where the disease can be successfully arrested by early detection, and where its effects are irreversible if undetected over a substantial period of time, liability should be imposed upon defendants though they did not violate the standard existing within the profession of ophthalmology."[35]

In the field of radiation protection, where allowable exposure limits have been established well below the level at which present data indicate that injury is likely to occur, it is very improbable that cost-benefit analysis would lead a court to reject these standards. Dramatically different epidemiological or medical results would be required. The court is hardly the arena for the introduction of such new theory. The test in Helling was not a new or experimental test; had it been the court's decision may well have been different. Before a scientific theory appears in court, it should have been tested in the peer review process which, although not perfect, provides the most nearly level field on which any clash of ideas can be resolved.

Epidemiology is frequently relied on to estimate the risk to populations associated with potentially harmful agents such as radiation.[36] The use of statistical methods to estimate characteristics of a population, in theory, is proper. It is when epidemiological studies are offered to establish causation for an individual that its value is doubtful. Here a balance must be struck between the usefulness of such evidence on the question of *potential* for causation and its inability to establish injury to a particular person. Judge Foley struck a very reasonable balance in the following holding:

"Epidemiological studies may not, as a matter of law, be singularly used to establish causation to the requisite degree of medical certainty. However, in conjunction with credible medical evidence and opinion, the statistical results of these studies can be a collateral, albeit not controlling, element of proof."[37]

Epidemiological evidence may be used by defendants to prove a *lack* of causation. Such proof was presented by the U.S. in Timothy vs. U.S.[38] However, the defendant, quite properly, did not base its defense exclusively on such reports; it also had the opinion of an eminent physician and professor with impressive clinical experience. The two types of evidence reinforce each other and result in a whole greater than the sum of the parts. A case in which the court found causation, even though all of the epidemiological studies indicated the opposite, is discussed below.[39]

When epidemiological evidence is presented, the expert giving the analysis should also testify regarding the strength of the causal inferences in the study. This can be done, for example, by measuring the study against the criteria, discussed by A. Bradford Hill,[40] of (1) strength of the association, (2) consistency of associations, (3) temporally correct association, (4) specificity of the association, and (5) coherence with existing knowledge. It is certainly sound strategy to assume that on cross-examination any weakness in the causal inferences will be brought out.

A dramatic change from the traditional judicial standards and procedures for establishing causation is under study. In 1983 legislation was enacted which directed the Secretary of Health and Human Services "to devise and publish radioepidemiological tables that estimate the likelihood that persons who have or have had any of the radiation-related cancers, and who have received specific doses prior to the onset of such disease, developed cancer as a result of these doses".[41] Such tables have been developed and published by the Ad Hoc Working Group of the National Institutes of Health.[42]

This approach to the causation question is based on a probabilistic approach and is referred to as probability of causation. It attempts to estimate the conditional probability that a cancer in a specific organ of an individual resulted from doses that individual received before the development of the cancer. To do this, statistical analysis of certain dose-response data was undertaken to estimate a baseline. Probability theory is then used to estimate relative excess risks.

It is too early to predict how this approach in general, and these tables in particular, will affect radiation litigation. The most likely use of them will be as a screen to identify claims which are clearly without merit.

Use of probability of causation will not eliminate litigation; it will at most change the emphasis of the dispute from the medical effect of a dose to the dose itself. The size of the dose will become the issue most vigorously contested since once that is established, the calculation of the probability of causation is mechanical; it requires no medical judgment or professional opinion.

VI. CONCLUSION

In the litigation which follows a radiation accident, a claimant calls on the legal system to adjudicate a dispute. Scientific questions are thrust upon the court. The legal system (through attorneys for the parties) then invites scientists to assist the court in resolving such questions. The invitation, however, does not allow the scientist to bring along his full kit. Experimentation, such as repeating the accident with dosimeters to gather more accurate data, is generally not allowed. Also, the scientist must give up his practice of choosing which questions he will pursue.

Perhaps to a scientist, adjudication appears too crude and cumbersome a method to resolve disputes which include scientific questions. That is too harsh a judgment. In fact, adjudication has much in common with the scientific method. They both require public disclosure of the evidence used to support a conclusion, both allow opponents to confront the evidence to test its stength and bias, and both allow a review of the evidence and the reasoning used to connect the evidence with the conlusion. The adjudicative process can be described as requiring open standards, open findings, and open precedent,[43] and a rational relationship (measured by the preponderance standard) between the findings and the decision. The scientific method includes these, but more than just a rational relationship is required. This difference results from the fact that society imposes on its adjudication institution the constraint that it must resolve disputes brought to it in a time acceptable to the political institutions. When radiation questions are adjudicated, that process and its rules and standards will supersede any from science which are not identical. The point that the rules and standards of law, not science, will control the adjudication of disputes which involve scientific questions was made quite dramatically in Wells vs. Ortho Pharmaceutical Corporation.[44] The issue in this case was whether a spermicide manufactured by the defendant and used by the mother of the plaintiff had caused her serious birth defects. The epidemiological evidence overwhelmingly supported the conclusion that spermicides are not teratogenic. The court found that causation had been proven in spite of this evidence. In discussing this case in an article in the New England Journal of Medicine, two scientists concluded that "the courts will not be bound by reasonable scientific standards of proof."[45]

Part of the process of educating the scientist to be an expert witness is for his lawyer to teach him that the court is not a forum in which scientists themselves will settle disputes, and to explain the legal standards which the court will apply as *it* resolves the dispute. The expert must present the scientific information in this context and make it accessible by eliminating unnecessary complexity. The power and persuasiveness of such testimony will be proportional to its simplicity, completeness, and clarity.*

The builders of the transcontinental railroad in the last century knew that to cover vast distances, it was wise to start at opposite boundaries and lay tracks toward a point of convergence. This same principle should be applied in attempting to get a court across the vast scientific landscape in a radiation case. The scientist must learn some law and the lawyer, some science. The point of convergence is a team which will be able to assist a nonscientist to correctly solve a scientific problem.

---

* This applies not only to the scientific content, but also to the language and sentence structure. For example, the sentence: "The individual member of the social community often receives his information via visual, symbolic channels" would be of no use in court because it would not be understood. However, the sentence suggested by Dr. Feynman as the equivalent would be understood easily: "People read."[46]

REFERENCES

1. **Vaucouleurs, G. De,** *Discovery of the Universe,* Faber & Faber Ltd., London, 1957, 44.
2. **Boffey, P. M.,** New Psychiatric Categories are Accepted, *The New York Times,* 14, July 2, 1986.
3. Helling vs. Carey, 519 P.2d 981, 983, (Washington, 1974).
4. Helling vs. Carey, 519 P.2d 981, 983, (Washington, 1974).
5. **Bazelon, D. L.,** Science, technology, and the court, *Science,* 208, 1, 1980.
6. **Bazelon, D. L.,** Science, technology, and the court, *Science,* 208, 1, 1980.
7. William Jack Epps vs. Duke Power Co., South Carolina Workers' Compensation Commission, Docket No. 68,532, October 31, 1986.
8. Canterburry vs. Spence, 464 F.2d 772 (D.C. Cir. 1972).
9. **Rhodes, R.,** Physics Anyone Could Understand, *The New York Times Book Review,* February 8, 1987, 39.
10. Johnston vs. U.S., 597 F. Suppl. 374 (D.C. Kansas 1984).
11. **Batsford, G. W. and Robinson, C. A., Jr.,** *Hellenic History,* 4th ed., Macmillan, New York, 1956, 423.
12. Fed. Rules Civ. Proc. Rule 8, 28 U.S.C.A.
13. Fed. Rules Civ. Proc. Rules 26 & 33, 28 U.S.C.A.
14. Committee on the Biological Effects of Ionizing Radiation, *The Effects on Population of Exposure to Low Levels of Ionizing Radiation,* National Academy Press, Washington, D.C., 1980, 26.
15. Federal Rules Civ. Proc., Rule 34, 28 U.S.C.A.
16. Federal Rules Civ. Proc., Rule 26 & 27 28 U.S.C.A.
17. Committee on the Biological Effects of Ionizing Radiation, *The Effects on Population of Exposure to Low Levels of Ionizing Radiation,* National Academy Press, Washington, D.C., 1980, 14.
18. **Cleary, E. W., Ed.,** *McCormick on Evidence,* 2nd ed., West Publishing, St. Paul, MN, 1972, 749.
19. 30 Am. Jur. 2d, Evidence § 1164.
20. Allen vs. U.S., 588 F. Suppl. 247 (D.C. Utah 1984), Reversed on other grounds ("discretionary function" defense applied), Allen vs. U.S., 816 F. 2d 1417 (10th Cir. 1987); Cert. Denied, ___ U.S. ___ (1988).
21. Allen vs. U.S., 588 F. Suppl. 247, (D. C. Utah 1984), Reversed on other grounds ("discretionary function" defense applied), Allen vs. U.S., 816 F. 2d 1417 (10th Cir. 1987); Cert. Denied, ___ U.S. ___ (1988), 415.
22. Vaux vs. Hamilton, 103 N.W. 2d 291 (N.D. 1960).
23. Fitzgerald vs. Manning, 679 F. 2d 341, 350 (4th Cir. 1982).
24. Bertram vs. Wunning, 385 S.W. 2d 803 (MO. App. 1965).
25. Bertram vs. Wunning, 417 S. W. 2d 120, (MO. App. 1967).
26. Johnston vs. U.S., 597 F. Suppl. 374, 412 (D.C. Kansas 1984).
27. Fed. Rules of Evidence, Rule 702.
28. Krumback vs. Dow Chemical Co., 676 P. 2d 1215 (Col. app. 1983), Cert. denied February 27, 1984.
29. Johnston vs. U.S., 597 F. Suppl. 374,412 (D.C. Kansas 1984).
30. Johnston vs. U.S., 597 F. Suppl. 374,412 (D.C. Kansas 1984), 425.
31. National Bureau of Standards, National Bureau of Standards Handbook 29, Washington, D.C., 26.
32. Roberts vs. U.S., page 113, Civil Action LV 1766 RDF, June 14, 1984 (D.C. Nevada 1984)
33. U.S. vs. Carroll Towing Co., 159 F. 2d 169 (2nd cir. 1947).
34. **Cleary, E. W., Ed.,** *McCormick on Evidence,* 2nd ed., West Publishing, St. Paul, MN, 1972, 766.
35. Helling vs. Carey 519 P. 2d 981, 985 (Washington 1974).
36. **Whittemore, A. S.,** Epidemiology in risk assessment for regulatory policy, *J. Chron. Dis.,* 39, 1157, 1986.
37. Roberts vs. U.S., pp. 116, Civil Action LV 1766 RDF, June 14, 1984 (D.C. Nevada 1984).
38. Timothy vs. U.S., 612 F. Suppl. 160, (D.C. Utah, Central Div. 1985).
39. Wells vs. Ortho Pharmaceutical Corp., 788 F. 2d 741 (11th Cir. 1986).
40. **Hill, A. B.,** The environment and disease: association or causation?, *Proc. R. Soc. Med.,* 58, 295, 1965.
41. Orphan Drug Act, Public Law 97-414, Section 7(b) (1983).
42. Ad hoc Working Group to Develop Radioepidemiological Tables, *Rep. Ad Hoc Working Group to Develop Radioepidemiological Tables,* NIH Publ. 85-2748, National Institutes of Health, U.S. Government Printing Office, Washington, D.C., 1985.
43. **Davis, K. C.,** *Administrative Law Text,* 3rd ed., West Publishing, St. Paul, MN, 1972, 342.
44. Wells vs. Ortho Pharmaceutical Corp., 788 F. 2d 741 (11th Cir. 1986).
45. **Mills, J. L. and Alexander, D.,** Teratogens and litogens, *N. Engl. J. Med.,* 315, 1234, 1986.
46. **Feynman, R. P.,** *Surely You're Joking, Mr. Feynman!* Bantam Books, New York, 256, 1986.

Appendix 1

SAMPLE PROCEDURES FOR EMERGENCY MANAGEMENT OF RADIATION ACCIDENT CASUALTIES AT _____ HOSPITAL

TABLE OF CONTENTS

Section 1

INTRODUCTION AND GENERAL GUIDELINES

The following pages contain a sample protocol for handling radiation accidents in the initial stages as a patient presents at a hospital for treatment. With some adaptation, most hospitals will be able to modify these procedures to have a workable plan to deal with such accidents.

The protocol describes a Radiation Emergency Area (REA) which is usually set up near or in the Emergency Room. The protocol also calls for a Radiation Emergency Coordination Committee (RECC) to oversee changes in the protocol. This function may be taken by the Nuclear Medicine Committee, Disaster Committee, or Radiation Safety Committee if it is more practical for a given hospital.

Having a protocol does not ensure that personnel are familiar with it; therefore, there is a section included to be used in case the protocol is to be used by somebody on an emergency basis. After the protocol has been modified to fit a given hospital it should be tried by having a drill. Only this will assure the implementation of a workable plan.

1.1   **PURPOSE**
        This manual is designed to give both general and specific instructions for the provision of effective care to victims of accidents involving radiation, for protection of patient and hospital staff from injury by radioisotopes, and for prevention of contamination of other hospital areas by the radioactive patient. It is not intended to be an exhaustive review of the literature listed in the bibliography.

1.2   **THE RADIATION EMERGENCY COORDINATING COMMITTEE (RECC)**
1.2.1   **Composition**
1.2.1.1 *Chairman:* Radiation Safety Officer
1.2.1.2 *Members:*
        Designee, Department of Medicine (Hematology)
        Designee, Administration
        Designees, Department of Radiology (Nuclear Medicine)
        Designee, Nursing Service
        Designee, Emergency Service
        Designee, Department of Surgery
        Designee, Radiation Safety Office.
1.2.2   **Responsibilities**
1.2.2.1 *Policy and Procedures*
        Written statements of policy and procedures for the admission and management of radiation casualties shall be prepared, distributed to involved individuals, tested periodically and reviewed annually.
1.2.2.2 *Meetings*
        The Committee will meet semiannually at the call of the Chairman. Minutes will be maintained and distributed to the members and to the hospital Director. The Committee will consider such matters as affect the institution's preparedness to admit and treat radiation casualties, including availability of trained specialists, maintenance of supplies and equipment, and status of training.
1.2.2.3 *Availability and Response*
        The Committee shall assure that a trained staff is available at all times to respond to authorized requests for consultation relating to, or for treatment of, radiation casualties.

1.3   **CONSULTATION OR TREATMENT**
1.3.1   **General**
        Requirements for consultation or treatment of radiation casualties may arise from cases presented by staff members, non-staff physicians, unannounced arrival of radiation casualties (emergency cases), inquiries or requests for assistance from non-medical persons, and industries and institutions having formal agreements for radiation medical support. It is expected that most cases will be presented from the last category.
1.3.2   **Cases Presented by Staff Members or Non-Staff Physicians**
        Staff members or physicians from the community having patients involved in radiation accidents will be referred to the Chairman, RECC, or to the Nuclear Medicine Staff Physician on call. The Chairman, in consultation with RECC, will advise the physician in accordance with the procedures of this document.
1.3.3   **Unannounced Arrival of Radiation Casualties at the Emergency Room**
        Personnel on duty at the Emergency Room shall act in accordance with the instructions contained in Section 2, entitled "Admission, Care and Treatment of Radiation Accident Patients". A copy of this manual is on file in the Emergency Room.

1.3.4   **Inquiries or Requests for Assistance from Non-Medical Persons**
Such inquiries or requests shall be directed to the Radiation Protection Officer or the Emergency Room Charge Nurse by either the telephone operator or the staff member receiving the inquiry or request.

1.4   **HOSPITAL ADMISSIONS** (see also Section 4)
Every reasonable effort will be made to admit patients who present a radiation or contamination hazard through the REA. Since the REA can be set up and staffed for admission of radiation casualties at short notice, advance notification of requirements for these facilities should be made. As used in this document, a radiation or contamination hazard will be assumed to exist if the radiation level emanating from a radiation casualty or his apparel is detectable (i.e., twice background) with a portable beta-gamma G-M survey meter.

1.4.1   **Preparation of Decontamination Suite**
Upon notification of intent to admit a radiation casualty, the hospital shall assume the responsibility of supervising the preparation of the Decontamination Suite in the REA. This preparation will be accomplished in accord with the procedure presented in Section 5.

1.5   **RADIATION PROTECTION AND MONITORING OF ATTENDANTS**
Section 6 of this document presents specific operational procedures for personnel working in and supporting activities in the Decontamination Suite. Every effort should be made to keep exposure of each employee as low as reasonably achievable (generally less than 125 mR) (see Section 2.3, Principles of Radiation Protection).

1.6   **TELEPHONE DIRECTORY OF ESSENTIAL PERSONNEL**
A directory of essential personnel is included in this document as Section 3. It shall be the responsibility of the RECC Chairman to keep this directory current.

1.7   **AUDIT OF REA SUPPLIES AND EQUIPMENT**
The Radiation Safety Office shall conduct an audit of the supplies and equipment maintained for use in the REA. The audit shall be conducted semiannually and following any actual use. Records of the findings of these audits shall be maintained. Findings that adversely affect the state of readiness of this procedure shall be corrected immediately. Significant deficiencies that cannot be corrected promptly shall be brought to the attention of the Chairman, RECC. An inventory of supplies maintained for use in the REA is shown in Section 7 of this manual.

1.8   **PUBLIC RELATIONS**
Radiation accidents are a rare and noteworthy event. Consequently, they will draw considerable public attention. To avoid unnecessary alarm, misinterpretation and misunderstanding, it is imperative that correct and concise information be given. All requests for information concerning the patient and the accident should be directed to the Public Relations Office of the Hospital, which will contact the following:

1.   Chairman, RECC
2.   Primary Staff physician of record
3.   Director, Hospital
4.   Medical director of company involved

The information on the radiation accident should be channeled by the Chairman, RECC, through the hospital Public Relations Office as the central source for news dissemination to the media.

1.9   **AMENDMENTS AND REVISIONS**
The Chairman, RECC, will submit recommendations for amendment and/or revision of this document to RECC in the course of evaluations made during implementation of its provisions, or as a result of his review of the document. He shall conduct an annual review of the document and report his findings to RECC during its first meeting of each calendar year. He shall issue copies of approved amendments and revisions to individuals or departments identified in paragraph 1.10.

1.10   **DISTRIBUTION**
Copies of this document and all subsequently published amendments and revisions shall be distributed by the Secretary as shown below:
Internal Medicine
Surgery

Nursing Service
Nuclear Medicine Department
RECC Members
Emergency Room
Radiation Safety Office,
Telephone Switchboard Office
Public Relations Office,
Housekeeping
Security Office
Radiology Department, Educational Director
Clinical Research Center
Administration

Section 2

ADMISSION, CARE AND TREATMENT OF RADIATION ACCIDENT PATIENTS

This section is composed of two parts. The first section provides administrative guidance on the admission of radiation accident patients. The latter sections provide guidance on (1) emergency treatment of such patients, (2) assessment of radiation and medical status, (3) principles of radiation protection, and (4) initial bioassay samples.

2.1   **ADMISSION**
             Guidance is provided for the unannounced arrival of accident patients under two circumstances: (1) Emergency Room personnel become aware of the patient's status as a "radiation accident patient" before the patient has been removed from the ambulance, and (2) the patient has been brought into the Emergency Room before his status as a "radiation accident patient" has been determined. In all cases, ascertain whether the patient is *contaminated:*

1.   Call the hospital Radiation Safety Office, Nuclear Medicine, or the Nuclear Medicine technologist on call and state the situation, asking for assistance.
2.   If the Radiation Safety Officer is not available, utilize the G-M radiation survey meter(s) kept in the Head Nurse's office. Turn meter to "batt" position; the indicator should move to the "batt" position on the scale. If it does, proceed to the next step (if not, plug it into a 110v outlet): move the dial to the × 100 position and wait until the meter has time to react. IF THE METER GOES OFF SCALE, MOVE AWAY FROM THE PATIENT UNTIL THE INDICATOR REGISTERS WITHIN THE RANGE SHOWN. If the indicator does not move, switch the dial to × 10. If there is still no movement, adjust the dial to × 1. Move the probe over the patient slowly, assuring that you do not touch his body. If you get a marked increase in the number of clicks, you must assume the patient is contaminated.
3.   If in doubt, admit the patient to the decontamination suite in the REA.

2.1.1   **Patient Still in the Ambulance**
             If minimal medical attention is required, treat the patient in the ambulance as adequately as possible, while an appropriate radiation decontamination area is being set up. Ask the Nuclear Medicine technologist on call to assess the level of radiation contamination and exposure rate at arm's length. Instruct the driver, attendants, and Emergency Room personnel who have been in contact with the patient to stay in the vicinity of the ambulance (but not inside the ambulance). Have security clear an area of about 8 ft around the ambulance and keep unnecessary personnel and vehicles away.
             Attend to the patient's emergency medical condition as required. Use surgical gloves and mask. If immediate lifesaving measures are not necessary, observe the patient from a distance until the radiation level is ascertained. All equipment and supplies used to attend to patient *MUST* stay in the vicinity of the ambulance. *DO NOT* carry anything back to the Emergency Room. If the medical condition of the patient is such that he must be removed from ambulance:
             Admit the patient to the Decontamination Suite of the REA via the _____ entrance (see Figure 3, in Appendix A, Floor Plan).
             Keys to the radiation emergency supply cabinet located in _____ are in the possession of the Emergency Room Charge Nurse and the Holding Unit Charge Nurse.
             Instruct driver to stay with ambulance until a radiation survey has been made of him, his equipment, and his vehicle.
             Bring necessary equipment and supplies to treat the patient from Emergency to the Holding Unit. *ALL* equipment, supplies and personnel entering REA *MUST* stay there until arrival of radiation monitoring personnel. Position a guard at the door. Pass Emergency Room supplies and equipment into area but *DO NOT* allow personnel and equipment to come out until checked for radioactivity.
             Personnel attending patient in area should work at arm's length to perform stabilizing lifesaving measures and then prompt decontamination (usually <30 min). Other personnel stand 8 ft away and approach the patient if necessary to assist with procedures.

2.1.2   **Radiation Status Discovered After Admission (i.e., on Obtaining Patient's History)**
             Immediately secure and label the entire area through which the patient has passed and in which he is located. Keep all personnel and equipment in the area. *DO NOT* allow anyone or anything to leave. Establish a control point through which only necessary personnel and equipment pass into this restricted area.

Attend to patient's emergency medical condition as required. Use surgical gloves and mask and gown when treating patient.

Request prompt assistance from the Radiation Safety Officer or Nuclear Medicine technologist. If possible, ascertain the means and route by which the patient was transported to the hospital.

2.2   EMERGENCY TREATMENT OF RADIATION ACCIDENTS

2.2.1   General

Emergency treatment of radiation accidents may have to be given before contact with or arrival of specialists having expertise in evaluation and management of these accidents. In this case, the management of the patient should take place in the following order:

1.   Resuscitation and stabilization - including basic life support and cardiopulmonary resuscitation as necessary.
2.   Initial decontamination (if not previously done)
3.   Evaluation of radiation and medical status
4.   Initial treatment of radiation injury

2.2.2   Resuscitation and Stabilization

Since radiation injury is not immediately life-threatening, primary attention should always be directed to maintenance of airway, breathing, and circulation; to traumatic life-threatening injuries; and to management of open wounds, etc.

2.2.3   Decontamination

Concomitantly, or as soon as possible, the patient should be decontaminated (see Section 8). In the initial decontamination:

1.   Survey for radioactivity and note levels of contamination on anatomical diagrams (see example at the end of Section 8)
2.   Remove and bag all clothing, shoes and personal articles.
3.   Remove obvious dirt and debris - bathe, if necessary, while protecting wounds.
4.   Flush all wounds with copious amounts of sterile water and/or saline.
5.   Blow nose into paper tissues to be saved for radioisotope analysis.
6.   Flush orifices with water or saline. Do not allow patient to swallow.

2.2.4   Evaluation of Radiation Exposure Status (See Figure 2 following Section 8)

In most cases this information will accompany any patients referred from industries using radioactive materials.

2.2.4.1   *History*

When did accident occur?
Is the cause of the accident known?
What type of radioactive isotopes were involved?
Was radioiodine present?
How long was the patient in the accident environment?
Who was with the patient?

>   *Note:*   If this information is not available with the patient, it will be determined as soon as the referring company reconstructs accident conditions.

2.2.4.2   *Radiation Dose Evaluation*

This will require the assistance of persons knowledgeable in radiation. This assistance can be by someone on location or by telephone. In any case, gather as much of the following information as possible:

Level of radiation in accident environment
Length of time exposed to the radiation field
Surface and air contamination in accident environment
Exposure recorded on patient's or area dosimeters
Level of residual contamination (beta, gamma) on patient using open window G-M tube (mark areas on Figure 2 following Section 8).
Elapsed time since the accident
Estimation of dose to the patient and to attendants

2.2.4.3   *Medical Assessment of Radiation Exposure*

An estimate of the severity of the patient's radiation exposure may be obtained by observing the following clinical symptoms and signs:

Nausea and vomiting: >100 rad (>1 Gy) (whole-body)
   Beginning within 2 h: >400 rad (>4 Gy) (whole-body)
   Beginning within 4 h: <200 rad (<2 Gy) (whole-body)
Skin erythema: >1000 rad (>10 Gy) if observed early
Diarrhea: >400 rad (>4 Gy) to abdomen
CNS symptoms (only reliable in the absence of cerebral trauma): >1000 rad (>10 Gy)

Lymphocyte count within 48 h

>1200/mm^3: good prognosis

300 to 1200/mm^3: guarded prognosis

300/mm^3: poor prognosis

2.2.5   Initial Treatment of Radiation Exposure and Internal Contamination

2.2.5.1   *Overexposure*

Since overexposure to external radiation results in a slowly unfolding course over a period of time, there is little in the way of specific treatment in very early stages. Treatment is symptomatic and should include making the patient comfortable and allaying the patient's fears. The patient may require antiemetics, fluids, sedatives, and analgesics.

2.2.5.2   Internal Contamination

1. If it is possible that the patient absorbed:
   (a)   Tritium (as tritiated water, HTO) — force fluids
   (b)   Iodine (^{131}I) — give saturated solution of KI (8 to 10 drops in water) for alert patients without head injury; inject 250 mg of potassium or sodium perchlorate intravenously for patients unable to take oral medicine.

2. If it is suspected that an appreciable amount of radioactivity has been ingested, stomach lavage, emetics (ipecac), or cathartics (MgSO) may be indicated. These should be followed by Gaviscon 30 cc and Phosphosoda 30 cc hourly to retard absorption of remaining radionuclides.

3. If exposure to transuranic nuclides (Plutonium-239, Americium-241, etc.) is documented, infuse 1 g of Zn-DTPA in 500 ml of 5% D/W over a 30-min period. (Investigational, available through REAC/TS, Oak Ridge Assoc. Univ., Oak Ridge, TN. See Section 3.3 for telephone number.)

2.3   PRINCIPLES OF RADIATION PROTECTION

Certain precautions to minimize exposure to attendants are necessary when dealing with a patient who has external contamination, specifically:

1. Initially, survey patient with the survey meter as described in Section 2.1.
2. Maintain maximum appropriate distance from the patient. Arm's length is usually adequate. If exposure levels are <10 mR/h at 1 ft, personnel may work safely at arm's length from the patient. If the exposure rate is uncertain or higher than 10 mR/h, attendants should stand 10 ft from the patient when close access is not essential.
3. Work efficiently to minimize exposure time.
4. Use the radiation shield (from Nuclear Medicine) only if directed by the Radiation Safety Officer.
5. Minimize the number of personnel near the patient.
6. If you expect to enter the Decontamination Suite, wear plastic apron and gown, or water-repellant coveralls, mask, cap, gloves, and dosimeters.
7. Rope off and control the area in which the patient is being treated (see floor plan diagram in Appendix A).
8. If radioiodine is a possible contaminant, all personnel assigned to the Decontamination room, Buffer Zone, and ambulance area should be given potassium iodide (130 mg) or a saturated solution of KI (8 to 10 drops) prior to arrival of the casualty. All persons, equipment, and supplies that enter this area must stay there until Nuclear Medicine technologists arrive to assist in the monitoring and decontamination of people and equipment.

2.4   INITIAL BIOASSAY SAMPLES

When a patient is known to have internal contamination, or when it is suspected, samples for radioactivity measurements should be obtained as soon as possible and labeled with name, date, time and type of specimen. Avoid cross-contamination of samples from external sources of contamination. Detailed instructions for procuring samples are given in Section 8.

2.4.1   Hospital Laboratory

1. Routine hematology: CBC with differential (1 lavender top tube)
2. Chemistries: SMA (1 red top tube)
3. Cytogenetics: 20 cc (heparinized) for chromosomes (keep samples chilled in a glass of ice) (2 green top tubes)
4. Radioisotope analyses: (1 red top, 2 lavender top tubes)
5. Culture swabs of wounds, nares, throat, and eyes before and after decontamination

2.4.2   Radioisotope Laboratory

The following samples will be sent to the Radiation Safety Officer:

Urine:

First urine — instruct patient to void when medically able. Save this and every subsequent urine specimen.

All urine — label with time, date, and patient name.

Feces:

First 4 days — every sample should be collected and refrigerated after being marked with name, date and time of collection.

Sputum or nose blow samples

Vomitus or lavage specimens

Tissue (note location)

Irrigation fluids

Cotton applicator smears of orifices, wounds, skin areas (note location)

Section 3

TELEPHONE DIRECTORY

3.1 **RADIATION EMERGENCY COMMUNICATIONS RESPONSIBILITIES**

(All telephones are area code _____)

3.1.1 **First notification of any radiation casualty sent to the BWH:**

Emergency Room Charge Nurse _____ or _____

3.1.2 **The Emergency Room Charge Nurse will then notify:**

1. Emergency Room Surgical Resident _____

2. Holding Unit _____

3. Hospital page operator who will
   notify by phone or pager

    a. Radiation Safety Officer,

             Days: _____

             Nights: _____ or Page _____

       or Nuclear Medicine Staff
   Physician on call _____ or Page _____

    b. Nuclear Medicine Technologist
   on call _____ or Page _____

    c. Security _____ or Page _____

    d. Administration _____ or Page _____

    e. Nursing Supervisor _____ or Page _____

    f. Office of Public Relations _____ or Page _____

    g. Housekeeping _____ of Page _____

3.2 **REFERENCE LIST OF TELEPHONE NUMBERS OF ESSENTIAL PERSONNEL**

3.2.1 **Administrator On Call** _____ (Day) (Director's Office)

    _____ (Night) (Page Center)

3.2.2 **Nursing Service**
a. Emergency Room Charge Nurse _____

3.3.3 **Radiation Emergency On Call Roster** _____

1. On Call Nuclear Medicine
   Staff Physician _____ or Page _____

2. On Call Nuclear Medicine
   Technologist _____ or Page _____

3.   Radiation Safety Officer   _____   or Page   _____
                                          _____   (Home)

3.2.4   **Security**   _____   or Page   _____

3.2.5   **Department of Surgery**
        Emergency Room Resident on Call   _____   or Page   _____

3.2.6   **Department of Medicine (Hematology)**
        Hematologist on Call   _____   or Page   _____

3.3   **EXTERNAL RADIOLOGICAL EMERGENCY ASSISTANCE (24 hours)**

Department of Energy   (202) 586-8100
Federal Emergency Management Agency   (202) 566-1600 (x3014)
Nuclear Regulatory Commission   (301) 951-0550

Radiation Emergency Assistance Center/Training Site (REAC/TS)
Oak Ridge, Tennessee (24 hours)

(615) 481-1000 (x1502 or beeper 241)

State Radiation Control Program   _____

Section 4

OPERATIONAL PHASES OF RADIATION ACCIDENT CASUALTY CARE

4.1 **UNANNOUNCED ADMISSIONS**

The procedure to be followed in the event that a victim of a radiation accident arrives unannounced at the Emergency Department is presented in Section 2.

4.2 **ANNOUNCED ARRIVAL OF RADIATION CASUALTIES**

Action involving the hospital will take place in five phases: (1) notification, (2) arrival, (3) treatment, (4) cleanup, and (5) definitive care.

4.2.1 **Notification Phase: Responsibilities (Job Descriptions in Appendix A)**

1. As soon as possible, industry personnel or attending police officers will alert the Emergency Room Charge Nurse of any intent to refer accident victims. This notification should contain the following information: (See form following this section).
    a. Probability of referral
    b. Number and names of patients
    c. Estimated time of arrival
    d. Condition of patient(s) and description of injuries
    e. Estimated radiation exposure
    f. Extent and nature of contamination (how much and which radioisotopes)
    g. Special needs for equipment and/or personnel
2. The Emergency Room Charge Nurse shall:
    a. Alert the hospital page operator who will in turn notify other involved staff members (Section 3)
    b. Contact the Emergency Room Resident
    c. Direct preparation of the REA (Section 5)
    d. Assure the availability of ancillary personnel
    e. Supervise preparation of all necessary equipment for radioisotope containment and decontamination.
4. Radiation Safety Officer/Nuclear Medicine Technologists:
    a. Check all dosimeters and monitoring equipment
    b. Prepare for contaminated sample collections/supplies
    c. Brief assembled staff on safety procedures to be followed during operational management of the patient
5. Emergency Room Personnel:
    a. Assist Housekeeping in preparation of the Decontamination Suite in the REA
    b. Assure that the required equipment is opened up and ready for use
    c. Prepare to give direct nursing care to patients
6. Security:
    a. Clear vehicle access to the Holding Unit
    b. Post guards at the Radiation Casualty entrance and the REA entrance as shown in Figure 3 in Appendix A.
    c. Clear access route to REA of unauthorized personnel
7. Surgery: Assure availability of an anesthesiologist and other surgeons as needed.

4.2.2 **Arrival Phase**

Security will direct the ambulance to REA entrance, secure the area around ambulance and hold the ambulance until cleared by the Radiation Safety Officer or Nuclear Medicine Technologist. The emergency room surgeon in charge, the Radiation Protection Officer, the Nuclear Medicine Technologist on call, and the radiation protection staff will meet the ambulance outside the REA. Technologist will evaluate the radiation and contamination status of the patient, ambulance personnel, and the ambulance. The Radiatior Safety Officer will advise on radiation safety precautions to be followed. The Emergency Room surgeon will ascertain the medical status of the patient. The patient will then be brought into the Decontamination Suite of the REA (Room _____) via the adjacent Radiation Casualty Entrance. Ambulance attendants will then meet beside the ambulance where the Nuclear Medicine Technologist and/or health physicist will monitor them and the ambulance and instruct them regarding their personal decontamination if required. When they have completed decontamination, they will be permitted to leave the REA.

Only persons and equipment necessary for patient care and treatment will be permitted in the Radiation Emergency Area (REA). After the arrival of the contaminated patient, all persons or items leaving the Holding Unit will be monitored for radioactive contamination at the point of egress. Personnel found to be contaminated will be decontaminated before leaving. Contaminated equipment and clothes will be packaged in polyethylene bags.

Should there be a number of patients, the customary mass casualty triage system will be used. The section of the emergency room nearest the REA would be prepared as an additional REA. Once the patient enters the REA, Housekeeping will roll up the yellow Herculite outside, and stow it inside. When indicated by the Nuclear Medicine Technologist, Security may restore the ambulance driveway to normal use.

4.2.3   **Decontamination and Treatment Phase** (See Section 8)

4.2.4   **Clean-Up Phase**

When the patient's surface radiation levels are minimized (or to twice background) he may be transferred from the REA. With fresh covering laid on the floor, a clean stretcher or wheelchair is brought in and, following transfer onto the vehicle, a final survey is made of the patient, linens, and vehicle before proceeding to other hospital areas.

After the patient has been moved from the Holding Unit to the main hospital, attending personnel will proceed with removal of protective apparel, personnel monitoring, and decontamination in accordance with procedures given in Section 6.4.

The Radiation Safety Officer will provide decontamination instruction and will monitor attending personnel.

The Radiation Safety Officer will decontaminate equipment and all facilities and will collect and dispose of nonsalvageable items.

As soon as is convenient following cleanup activities, all personnel who were involved in the care or treatment of the patient will attend a postaccident conference convened by the Radiation Safety Officer. The conference will cover subjects such as the following:

1.   medical and operational review of the event;
2.   exposures of attending personnel, if any;
3.   recommendations for future handling of radiation casualties.

Following the postaccident conference, the Radiation Safety Officer will submit a complete report of events to the RECC, to concerned regulatory authorities, and to the Medical and Hospital Director and management of the company in which the accident occurred.

Upon admission of the accident victim(s) to a nursing care unit room, precautionary notices will be placed in the medical record and on the room door in accord with standard hospital practice appropriate to the nature and quantity of radioactive materials remaining.

RADIATION ACCIDENT MESSAGE RECEIPT

To be used by ER head nurse or Nursing Supervisor when receiving the report of a radiation accident:

DATE: _____ TIME: _____ Supervisor _____ R.N.

Person making notification _____ Telephone _____

EXPECTED TIME OF ARRIVAL: _____

	Casualty #1	Casualty #2
Medical problems:	_____	_____
	_____	_____
	_____	_____
	_____	_____
First aid measures given:	_____	_____
	_____	_____
	_____	_____
	_____	_____

Radiation injury	Circle One	Circle One
1. Exposure?	yes / no	yes / no
	_____ mR/h	_____ mR/h
2. Skin contamination?	yes / no	yes / no
Which isotopes?	_____	_____
3. Inhalation?	yes / no	yes / no
Which isotopes?	_____	_____
4. Ki given?	yes / no	yes / no
5. Decontaminated?	yes / no	yes / no

READ THIS BACK TO THE CALLER

Section 5

PREPARATION OF THE RADIATION EMERGENCY AREA

5.1 **PURPOSE**

To outline procedures for preparing to receive a radiation casualty

5.2 **DEFINITIONS**

5.2.1 **Decontamination Suite**

Room _____ in the Emergency Room can be modified to permit its use for decontamination and initial treatment of patients exposed to accidents involving radioisotopes.

5.2.2 **Radiation Emergency Area (REA)**

This designation is given to Room _____ (Decontamination Suite), Room _____ and the adjacent floor passage area (the *Buffer Zone*. During reception and care of a radiation casualty, the Radiation Emergency Area is identified by rad-tape or signs and is off-limits to personnel without dosimeters.

5.3 **PROCEDURES**

- A verbal communication, from either the accident site or the Radiation Safety Officer, will be received by the Emergency Room Charge Nurse stating that the hospital will be receiving a radiation casualty, with information stating the condition of the patient, estimated time of arrival, nature of exposure and other details listed in Section 4.
- The charge nurse who receives the communication in the Emergency Room will be responsible for appropriate notifications (see Section 3). The hospital housekeeping department will be requested to assist with area preparations. At this time, hospital security will be directed to cordon off the ambulance driveway receiving site and to control patient, employee, and spectator traffic.
- The radiation emergency supplies located in _____ will be opened by the charge nurse and appropriate supplies transferred to the Decontamination Suite (see Section 7, Supply Inventory). Keys to the closet are held by the radiation safety office and the Emergency Room Charge Nurse.
- If time permits, before patient arrival the decontamination room floor will be covered. A mobile stretcher is positioned lengthwise in the Decontamination room to accommodate the decontamination tub with its attached drainage tube. A plastic container will be positioned just underneath the tub drain to receive the drainage tube. Two or three linen disposal bags lined with plastic should be secured in mobile frames.
- The showerhead attached to a hose and faucet will be tested by the charge nurse to ensure its functional status and comfortably warm water temperature.
- The Radiation Safety Officer will initiate the appropriate measures for redirecting air circulation if necessary.
- The Buffer Zone (the area immediately outside the Decontamination Suite), will be identified with special rad-tape provided for this purpose.
- Two tables in the Buffer Zone and one in the Decontamination Suite will be needed to hold supplies. Sample containers will be numbered to facilitate recording of location.
- A nurse and a Nuclear Medicine technologist will be positioned outside the Buffer Zone to assist with appropriate body coverings and equipment (ring TLD and pen dosimeters, caps, masks, coveralls or gowns, gloves, and plastic aprons).

5.4 **RADIATION CASUALTY TREATMENT TEAM**

Job descriptions for personnel required during radiation decontamination are described in Appendix A.

5.5 **CLEANUP PROCEDURES**

When the decontaminated patient has been transferred from the Radiation Emergency Area, cleanup procedures will be supervised by the Radiation Safety Officer. Housekeeping, with the assistance of the Nuclear Medicine technologist and the Radiation Safety Officer, will safely package all radioactive materials in plastic bags. These will be removed from the premises and taken to the hospital radiation waste disposal area. A thorough washdown of the area will ensue, and normal usage will be resumed when approved by the Radiation Safety Officer.

Section 6

USE OF PROTECTIVE CLOTHING AND DOSIMETERS

To prevent personnel from becoming contaminated with radioactive material and to minimize the possibility of internal contamination, protective clothing will be issued to all persons who enter the decontamination room.

6.1 **STANDARD PROTECTIVE CLOTHING**

Standard protective clothing includes a scrub suit (for females), a water repellant jumpsuit gown, 2 pairs of surgical gloves, a surgical mask and cap, and a vinyl apron. Ring and badge dosimeters should be in place before putting on the gown or jumpsuit.

6.2 **CONDITIONS REQUIRING PROTECTIVE CLOTHING**

1. All personnel in the Decontamination Suite require protective clothing, regardless of the degree of contamination present on the patient or his clothing. Standard protective clothing will suffice in all cases where gross decontamination has been performed (i.e., where very little ''loose'' contamination is confined to a relatively small area.)

   Personnel in the Buffer Zone not in direct contact with the patient or contaminated supplies need wear only latex gloves unless otherwise directed by the Radiation Safety Officer.

2. Without specific instructions to the contrary, standard protective clothing may be assumed to suffice. If greater protection is required, taping of protective clothing at wrists and ankles may be required. For this purpose, tape is available. Hoods may also be suggested. Respiratory protection is rarely necessary unless alpha emitters (such as plutonium or americium) is present. Face masks and air packs, if necessary, will be supplied at the time of the accident by the site where the accident occurred.

6.3 **REMOVING CONTAMINATED PROTECTIVE CLOTHING**

1. Upon completion of their activities in the Decontamination Suite, personnel will proceed to the door, have their gloves monitored and, if not contaminated, they will take off the protective clothing down to their scrub suit and deposit garments in a plastic bag, in the following order:

   a. Remove surgical mask and cap or hood,

   b. Remove apron and gown or jumpsuit, turning them inside out;

   c. Step out of the contamination area onto the mat or step-off pad with the first uncovered shoe.

   d. Remove mask, cap and finally gloves.

2. After removal of these items, personnel proceed into the buffer zone (without crossing the rope between the Buffer Zone and the uncontrolled hospital area) to have their dosimeters collected and to be monitored for any remaining contamination.

6.4 **CLEARANCE PROCEDURES**

1. In case no contamination is found, personnel may proceed to the change area and put on their normal clothing.

2. In case persons are found to be contaminated, they will use a clean washcloth, and if necessary, take a shower, be monitored again, and, if free from contamination be supplied with disposable garments; then proceed as described above. The Radiation Safety Officer should be consulted if there is difficulty with decontamination.

6.5 **USE OF DOSIMETERS**

1. Dosimeters will be supplied at the Control Point to all personnel entering the Radiation Emergency Area.

2. Dosimeters are of three types.

   a. Direct reading dosimeters (''pen-dosimeters''), which are supplied to all personnel in the Decontamination Suite;

   b. Ring dosimeters (TLD type), which are supplied only to the physician, nurses, and monitoring technologist A who directly contact the patient.

   c. Badge dosimeters (film of TLD type), supplied to all personnel within Control Area and Decontamination Suite.

3.   Dosimeters are to be worn as follows:

   a.   Film or TLD type are worn above the sternum, clipped to the scrub suit; i.e., under the outer layer of the protective clothing.

   b.   On the ring finger of the right and left hand under the glove, the TLD chip faces inward (ring dosimeters).

   c.   Pen dosimeters to be worn on collar, outside protective clothing so that they are accessible during patient treatment.

4.   Upon leaving the Radiation Emergency Area, the wearer should surrender his dosimeters to the Nuclear Medicine Technologist, or the Radiation Safety Officer who will record the reading of the pen dosimeter (Figure 1) and retain the film or TLD dosimeters for later processing.

5.   The Radiation Safety Office must assure that the records clearly show the serial number of each dosimeter worn by each individual who occupied the Radiation Emergency Area and duration of time each individual spent in the REA.

6.6   GUIDE TO SAFE EXPOSURES FOR PERSONNEL ATTENDING A RADIATION CASUALTY (REFERENCE: NCRP-39, "BASIC RADIATION PROTECTION CRITERIA")

1.   Routine Emergencies: Those casualties usually partly decontaminated at the accident scene.

   Aim: To hold your exposure to 125 mR, the recommended quarterly exposure limit for non-occupationally exposed people.

   Survey meter reading at 1.5 feet (mR/h):   2.5   5   10   25   100

   Time you may work at 1.5 feet (h):   50   25   12.5   5   1.25

   Thus, if the radiation level at arm's length is 100 mR or less, you have plenty of time for further decontamination or emergency care.

   (Calculations were approximated from a point source.)

2.   Short-handed Emergencies

   Aim: To hold your exposure to 1250 mR, the recommended quarterly exposure limit for occupationally exposed workers. It would be wise to exclude females under age 45.

   Survey meter reading at 1.5 feet (R/h):   0.1   0.5   1   5   10

   Time you may work at 1.5 feet (h):   10   2.5   1.25   0.25   0.12

3.   Life-Saving Emergencies

   You may receive up to 25 R *per incident* as whole-body radiation (100 R to the hands).

   You may receive up to 100 R whole-body or 200 R to the hands in a once-in-a-lifetime situation.

PERSONNEL DOSIMETRY LOG

Name/Social Security Number	Date/Time Issued	Ring TDL Number	Pocket TDL Number	Pen Dosimeter	Reading Pen Dosimeter Initial	Reading Pen Dosimeter Final	Remarks

_____ Signature

_____ Date

FIGURE 1. Sample of personnel dosimetry log used by the Radiation Safety Officer to record vital information on personnel leaving the REA.

Section 7

SUPPLY INVENTORY

7.1	**SPECIFIC RADIATION-RELATED ITEMS**	
	Gamma dose rate survey instrument (ion chamber such as Eberline PIC 1 mR/h to 1000 R/h	1
	Beta-gamma monitor, Geiger-Mueller type (located in Emergency Room head nurse's office)	
	Alpha meter (if near a weapons facility)	1
	Self-reading pocket dosimeters, (0 to 1 R range)	10
	Thermoluminescent dosimeters, whole-body type	10
	Thermoluminescent dosimeters, ring type	6
	Charger for self-reading dosimeters	1
	Decontamination tabletop tub, side panels, and hose	1
	Plastic containers for water collection	2 or 3
	Lead container, high activity samples	1
	Long-handled forceps	1
	Kit, decontamination and sample taking (see Sections 7.2, 7.3)	1
	Hose, low pressure, with shower head and valve	1
	Floor covering (barbecue cloth)	2 rolls
	Masking tape, 2 in.	1 roll
	Duct tape 2 in.	2 rolls
	Set, radiation warning signs, tape, and rope	1
	Batteries, 9 volt, size C and D, for instruments	4
	Disposable protective clothing packs (head covers, gowns, jumpsuits, gloves, and masks)	10
	Plastic shoe covers	20
	Scrub suits	5
	Poly bags (large)	10
	Poly bags (small)	20
	Signs, "Caution Radiation Area"	4
	Signs, "Caution Radioactive Material"	4
	Stickers, "Contaminated Material"	10
	Barrier Tape	3 rolls
	Tape "radioactive" for labeling samples and plastic bags	2
	Notebook	1
	Body charts	12
	Pencils	6
7.2	**DECONTAMINATION KIT**	
	Absorbent cotton balls, extra large	1 box
	Sponge-holding forceps	1
	Plastic beaker, large (to contain used sponges)	2
	Prep sponges (for large area decontamination)	6
	Surgical hand brushes	6
	Wash bottle (to hold water for decontamination)	1
	Sterile gauze pads, 4X4 in., in box	1 box
	Solution bowl, plastic	1
	Plungerless syringes, 50cc, sterile	1
	Cotton tipped applicators	1 pkg
	Sodium hypochlorite (bleach)	1 bottle
7.2.1	**Miscellaneous Materials**	
	Nivea® cream, jar (apply on dry skin after compete decon)	1
	Prep kit (for clipping and shaving)	1
	Nail clippers, pair	1
	Scissors, heavy duty	1

Medical and Radiation Status Sheets	5
Plastic bags, assortment (to hold decon materials after use)	1
Tags, with wire, to indicate contents of bags	10
Tissue paper, box	1

7.3	**SAMPLE TAKING KIT**	
	Alcohol wipes, sterile, prepackaged	1 box
	Tissue paper box (for nose blows)	1 box
7.3.1	**Small Specimens (hair, nails, tissue samples, sputum)**	
	Bottles, wide mouth, 100 ml	5
	Sample rack with sample tubes	2
7.3.2	**Excreta, Irrigation Fluids, Vomitus**	
	Jar, plastic for feces samples	2
	Urine: specitainers, 2500 ml	2
	Bottles, wide mouth, 500 ml, for collection of irrigation fluids	2
7.3.3	**Miscellaneous Items**	
	Plastic bags, assorted sizes	10
	Tags, with wire	20
	Numbered labels, self-sticking	1 roll

7.4	**SUPPLIES TO BE FURNISHED BY EMERGENCY DEPARTMENT/ HOLDING UNIT**	
	Vacutainers® green, red, gray, lavender	6 each
	Suture Kit	as needed
	Sterile culture swabs	as needed
	Sterile urine sample container	2
	Surgical gloves, assorted sizes, sterile	12
	Crash chart (as needed) Supplies specific to injuries	
	Hydrogen peroxide	
	Surgical soap	
	Potassium iodide tablets (130 mg)	12

Section 8

PROCEDURES FOR PATIENT DECONTAMINATION AND SAMPLE TAKING

These procedures cover the use of the Decontamination and Sample Taking Kits. The kits provide some of the necessary items for the cleansing of a patient contaminated with radioisotopes and the collection of specimens of this contamination. Other materials will be supplied through the Emergency Department. Section 7 provides a list for each of the two kits. Following use, the lists should be consulted for replenishment.

The collection of specimens is a prerequisite for a thorough evaluation of the medical and radiation status of the patient. Several alpha and beta emitting radionuclides may not be detected by the Geiger type meter, hence laboratory analysis of samples is necessary for documenting their absence, or, if found, their identities. Mixtures of gamma emitters may be resolved into their specific components. Thus, sampling should be performed before and after patient decontamination. This section contains a copy of a "Patient Radiation and Medical Status Report Sheet", which is most useful if completed at the accident scene and sent to the hospital with any injured patient.

8.1 PATIENT DECONTAMINATION PROCEDURES
8.1.1 Principles

1. The objectives of decontamination are:
   A. to prevent injury caused by the presence of radioactive substances on the body;
   B. to prevent the spread of contamination over and into the patient;
   C. to protect attending personnel from becoming contaminated themselves or (in extreme cases) from being exposed to a source of radiation.
2. Although decontamination should be started as soon as possible, primary attention should be given to the alleviation of life-threatening conditions created by traumtic inury.
3. Decontamination is essentially the physical removal of radioactive dirt or liquid from the skin, wounds, or body orifices. Most decontaminants contain detergents or other chemical agents to facilitate this removal. Therefore, most decontaminants are suitable for decontamination of the intact skin and may not always be appropriate for wound cleansing or irrigation of body orifices. Removal of clothes and shoes will remove most contamination.
4. Decontamination is performed:
   A. generally from the highest level of contamination *outside* the wound to the lowest unless the wound and contamination are congruent (e.g., burns); usually, this means head and hands first;
   B. by showering only if patient is ambulatory and in the absence of an open wound or burn;
   C. starting with the simplest procedure (e.g., soap and water) to more complicated procedures;
   D. with due regard to contamination of wounds, body orifices, etc. (see below for specific guidelines).
5. Usually, the effect of decontamination is greatest in the earliest stages, i.e., most of the radioactive material is removed during the first decontamination effort. Continued decontamination may show diminishing effectiveness. At some point, a decision has to be made to either accept some residual contamination, or proceed with the use of more potent decontaminants (more specific guidelines below).

8.1.2 Measures to be Taken before Decontamination

1. Assuming that gross decontamination has been performed at the accident site, it can be expected that the residual contamination is minor, and/or that serious contamination is localized, e.g., around and in a wound. Before decontamination, the following steps should be taken:
   A. Judge whether the patient's medical condition requires immediate intervention; if so, proceed, covering the contaminated area with a plastic drape or a towel.
   B. When appropriate, obtain a briefing from the ambulance personnel or industrial health physicist as to the contamination status of the patient and as to the specific measures to be taken by attending personnel with regard to their protection. Confirm this in consultation with the Radiation Safety Officer.
   C. Monitor the patient with the radiation survey instrument by scanning the entire body (holding the probe about 2 inches from the skin) and record the findings on the Body Chart; decide in which order skin decontamination shall be performed.

       D.   Inspect wounds, inquire about their decontamination at the accident site, and decide whether further wound decontamination or treatment can safely be postponed until completion of skin decontamination.

       E.   Initial samples should be taken (see paragraph 8.2 for further details).

       F.   Proceed with decontamination of the patient.

  2.   In case no decontamination has been performed at the accident site (most likely because of an urgent need for emergency surgical treatment):

       A.   Perform a gross decontamination by removing all clothing and obvious dirt and debris; if airway/circulation support is necessary, cover the contaminated area with a plastic drape and proceed.

       B.   At the same time, obtain a briefing from the Radiation Safety Officer or health physicist as to the measures to be taken by attending personnel with regard to their protection.

       C.   After the emergency treatment, proceed with the applicable steps described under 8.1.2,1B to E above.

8.1.3   Decontamination Techniques

  A.   General

Three general rules apply to the performance of decontamination:

1. Most radioactive contaminants are on clothing and shoes, hence prompt removal of clothing is essential; residual contamination is most often on hands, head and neck.
2. Check the effectiveness of the technique applied by monitoring periodically;
3. Avoid the spread of radioactive materials from the area being decontaminated to areas of lesser contamination.

Except when prohibitive degrees of contamination are present on/in any of the locations listed below, or when wound care is urgent, decontamination is performed in the following order:

1. Head, face and hands (to prevent internal contamination);
2. Wounds and adjacent skin;
3. Other skin areas.

  B.   Decontamination of Wounds

1. Use aperture drape to isolate the contaminated area;
2. Take and label sample (see paragraph 8.2.2.A);
3. Depending on surface and depth of wound, irrigate wound with sterile saline. Use gauze pads and sterile saline or use culture swabs to cleanse wound; collect all materials used, and place in labeled containers;
4. Remove obviously necrotic and devitalized tissue as indicated surgically; keep all tissue specimens removed (see paragraph 8.2);
5. Decontaminate skin adjacent to wound as described below (see paragraph 8.1.3.D);
6. Monitor wound; record result on body chart;
7. If contamination persists, consult with Radiation Safety Officer to determine further courses of action;
8. If wound is free of radioactivity, treat wound as indicated by normal practice.

  C.   Decontamination of Body Orifices

1. Take samples of activity in nares, ear canals, throat and other orifices as indicated (see paragraph 8.2.2.A);
2. If nose swab or nose-blown tissue indicates significant radioactivity in nasal canal, irrigate;
3. Gently clean orifice using wetted swabs;
4. Decontaminate area surrounding orifices as described below;
5. Collect all materials used and label containers.

  D.   Decontamination of Skin

1. Take swab sample of area (see paragraph 8.2.2.A);
2. Protect adjacent area by covering with plastic drape or towels;
3. Cleanse skin area;
    a.   Around wounds and orifices: using warm water, and large absorbent balls, cover entire contaminated surface with water repeatedly renewing cotton balls: remove water after 2 to 3 min by wiping repeatedly with wetted cotton balls; monitor; record result.

b.   Other skin areas:
Wash thoroughly with surgical soap and warm water, using either cotton balls, pre-op sponges, or sanitary napkins; cover area with a good lather; rinse off after 2 to 3 min with running water; monitor; record result on body chart. Do not abrade the skin. Minimal residual contamination can be treated with other decontaminants (see paragraph 8.1.3.D.5).

4.   If contamination persists: repeat step (3) once.

5.   If contamination still persists: try gentle application of diluted bleach (sodium hypochlorite) or hydrogen peroxide. Repeat a few times using new cotton balls; remove decontaminants with water; monitor; record result on body chart.

6.   After complete decontamination: dry skin and apply skin moistening cream.

7.   If residual contamination is present: consult with the Radiation Safety Officer to decide whether further efforts are indicated; if it is decided to accept residual contamination, dry the skin and apply Saran Wrap®, mark area involved, and record on body chart;

8.   Collect all materials used and label containers:

9.   Final samples should be taken of all previously decontaminated areas;

10.   Attending personnel should remove outer aprons and gloves before transferring patient.

8.2   PROCEDURES FOR SAMPLE TAKING

8.2.1   Principles

A.   The objectives of collecting specimens from a radiation accident victim are:

1.   To evaluate the location and identity of the radioactive contaminants on and in the body;

2.   To obtain data with regard to the patient's exposure to external and internal radiation;

3.   To supply information on the potential injury by the radiation;

4.   To insure that all radioactivity has been removed;

5.   To gather information useful for accident reconstruction and analysis.

B.   To meet these objectives, the following types of specimens are collected routinely:

1.   Materials containing the external contaminant (swabs, tissue samples, contaminated cleansing fluids, etc.);

2.   Specimens containing internal contaminant (feces, urine, blood, sputum, etc.);

3.   In case of neutron irradiation: materials in which neutron-induced radioactivity may be present (watches, metal jewelry, hair, nail clippings);

4.   Hematological specimens (whole blood in heparinized, EDTA, oxalated, and uncoated tubes; blood smears).

C.   As the analysis of radioactive of radioactive samples with regard to their composition is only possible in samples with a relatively high radioactivity, care should be taken to collect and store these samples separately from the usually bulky samples with rather low radioactivity (such as cleansing fluids, drapes, towels, etc.).

D.   A sample which is not identifiable as to its source (location, time taken) may be practically worthless: therefore, take care to properly collect, store, and mark all samples.

8.2.2   Sample Taking Techniques and Indications

A.   External Contamination
Before decontamination, the following samples should be obtained:

1.   Skin samples: use culture swabs; moisten with a few drops of water, rub over a skin area of about 100 cm^2 (4 × 4 in.). Place swab in sample tube, record location and time and area smeared (if other than 100 cm^2) on body chart.

2.   Wound samples: use either one of the following methods:

a.   Large wounds with visible blood or wound fluid: obtain a few mls using dropper; transfer to a red top tube and label;

b.   Superficial wounds: rub gently with culture swab, return to tube, label;

c.   Wounds with visible dirt or debris: remove with applicator or use tweezers, and transfer sample to a red top tube; label.

B.   Internal Contamination

1.   Body orifices: wet culture swab with a few drops of water, swab, store in holder, label; ask patient to blow his nose into tissue and place in sample tube or container.

2.   Obtain blood samples as listed in Section 2.4.1

3.   In all cases where internal contamination is suspected: collect all urine and feces in containers supplied, record time of voiding.

C.   External Exposure
In all cases of exposure or contamination being known or suspected:
1.   Obtain a blood smear for differential;
2.   Obtain a leukocyte count and absolute lymphocyte count;
3.   Obtain 30 ml of blood in vacutainers (2 green, 1 red top tubes).
Record date and time these samples were taken.
See 2.4.1 and 2.4.2.

PATIENT RADIATION AND MEDICAL STATUS RECORD
(To Accompany Patient Going to Hospital)

Name of patient: _____

Date, time of incident: _____

Brief description of incident:

General medical condition (list all known problems):

First aid measures performed at plant:

Potassium iodide or perchlorate given (circle one): Yes / No _____

Radiation (circle one):   exposure / contamination / both

Approximate absorbed dose: whole body _____ Rems
local (see body chart): _____

Possible contaminants:

Dosimeters sent to: Name _____ location: _____

External Exposure?	Yes / No		Internal contamination?	
Symptoms observed:		Time	sampling: nose blow	Yes / No
nausea	Yes / No	_____	mouth	Yes / No
vomiting	Yes / No	_____	urine	Yes / No
skin erythema	Yes / No	_____	feces	Yes / No
blood samples taken	Yes / No	_____		

Skin Contamination?

sampling: skin areas   Yes / No
clothing   Yes / No
decontamination
procedure: Yes / No

_____

_____

Location of residual contamination at
time of transfer: _____

_____

Wound contamination?

samples taken: Yes / No
residual contamination: Yes / No

_____

_____

Neutron irradiation only:
(circle those specimens taken)

belt buckle   nail clippings
ring, hair   buttons

Signed, _____

INDICATE CONTAMINATED AREAS AS TO LOCATION,
DEGREE OF CONTAMINATION, DECON EFFORT
INDICATE LOCATION OF WOUNDS

Survey No. _____   Surveyed by _____

Time _____   Date _____

Meter Used _____   Skin to Probe Distance _____

S/N _____

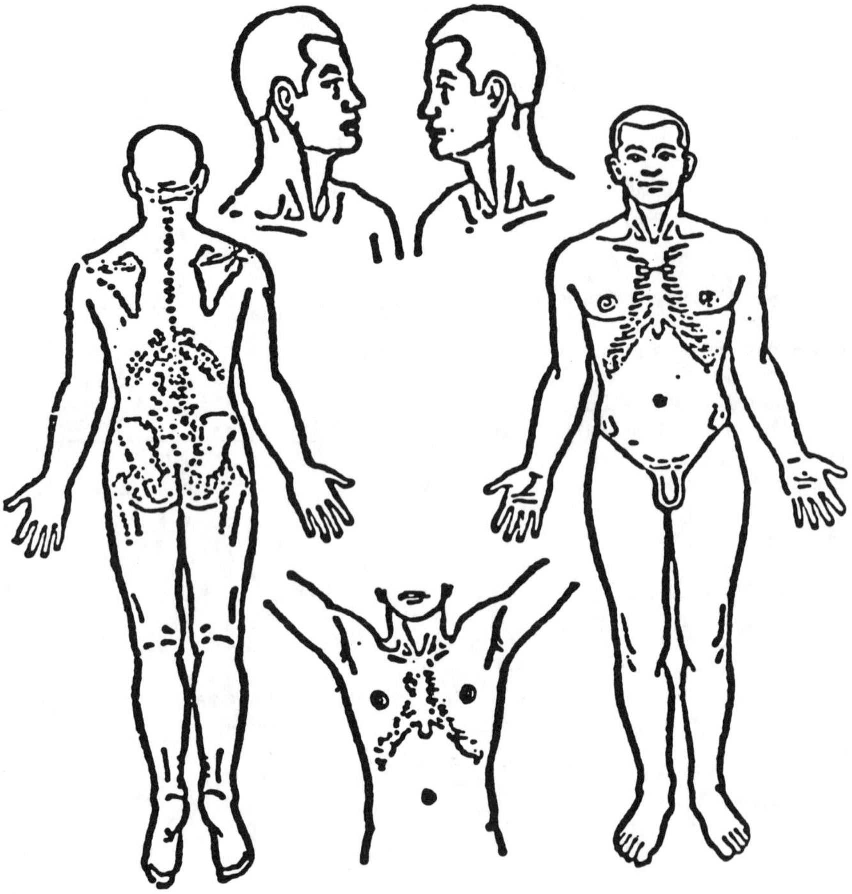

1. _____   6. _____
2. _____   7. _____
3. _____   8. _____
4. _____   9. _____
5. _____   10. _____

FIGURE 2.   Sample of information sheet used by medical personnel at the hospital or, if possible, at the scene of a radiation accident to determine levels of contamination at various areas of the body. See Section 2.2.

Appendix A

RADIATION ACCIDENT EMERGENCY STAFF JOB DESCRIPTIONS

I.   Personnel
    A.   Nurse A — first assistant to Surgeon
    B.   Nurse B — inside Decontamination Suite
    C.   Nurse C — at door of Decontamination Suite
    D.   Surgeon
    E.   Nuclear Medicine Technician A
    F.   Radiation Safety Officer
    G.   Nursing Supervisor (Nurse D)
    H.   Housekeeping Personnel
    I.   Security Personnel
II.   Floor Plan of Staff Assignments in the REA

I. PERSONNEL

A. NURSE A

Location: Decontamination Room

Radiation Protection Measures: Full protective clothing; ring, TLD and pen dosimeters; plastic apron

Responsibilities:
1.   Direct nursing care of patient
2.   Physician assistance

Duties:
1.   Assist physician as needed in restoring patient's medical stability; take vital signs, draw initial blood samples
2.   Offer continued reassurance to patient as to his radiation exposure and medical care
3.   Remove outer clothing, including shoes and socks
4.   Sample skin, orifices, any areas known to be contaminated, number all containers (if necessary)
5.   Proceed with decontamination process
6.   Assist physician with treatment of injuries
7.   Assist with patient transfer to clean stretcher

B. NURSE B

Location: Decontamination Room

Radiation Protection Measures: Full protective clothing; TLD, pen dosimeters; plastic apron

Responsibilities:
1.   Interface with Buffer Zone nurse
2.   Assist Nurse A

Duties:
1.   Back-up nurse ready to assist Nurse A and surgeon if needed
2.   Assist with sampling procedure; give samples to Nurse C
3.   Relay status reports, instructions from physician and nurse to those in Buffer Zone

C. NURSE C

Location: doorway of Decontamination Room

Radiation Protection Measures: Plastic gloves, TLD badge

Responsibilities: Assisting Radiation Emergency Area staff as needed

Duties:
1.   Fulfill special requests of Surgeon or Nurse A and B
2.   Hand equipment, instruments, etc. to personnel within the Decontamination Suite
3.   Receive sample containers, place in rack for monitoring
4.   Record on body chart location and container number of samples taken
5.   Record vital signs and other medical information as appropriate

D. SURGEON

Location: Decontamination Room

Radiation Protection Measures: Full protective clothing, ring, TLD, pen dosimeters; plastic apron

Responsibilities:
1. Medical needs of the patient; trauma care
2. Determination of the need for other specialists

Duties:
1. Perform life-saving measures as needed; judgment of general medical condition
2. Reassure patient
3. Determine priorities of care, with respect to seriousness of injuries
4. Direct removal of clothing
5. Direct and assist with preliminary and final sampling for radioactivity
6. Direct preliminary and final decontamination
7. Assess and treat specific injuries
8. Assist with patient transfer to clean stretcher
9. Transfer senior staff responsibility for the patient at completion of decontamination, if appropriate

E. NUCLEAR MEDICINE OR RADIATION TECHNICIAN (A)

Location: Decontamination Room

Radiation Protection Measures: Full protective clothing; ring, TLD, pen dosimeter; plastic apron

Responsibilities:
1. Determine levels of patient contamination during treatment and decontamination
2. In the absence of the Radiation Safety Officer, assume responsibility for protection of staff from excessive exposure

Duties:
1. Make sure RM 14 (or other survey instrument being used) is covered with Saran Wrap® and operating correctly prior to patient arrival
2. Survey patient when first admitted to decontamination room
   a. Complete body survey, front and back
   b. Announce all readings in mR/h (if instrument only records in cpm, calculate the mRem equivalent
3. Continue to survey patient at each stage of decontamination, keeping personnel informed audibly as to meter readings; ensure that readings are being recorded
4. Perform final survey when patient is ready for transfer
5. After patient has left, assist with monitoring of personnel, equipment and physical area involved with decontamination

F. RADIATION SAFETY OFFICER

Location: Buffer zone (may need to go into decontamination room if technician A is not present

Radiation Protection Measures: TLD and pen dosimeters; protective clothing

Responsibilities:
1. Overall decontamination management
2. Interpretation of radiation level measurements
3. Reassurance of staff

Duties:
1. Receive accident report from attendant with victim
2. Determine the need for specialized protection (e.g., lead shield, additional anti-contamination clothing)
3. Record radiation survey data; calculate potential exposures to staff; determine if rotation of personnel is needed; maintain visible progress chart
4. Reassure staff as to their safety
5. Supervise containment procedures
6. Advise on any problems which may arise in regard to exposures or contamination of the victim, personnel or ambulance
7. Supervise the work of the nuclear medicine or radiation technicians
8. Responsible for final release of patient, staff and area after personnel clean up
9. Final interrogation of patient regarding details of the accident
10. Prepare report for Public Relations

G. CHARGE NURSE/NURSING SUPERVISOR (NURSE D)

Location: adjacent to REA

Radiation Protection Measures: None

Responsibilities:
1. Organization and implementation of logistical support
2. Direction of immediate support function
3. Liaison with hospital

Duties:
1. Mobilize all pertinent hospital personnel
2. Supervise logistical preparations, including supplies and equipment, set up of REA, appropriate protective clothing and dosimetry for personnel
3. Direct overall nursing and administrative functions
4. Anticipate additional supplies and equipment that may be needed (e.g., stretcher, splinting, etc.)
5. Assist in setting up special equipment if needed
6. Assist as needed with sample containers — make sure they get recorded and labeled properly
7. Ensure continued security in the REA during the entire patient admission to the Unit
8. Ensure that all supplies and equipment are inventoried and restocked

H. HOUSEKEEPING PERSONNEL

Radiation Protection Measures: None

Responsibilities:
1. To prepare, under supervision, the decontamination room and Buffer Zone for a contaminated casualty
2. To assist with the cleanup of the decontamination room and Buffer Zone, under the direction of the Radiation Officer

Duties:
1. Remove unnecessary furniture from decontamination room
2. Bring radiation emergency supplies to REA
3. If time permits, cover floor of REA and pathway to ambulance; tape outside edges and step off mats as directed
4. Place decontamination tub onto stretcher and secure with straps; hook tubing to tub and direct it into plastic container
5. Attach flexible hosing and shower head to water outlet
6. Rope off Buffer Zone area and tape signs in appropriate locations
7. After casualty has entered decontamination room, roll up floor covering pathway to ambulance
8. After casualty has been transferred, assistance may be required for cleanup procedures. This will be under the direct supervision of the Radiation Safety Officer. Plastic gloves and booties may be appropriate for the situation

I. SECURITY PERSONNEL

Radiation Protection Measures: None

Responsibilities:
1. To secure area around the Buffer Zone and at the special entrance to the Decontamination Room

Duties:
1. Rope off outside special entrance for ambulance drop-off
2. Restrict ambulance and attendants within the roped-off area until dismissed by the Radiation Safety Officer

II. FLOOR PLAN OF STAFF ASSIGNMENTS IN THE REA

A diagram of the treatment area should be included here. An example is provided in Figure 3.

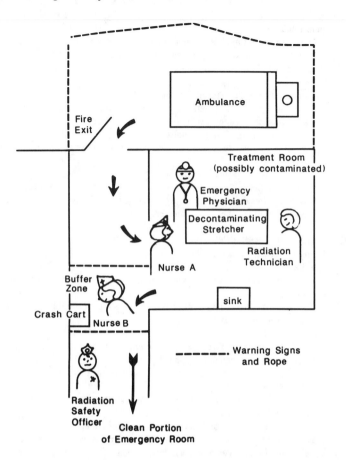

FIGURE 3.   Stylized map of radiation emergency room.

Appendix 2

DIRECTORY OF FEMA OFFICES (FIGURE 1)

National Office
    Federal Emergency Management Agency   (202) 646-2500
    500 C Street SW
    Washington, DC 20472

    Emergency Information and Coordination   (202) 566-1600
      Center (EICC) (24 h)   ext. 3014

Regional Offices

    FEMA Region I   (617) 223-9540
    442 J.W. McCormack   FTS 223-9540
    Boston, MA 02109 (Maynard, MA)

    FEMA Region II   (212) 238-8200
    26 Federal Plaza, Room 1337   FTS 649-8200
    New York, NY

    FEMA Region III   (215) 931-5500
    Liberty Square Bldg., 2nd Floor   FTS 489-5500
    105 S. 7th St.
    Philadelphia, PA 19106

    FEMA Region IV   (404) 853-4200
    1371 Peachtree St. NE, Suite 700   FTS 230-4200
    Atlanta, GA 30309

    FEMA Region V   (312) 408-5500
    175 W. Jackson Blvd., 4th Floor   FTS 363-5500
    Chicago, IL 60604

    FEMA Region VI   (817) 898-9399
    Federal Regional Center, Room 206   FTS 749-9399
    Denton, TX 76201-3698

    FEMA Region VII   (816) 283-7063
    911 Walnut St., Room 300   FTS 759-7063
    Kansas City, MO 64106

    FEMA Region VIII   (303) 235-4811
    Federal Regional Center, Building 710   FTS 322-4811
    Box 25267
    Denver, CO 80225-0267

    FEMA Region IX   (415) 923-7100
    Bldg. 105., Presidio at San Francisco   FTS 469-7100
    San Francisco, CA 94129

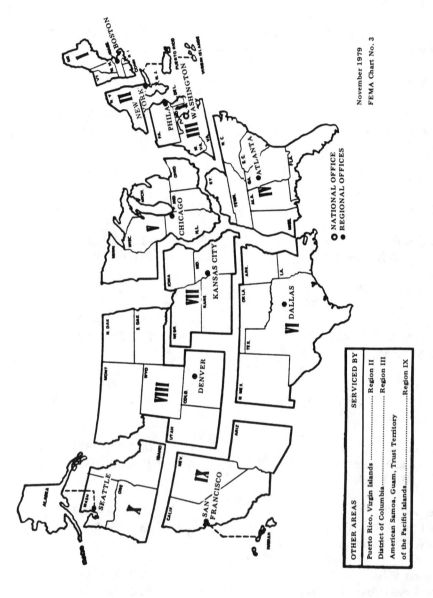

FIGURE 1.   Map of FEMA regions.

FEMA Region X
Federal Regional Center
Bothell, WA 98021-9796

(206) 481-8800
FTS 390-4600

U.S. DEPARTMENT OF ENERGY RADIOLOGICAL ASSISTANCE REGIONS AND COORDINATING OFFICES (FIGURE 2)

Department of Energy, Emergency Operations Center (24 h)	(202) 586-8100
Region 1	(516) 282-2200
Region 2	(615) 576-1006
Region 3	(803) 725-3333
Region 4	(505) 844-4667
Region 5	(312) 972-4800
Region 6	(208) 526-1515
Region 7	(415) 273-4237
Region 8	(509) 373-3800

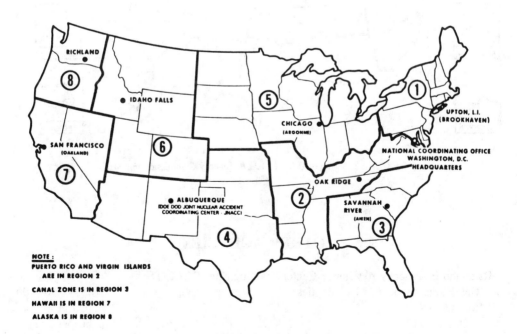

FIGURE 2.   Map of U.S. Department of Energy regions.

U.S. NUCLEAR REGULATORY COMMISSION (FIGURE 3)

Emergency Operations (24 h)	(301) 951-0550
Region I, Office of Inspection and Enforcement, USNRC, 475 Allendale Rd, King of Prussia, PA 19406	(215) 337-5000
Region II, Office of Inspection and Enforcement, USNRC, 101 Marietta St., Atlanta, GA 30323	(404) 331-4503
Region III, Office of Inspection and Enforcement, USNRC, 799 Roosevelt Rd., Glen Ellyn, IL 60137	(312) 790-5500
Region IV, Office of Inspection and Enforcement, USNRC, 611 Ryan Plaza Drive, Suite 1000, Arlington, TX 76012	(817) 860-8100
Region V, Office of Inspection and Enforcement, USNRC, 1990 N. California Blvd., Suite 202, Walnut Creek Plaza, Walnut Creek, CA 94596	(415) 943-3700

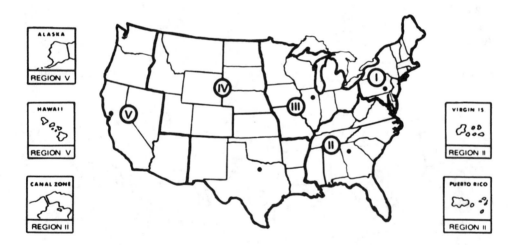

FIGURE 3.   Map of U.S. Nuclear Regulatory Commission regions.

OTHER AGENCIES

Radiation Emergency Assistance Center Training Site (REAC/TS)
   Oak Ridge Associated Universities   (615) 481-1000
   REACT/TS   (ext. 1502 or
   P.O. Box 117   beeper 241)
   Oak Ridge, TN 37830

Appendix 3

EQUIPMENT AND SERVICES LIST

This represents a partial list of suppliers. A more complete listing can be found in the Nuclear News Buyer's Guide available from the American Nuclear Society, 555 N. Kensington Avenue, LaGrange Park, Illinois 60525.

BADGE SERVICES
F = Film
T = TLD
Eberline Analytical Corp., Albuquerque, New Mexico (T)
Harshaw/Filtrol Partnership, Solon, Ohio (T)
R. S. Landauer, Jr. & Co., Glenwood, Illinois (F, T)
Radiation Service Organization, Laurel, MD (F,T)
Teledyne Isotopes, Westwood, NJ (T)

CLOTHING, PROTECTIVE, ANTICONTAMINATION
C   Coveralls
D   Disposable
G   Gloves
H   Head Coverings
L   Lab Coats
SC   Shoe Covers

Bortek Systems, Royersford, PA (C, D, G, H, L, SC)
Disposables, Inc., Manhasset, NY (C, D, H, L, SC)
Euclid Garment Mfg., Co., Kent, OH (C, G, H, L, SC)
Frham Safety Products, Inc., Nashville, TN (C, D, G, H, L, SC)
INS Corp. (Div. of UniFirst Corp.), Springfield, MA (C, D, G, H, L, SC)
Mohawk Industrial & Nuclear Supply, Inc., Manchester, CT (D)
Syracuse Safety Services, Inc., Syracuse, NY (C, D, G, H, L, SC)

CLOTHING, PROTECTIVE, OTHER THAN ANTICONTAMINATION
B   Bibs & Aprons
C   Coveralls
FS   Face Shields
F   Footwear
GG   Gloves, Grinding
GW   Gloves, Welding
GS   Goggles/Spectacles
HH   Hard Hats
HL   Hat Liners (Winter)
HP   Hearing Protection Devices
RW   Rainwear
SS   Splash Sleeves

Bortek Systems, Royersford, PA (C, FS, F, GS, HL, RW, SS)
Euclid Garment Mfg., Co., Kent, OH (B, C, F, RW, SS)
Frham Safety Products, Inc., Nashville, TN (B, C, FS, F, GG, GW, GS, HH, HL, HP, RW, SS)

Herculite Products, Inc., New York, NY (B)

Mohawk Industrial & Nuclear Supply, Inc., Manchester, CT (B, C, FS, F, GG, GS, HH, HL, HP, RW, SS)

Syracuse Safety Services, Inc., Syracuse, NY (B, C, FS, F, GG, GW, GS, HH, HL, RW, SS)

CONSULTING AND TRAINING
Health Physics:
  Porter Consultants, Ardmore, PA
Medical:
  Radiation Emergency Management Services, Albuquerque, NM

COUNTERS, DETECTORS, RADIATION
A   Alpha
B   Beta
G   Gamma
N   Neutron
C   Combinations of Above
ER   Dose Rate, Emergency Range
GM   Geiger-Muller Type
IC   Ion Chamber Type
PC   Proportional Chambers
SL   Scintillation Counters, Liquid
SR   Scintillation Counters, Radioimmunoassay
ST   Scintillation Counters, Solid-State
SS   Solid State Semiconductor Type
DT   Desk-Top
FS   Floor-Standing
FL   Flow
M   Modular
P   Portable

Baird Corp., Bedford, MA (A, B, G, C, GM, PC, ST, DT, M, P)

Eberline Instrument Corp., Santa Fe, NM (A, B, G, N, C, GM, IC, PC, ST, SS, DT, FS, P)

EG&G Ortec, Inc., Oak Ridge, TN (A, B, G, N, C, GM, IC, PC, SL, ST, SS, DT, FS, FL, M, P)

Victoreen, Inc., Cleveland, OH (A, B, G, N, C, GM, IC, PC, SL, ST, DT, FS, FL, M, P)

Xetex, Inc., Mountain View, CA (A, B, G, N, C, GM, IC, PC, ST, SS, DT, FS, FL, M, P)

MATS, ADHESIVE, CONTAMINATION CONTROL
Bortek Systems, Royersford, PA
Euclid Garment Mfg., Co., Kent, OH
Frham Safety Products, Inc., Nashville, TN
Mohawk Industrial and Nuclear Supply, Inc., Manchester, CT

MONITORS, RADIATION, PERSONNEL
AL   Audible Alarm (Electronic)
D   Doorway

FB   Film Badges, Films
HF   Hand and Foot
PI   Pocket Ion Chambers
TL   Thermoluminescent Dosimeters
WB   Whole-Body

Canberrra Industries/RMC, Meriden, CT (WB)
Dosimeter Corp., Cincinnati, OH (AL, PI, WB)
Eberline Instrument Corp., Santa Fe, NM (D, HF, PI, WB)
Helgeson Scientific Services, Inc., Pleasanton, CA (HF, WB)
Victoreen, Inc., Cleveland, OH (PI, TL)

SIGNS, WARNING, RADIATION
Atomic Products Corp, Shirley, NY
Bortek Systems, Royersford, PA
Frham Safety Products, Inc., Nashville, TN
Mohawk Industrial & Nuclear Supply, Inc., Manchester, CT
Radiation Service Organization, Laurel, MD

TAGS & LABELS (WARNING, INVENTORY, ETC.)
Bortek Systems, Royersford, PA
Mohawk Industrial & Nuclear Supply, Inc., Manchester, CT
Radiation Services Organization, Laurel, MD

TAPE
C   Cloth, Nuclear
F   Foam
MS   Moisture-Sensitive
RS   Reinforced Strapping, Nuclear
WL   Warning, Luminescent

Bortek Systems, Royersford, PA (C, WL)
Frham Safety Products, Inc., Nashville, TN (C, MS, RS)
Mohawk Industrial & Nuclear Supply, Inc., Manchester, CT (C, MS, RS, WL)
Syracuse Safety Services, Inc., Syracuse, NY (C, F, MS, RS, WL)

SHIELDING MATERIALS, RADIATION
A   Aggregates, High-Density Concrete
B   Blankets
CB   Blocks, Concrete, Lead-Core
BM   Blocks, Modular
BC   Bricks, Composite
BL   Bricks, Lead
CM   Castable Shielding Materials
CC   Castings, Composite
CL   Castings, Lead
CS   Collars, Streaming
CW   Container Wraps
CR   Criticality Control
FS   Frisker Shields
GN   Gamma/Neutron Composite

PW   Pipe Wraps
PC   Plugs, Closures
TN   Thermal Neutron Materials
WP   Wall Panels

Aarval Lead Products, Plymouth, MN
Advanced Refractory Technologies, Buffalo, NY (B, BM, BC, CM, CR, TN)
Amer Industrial Technologies, Inc., Wilmington, DL (A, CB, BM, BL, CM, CC, CL, CS, CW, GN, PW, PC, WP)
Mohawk Industrial & Nuclear Supply, Inc., Manchester, CT (B, BC)
Nuclear Sources & Services, Inc., Houston, TX (BL, CL, GN, PC, TN)
Reactor Experiments, Inc., San Carlos, CA (A, B, BM, BC, BL, CM, CC, CL, CS, CW, CR, GN, PC, TN, WP)

ADDRESSES OF SOURCES

AARVAL LEAD PRODUCTS, P.O. Box 41276, Plymouth, MI 55447
(612/541-1200 or 800/328-3361)

ADVANCED REFRACTORY TECHNOLOGIES, INC., 699 Hertel Ave., Buffalo, NY 14207
(716/875-4091)

AMER INDUSTRIAL TECHNOLOGIES, INC., 1000 S. Madison St., Wilmington, DL 19801
(Telex:510-666-2005)

ATOMIC PRODUCTS CORP., P.O. Box R, Shirley, NY 11960-0917
(516/924-9000; Telex 797566)

BAIRD CORP., 125 Middlesex Turnpike, Bedford, MA 01730
(617/276-6204)

BORTEK SYSTEMS, P.O. Box 355, Royersford, PA 19468
(215/948-9696)

CANBERRA INDUSTRIES, INC./RMC, One State Street, Meriden, CT 06450
(203/238-2351)

DISPOSABLES, INC., 14 Locust Street, Manhasset, NY 11030
(516/627-4554)

DOSIMETER CORP., 11286 Grooms Rd., Cincinnati, OH 45242
(513/489-8100)

EBERLINE INSTRUMENT CORP., P.O. Box 2108, Airport Rd., Santa Fe, NM 87504-2108
(505/471-3232)

EBERLINE ANALYTICAL CORP., Thermo Analytical Corp., 5635 Kircher Blvd. N.E., Albuquerque, NM 87109
(505/345-9931)

EG&G ORTEC, INC. (Sub. of EG&G), 100 Midland Road, Oak Ridge, TN 37830
(615/482-4411, ext 530)

EUCLID GARMENT MFG., CO., 333 Martinel Dr., P.O. Box 535, Kent, OH 44240-0535
(216/673-7413)

FRHAM SAFETY PRODUCTS, INC., P.O. Box 101177, 1100 Elm Hill Pike, Suite 145,
Nashville, TN 37210
(615/254-0841)

HARSHAW/FILTROL PARTNERSHIP, 6801 Cochran Rd., Solon, OH 44139
(216/349-6590)

HELGESON SCIENTIFIC SERVICES, INC., 5587 Sunol Blvd., Pleasanton, CA 94566
(415/846-3453, TWX: 910 4826460)

HERCULITE PRODUCTS, INC. (Sub. of Health-Chem Corp.), 1107 Broadway, New York,
NY 10010
(212/691-7550)

INS CORP. (Div. of UniFirst Corp.), 295 Parker St., P.O. Box 201, Springfield, MA 01151
(413/543-6911)

R.S. LANDAUER, JR. & CO., Div. of Tech/Ops., Inc., 2 Science Road, Glenwood, IL
60425-1586
(312/755-7000)

MOHAWK INDUSTRIAL & NUCLEAR SUPPLY, INC., 5 Glen Road, Manchester, CT
06040
(203/643-5107 or 1-800/243-4678)

PORTER CONSULTANTS, INC., 125 Argyle Road, Ardmore, PA 19003
(215/896-5353)

RADIATION EMERGENCY MANAGEMENT SERVICES, 3004 LaMancha Street NW,
Albuquerque, NM 87104
(505/243-0236)

RADIATION SERVICE ORGANIZATION, P.O. Box 1526, Laurel, MD 20707
(301/792-7444)

REACTOR EXPERIMENTS, INC., 963 Terminal Way, San Carlos, CA 94070
(415/592-3355)

SYRACUSE SAFETY SERVICES, INC., 1108 Spring St., Syracuse, NY 13208
(1-800/428-8772)

TELEDYNE ISOTOPES, 50 Van Buren Ave., Westwood, NJ 07675
(201/664-7070)

VICTOREEN, INC., (Sub. of Sheller-Globe Corp.), 10101 Woodland Ave., Cleveland, OH 44104
(216/795-8200)

XETEX, INC., 600 National Ave., Mountain View, CA 94043-2257
(415/964-3261)

Appendix 4

CONVERSION TABLES

TABLE 1
Conventional and International (SI) Unit Conversions

Factor	Prefix	Symbol	Factor	Prefix	Symbol
10^{18}	exa	E	10^{-1}	deci	d
10^{15}	peta	P	10^{-2}	centi	c
10^{12}	tera	T	10^{-3}	milli	m
10^{9}	giga	G	10^{-6}	micro	μ
10^{6}	mega	M	10^{-9}	nano	n
10^{3}	kilo	k	10^{-12}	pico	p
10^{2}	hecto	h	10^{-15}	femto	f
10^{1}	deka	da	10^{-18}	atto	a

From *Medical Effects of Ionizing Radiation*, Mettler, F. A. and Moseley, R. D., Eds., Grune & Stratton, New York, 1985. With permission.

TABLE 2
Conversion of Exposure Units

Coulomb/kilogram		Roentgen (R)
10 Ckg^{-1}	=	38,000 R
1 Ckg^{-1}	=	3,880 R
10^{-1} Ckg^{-1}	=	388 R
10^{-2} Ckg^{-1}	=	38.8 R
10^{-3} Ckg^{-1}	=	3.88 R
10^{-4} Ckg^{-1}	=	0.388 R (388 mR)
10^{-5} Ckg^{-1}	=	3.88×10^{-2} R (38.8 mR)
10^{-6} Ckg^{-1}	=	3.88×10^{-3} R (3.88 mR)
10^{-7} Ckg^{-1}	=	3.88×10^{-4} R (388 μR)
10^{-8} Ckg^{-1}	=	3.88×10^{-5} R (38.8 μR)
10^{-9} Ckg^{-1}	=	3.88×10^{-6} R (3.8 μR)
10^{-11} Ckg^{-1}	=	3.88×10^{-7} R (388 nR)
10^{-12} Ckg^{-1}	=	3.88×10^{-8} R (38.8 nR)

From *Medical Effects of Ionizing Radiation*, Mettler, F. A. and Moseley, R. D., Eds., Grune & Stratton, New York, 1985. With permission.

TABLE 3
Conversion of Absorbed Dose Units

SI units		Conventional
100 Gy (10^2 Gy)	=	10,000 rads (10^4 rad)
10 Gy (10^1 Gy)	=	1,000 rads (10^3 rad)
1 Gy (10^0 Gy)	=	100 rads (10^2 rad)
100 mGy (10^{-1} Gy)	=	10 rads (10^1 rad)
10 mGy (10^{-2} Gy)	=	1 rad (10^0 rad)
1 mGy (10^{-3} Gy)	=	100 mrads (10^{-1} rad)
100 μGy (10^{-4} Gy)	=	10 mrads (10^{-2} rad)
10 μGy (10^{-5} Gy)	=	1 mrad (10^{-3} rad)
1 μGy (10^{-6} Gy)	=	100 μrad (10^{-4} rad)
100 nGy (10^{-7} Gy)	=	10 μrad (10^{-5} rad)
10 nGy (10^{-8} Gy)	=	1 μrad (10^{-6} rad)
1 nGy (10^{-9} Gy)	=	100 nrad (10^{-7} rad)

From *Medical Effects of Ionizing Radiation*, Mettler, F. A. and Moseley, R. D., Eds., Grune & Stratton, New York, 1985. With permission.

TABLE 4
Conversion of Dose Equivalent Units

100 Sv (10^2 Sv)	=	10,000 rem	(10^4 rem)
10 Sv (10^1 Sv)	=	1,000 rem	(10^3 rem)
1 Sv (10^0 Sv)	=	100 rem	(10^2 rem)
100 mSv (10^{-1} Sv)	=	10 rem	(10^1 rem)
10 mSv (10^{-2} Sv)	=	1 rem	(10^0 rem)
1 mSv (10^{-3} Sv)	=	100 mrem	(10^{-1} rem)
100 μSv (10^{-4} Sv)	=	10 mrem	(10^{-2} rem)
10 μSv (10^{-5} Sv)	=	1 mrem	(10^{-3} rem)
1 μSv (10^{-6} Sv)	=	100 μrem	(10^{-4} rem)

TABLE 4 (continued)
Conversion of Dose Equivalent Units

100 nSv (10^{-7} Sv)	=	10 μrem	(10^{-5} rem)
10 nSv (10^{-8} Sv)	=	1 μrem	(10^{-6} rem)
1 nSv (10^{-9} Sv)	=	100 nrem	(10^{-7} rem)

From *Medical Effects of Ionizing Radiation*, Mettler, F. A. and Moseley, R. D., Eds., Grune & Stratton, New York, 1985. With permission.

TABLE 5
Conversion of Radioactivity Units

100 TBq (10^{14} Bq)	=	2.7 kCi (2.7×10^3 Ci)
10 TBq (10^{13} Bq)	=	270 Ci (2.7×10^2 Ci)
1 TBq (10^{12} Bq)	=	27 Ci (2.7×10^1 Ci)
100 GBq (10^{11} Bq)	=	2.7 Ci (2.7×10^0 Ci)
10 GBq (10^{10} Bq)	=	270 mCi (2.7×10^{-1} Ci)
1 GBq (10^9 Bq)	=	27 mCi (2.7×10^{-2} Ci)
100 MBq (10^8 Bq)	=	2.7 mCi (2.7×10^{-3} Ci)
10 MBq (10^7 Bq)	=	270 μCi (2.7×10^{-4} Ci)
1 MBq (10^6 Bq)	=	27 μCi (2.7×10^{-5} Ci)
100 kBq (10^5 Bq)	=	2.7 μCi (2.7×10^{-6} Ci)
10 kBq (10^4 Bq)	=	270 nCi (2.7×10^{-7} Ci)
1 kBq (10^3 Bq)	=	27 nCi (2.7×10^{-8} Ci)
100 Bq (10^2 Bq)	=	2.7 nCi (2.7×10^{-9} Ci)
10 Bq (10^1 Bq)	=	270 pCi (2.7×10^{-10} Ci)
1 Bq (10^0 Bq)	=	27 pCi (2.7×10^{-11} Ci)
100 mBq (10^{-1} Bq)	=	2.7 pCi (2.7×10^{-12} Ci)
10 mBq (10^{-2} Bq)	=	270 fCi (2.7×10^{-13} Ci)
1 mBq (10^{-3} Bq)	=	27 fCi (2.7×10^{-14} Ci)

From *Medical Effects of Ionizing Radiation*, Mettler, F. A. and Moseley, R. D., Eds., Grune & Stratton, New York, 1985. With permission.

TABLE 6
Absorbed Dose Estimates (mSv/MBq) from Various Radionuclides in Critical Organ or Lung (50-Year Commitment)

		Dose in Organ	
Radionuclide	Critical organ	Critical organ	Lung
Americium 241	Bone	8.1×10^6	5.7×10^5
Americium 243	Bone	8.1×10^6	5.4×10^5
Arsenic 74	Total body	2.7	97.3
Arsenic 77	Total body	0.11	7.57
Barium 140	Bone	132	351
Cadmium 109	Liver	143	405
Calcium 45	Bone	200	64.8
Calcium 47	Bone	32.4	67.5
Californium 252	Bone	3.0×10^6	1.37×10^6
Carbon 14	Total body	0.162	54
Cerium 141	Liver	89.1	111
Cerium 144	Bone	4320	4590
Cesium 137	Total body	8.1	405
Chromium 51	Total body	0.189	7.29
Cobalt 57	Total body	0.243	43.2
Cobalt 58	Total body	1.35	167.4
Cobalt 60	Total body	4.05	702

TABLE 6 (continued)
Absorbed Dose Estimates (mSv/MBq) from Various Radionuclides in Critical Organ or Lung (50-Year Commitment)

| Radionuclide | Critical organ | Dose in Organ | |
		Critical organ	Lung
Curium 242	Liver	1.45×10^5	1.57×10^5
Curium 243	Liver	4.05×10^6	5.67×10^5
Curium 244	Liver	2.97×10^6	5.67×10^5
Europium 152	Kidney	1.86×10^4	2970
Europium 154	Bone	9180	7.83×10^4
Europium 155	Kidney	2511	513
Fluorine 18	Total body	0.019	0.81
Gallium 72	Liver	6.48	12.7
Gold 198	Total body	0.27	23.5
Hydrogen 3	Total body	0.54	—
Indium 114m	Kidney, spleen	1674	459
Iodine 125	Thyroid	1458	—
Iodine 131	Thyroid	1755	—
Iron 55	Spleen	324	6.21
Iron 59	Spleen	1890	200
Lead 210	Kidney	3.24×10^5	2.48×10^4
Mercury 197	Kidney	5.94	2.43
Mercury 203	Kidney	81	83.7
Molybdenum 99	Kidney	46	2.54
Neptunium 237	Bone	7.56×10^6	4.86×10^5
Neptunium 239	Colon	6.21	7.29
Phosphorus 32	Bone	27	151
Plutonium 238	Bone	7.02×10^6	5.67×10^5
Plutonium 239	Bone	8.10×10^6	5.4×10^5
Polonium 210	Spleen	2.97×10^5	4.05×10^4
Potassium 42	Total body	0.22	15.1
Promethium 147	Bone	594	459
Promethium 149	Bone	11.9	19.2
Radium 224	Bone	2970	1.89×10^4
Radium 226	Bone	2.7×10^6	1.11×10^5
Rubidium 86	Total body	2.43	178
Ruthenium 106	Kidney	216	5940
Scandium 46	Liver	189	405
Silver 110m	Total body	2.16	891
Sodium 22	Total body	4.86	0.32
Sodium 24	Total body	0.46	0.62
Strontium 85	Total body	5.94	89.1
Strontium 90	Bone	8.6×10^4	1107
Sulfur 35	Testis	1.1×10^4	0.02
Technetium 99m	Total body	0.0027	0.17
Technetium 99	Kidney	35.1	35.1
Thorium 230	Bone	7.83×10^6	4.86×10^5
Thorium 232	Bone	7.83×10^6	4.86×10^5
Uranium 235	Kidney	4.6×10^4	4.6×10^5
Uranium 238	Kidney	4.32×10^4	4.32×10^5
Uranium natural	Kidney	4.6×10^4	4.6×10^5
Yttrium 90	Bone	32.4	46
Zinc 65	Total body	17.8	74.5
Zirconium 95	Total body	0.81	294

Note: To obtain values in rems/mCi of radionuclide in organ, multiply values in table by 3.7.

From *Medical Effects of Ionizing Radiation,* Mettler, F. A. and Moseley, R. D., Eds., Grune & Stratton, New York, 1985. With permission.

TABLE 7
Specific Gamma Ray
Constants

Nuclide	Γ^a	Nuclide	Γ^a
Actinium 227	~2.2	Lanthanum 140	11.3
Antimony 122	2.4	Lutecium 177	0.09
Antimony 124	9.8	Magnesium 28	15.7
Antimony 125	~2.7	Manganese 52	18.6
Arsenic 72	10.1	Manganese 54	4.7
Arsenic 74	4.4	Manganese 56	8.3
Arsenic 76	2.4	Mercury 197	~0.4
Barium 131	~3.0	Mercury 203	1.3
Barium 133	~2.4	Molybdenum 99	.9
Barium 140	12.4	Neodymium 147	0.8
Beryllium 7	~0.3	Nickel 65	~3.1
Bromine 82	14.6	Niobium 95	4.2
Cadmium 115m	~0.2	Osmium 191	~0.6
Calcium 47	5.7	Palladium 109	0.03
Carbon 11	5.9	Platinum 197	~0.5
Cerium 141	0.35	Potassium 42	1.4
Cerium 144	~0.4	Potassium 43	5.6
Cesium 134	8.7	Radium 226	8.25
Cesium 137	3.3	Radium 228	~5.1
Chlorine 38	8.8	Rhenium 186	~0.2
Chromium 51	0.16	Rubidium 86	0.5
Cobalt 56	17.6	Ruthenium 106	1.7
Cobalt 57	0.9	Scandium 46	10.9
Cobalt 58	5.5	Scandium 47	0.56
Cobalt 60	13.2	Selenium 75	2.0
Copper 64	1.2	Silver 110m	14.3
Europium 152	5.8	Silver 111	~0.2
Europium 154	~6.2	Sodium 22	12.0
Europium 155	~0.3	Sodium 24	18.4
Gallium 67	~1.1	Strontium 85	3.0
Gallium 72	11.6	Tantalum 182	6.8
Gold 198	2.3	Technetium 99m	0.60
Gold 199	~0.9	Tellurium 121	3.3
Hafnium 175	~2.1	Tellurium 132	2.2
Hafnium 181	~3.1	Thulium 170	0.025
Indium 114m	~0.2	Tin 113	~1.7
Iodine 124	7.2	Tungsten 185	~0.5
Iodine 125	~0.7	Tungsten 187	3.0
Iodine 126	2.5	Uranium 234	~0.1
Iodine 130	12.2	Vanadium 48	15.6
Iodine 131	2.2	Xenon 133	0.1
Iodine 132	11.8	Ytterbium 175	0.4
Iridium 192	4.8	Yttrium 88	14.1
Iridium 194	1.5	Yttrium 91	0.01
Iron 59	6.4	Zinc 65	2.7
Krypton 85	~0.04	Zirconium 95	4.1

a $\Gamma = R - cm^2/h - mCi$ or $\Gamma/10 = R/h$ at 1 m/Ci.

The following gives examples of the use of specific gamma ray constants (Γ). The constant gives the exposure in R/mCi/h at 1 cm or the constant divided by 10 gives exposure in R/h at 1 m from 1 Ci. The specific gamma ray constant can be used to find the exposure rate (R/h) for a source of activity A (mCi) at any distance d (cm) by using the following formula:

TABLE 7 (continued)
Specific Gamma Ray Constants

$$\text{Exposure rate} = \frac{\Gamma A}{d^2}$$

As an example, to calculate the exposure rate at 92 cm (3 ft) from a 1 Ci(1000mCi) source of cobalt 60, the calculation would be as follows:

$$\text{Exposure rate} = \frac{13.2 \times 1000}{(92)^2} = \frac{13,200}{8464} = 1.56 \text{ R/h}$$

From *Medical Effects of Ionizing Radiation*, Mettler, F. A. and Moseley, R. D., Eds., Grune & Stratton, New York, 1985. With permission.

TABLE 8
Radionuclides Listed Alphabetically

Radionuclide	Physical half-life	Effective half-life	Radiation
Americium 241	458 years	139 years	α, e^-, γ
Americium 243	7950 years	194 years	α, γ
Antimony 122	67 h	—	β^-, β^+, γ
Antimony 124	60 d	—	β^-, γ
Antimony 125	2.7 years	—	β^-, e^-, γ
Argon 37	35 d	—	γ
Arsenic 74	18 d	17 d	β^-, β^+, γ
Arsenic 76	26.5 h	—	β^-, γ
Arsenic 77	39 h	24 h	β^-, γ
Barium 131	12 d	—	γ, e^-
Barium 133	7.2 years	—	γ, e^+
Barium 137m	2.55 min	—	γ, e^-
Barium 140	13 d	11 d	β^-, e^-, γ
Beryllium 7	53 d	—	γ
Bismuth 207	30 years	—	e^-, γ
Bismuth 210	5.01 d	—	α, β^-, γ
Bromine 82	35.34 h	—	β^-, γ
Cadmium 109	453 d	140 d	e^-, γ
Cadmium 115	53.5 h	—	β^-, γ
Cadmium 115	43 d	—	β^-, γ
Calcium 45	165 d	162 d	β^-
Calcium 47	4.5 d	4.5 d	β^-, γ
Californium 242	2.6 years	2.2 years	γ, α, N
Carbon 11	20.3 min	—	β^+, γ
Carbon 14	5730 years	12 d	β^-
Cerium 141	33 d	30 d	β^-, e^-, γ
Cerium 144	284 d	280 d	β^-, e^-, γ
Cesium 131	9.70 d	—	γ
Cesium 134	2.05 years	—	β^-, γ
Cesium 137	30.0 years	70 d	β^-, e^-, γ
Chlorine 36	3.1×10^5 years	—	β^-, γ
Chromium 51	27.8 d	27 d	e^-, γ
Cobalt 57	270 d	9 d	e^-, γ
Cobalt 58	71.3 d	8 d	β^+, γ
Cobalt 60	5.26 years	10 d	β^-, γ
Copper 64	12.8 h	—	$\beta^-, e^-, \beta^+, \gamma$
Curium 242	163 d	155 d	α, N, γ
Curium 243	32 years	27.5 d	α, γ

TABLE 8 (continued)
Radionuclides Listed Alphabetically

Radionuclide	Physical half-life	Effective half-life	Radiation
Curium 244	17.6 years	16.7 years	α,N,γ
Dysprosium 159	144 d	—	e⁻,γ
Erbium 169	9.4 d	—	β⁻,e⁻,γ
Europium 152	13 years	3 years	β⁻,β⁺,e⁻,γ
Europium 154	16 years	3 years	β⁻,e⁻,γ
Europium 155	2 years	1.3 years	β⁻,e⁻,γ
Fluorine 18	2 h	2 h	β,γ
Gadolinium 153	242 d	—	e⁻,γ
Gallium 67	78.1 h	—	γ
Gallium 68	68.3 min	—	β⁺,γ
Gallium 72	14.1 h	12 h	β,γ
Germanium 71	11.4 d	—	γ
Gold 195	183 d	—	e⁻,γ
Gold 198	2.7 d	2.6 d	β⁻,e⁻,γ
Gold 199	75.6 h	—	β⁻,e⁻,γ
Hafnium 181	42.5 d	—	β⁻,e⁻,γ
Holmium 166	26.9 h	—	β⁻,e⁻,γ
Hydrogen 3	12 years	12 d	β⁻
Indium 111	2.8 d	—	γ
Indium 113m	100 min	—	e⁻,γ
Indium 114	72 s	—	β⁻,β⁺,γ
Indium 114m	49 d	27 d	e⁻,γ(DR)
Iodine 123	13 h	—	γ
Iodine 125	60 d	42 d	e⁻,γ
Iodine 129	1.7 × 10⁷ years	—	β⁻,e⁻,γ
Iodine 130	12.4 h	—	β⁻,γ
Iodine 131	8.05 d	8 d	β⁻,e⁻,γ
Iridium 192	74 d	—	β⁻,e⁻,
Iridium 194	17.4 h	—	β,X,
Iron 52	8.3 h	—	β⁻,
Iron 55	2.6 years	1 years	
Iron 59	45 d	42 d	β⁻,
Krypton 81m	13.0 s	—	
Krypton 85	10.76 years	—	β⁻,
Lanthanum 140	40.22 h	—	β⁻,
Lead 210	2 years	1.3 years	α,β⁻,e⁻,
Lutetium 177	6.7 d	—	β⁻,e⁻,
Magnesium 28	21 h	—	β⁻,e⁻,
Manganese 54	303 d	—	e⁻,
Mercury197	2.7 d	2.3 d	e⁻,
Mercury 197m	24 h	—	e⁻,
Mercury 203	4 d	11 d	β⁻,e⁻,
Molybdenum 99	67 h	1.5 d	β⁻,
Neodymium 147	11.1 d	—	β⁻,e⁻,
Neptunium 237	2 × 10⁶ years	200 years	α, (DR)
Neptunium 239	2.3 d	2.3 d	β,
Nickel 63	92 years	—	β⁻
Niobium 95	35 d	—	β⁻,
Nitrogen 13	10 min	—	β⁺,
Osmium 191	15 d	—	β⁻,e⁻,γ
Oxygen 15	124 s	—	β⁺,γ
Palladium 103	17 d	—	γ
Palladium 109	13.47 h	—	β⁻,e⁻,γ
Phosphorus 32	14 d	14 d	β⁻
Plutonium 238	88 years	63 years	γ,α
Plutonium 239	2.4 × 10⁴ years	197 years	γ,α

TABLE 8 (continued)
Radionuclides Listed Alphabetically

Radionuclide	Physical half-life	Effective half-life	Radiation
Polonium 210	138 d	46 d	α,γ
Potassium 42	12 h	12 h	β⁻,γ
Praseodymium 142	19.2 h	—	β⁻,γ
Praseodymium 143	13.6 d	—	β⁻
Praseodymium 144	17.3 min	—	β⁻,γ
Promethium 147	2.6 years	1.6 years	β⁻
Promethium 149	2.2 d	2.2 d	β⁻,γ
Protactinium 233	27.0 d	—	β⁻,e⁻,γ
Protactinium 234	6.75 h	—	β⁻,e⁻,γ
Radium 224	3.6 d	3.6 d	γ,α(DR)
Radium 226	160 years	44 years	α,e⁻,γ(DR)
Rhenium 186	90 h	—	β⁻,e⁻,γ
Rhodium 106	30 s	—	β⁻,γ
Rubidium 82	1.3 min	—	β⁺,γ
Rubidium 86	19.0 d	13.2 d	β⁻,γ
Ruthenium 97	2.9 d	—	e⁻,γ
Ruthenium 103	39.6 d	—	β⁻,γ
Ruthenium 106	367 d	2.5 d	β⁻(DR)
Samarium 151	87 years	—	β⁻,e⁻,γ
Samarium 153	47 h	—	β⁻,e⁻,γ
Scandium 46	84 d	40 d	β⁻,γ
Selenium 75	120.4 d	—	e⁻,γ
Selenium 77m	17.5 s	—	γ
Silver 110	24.4 s	—	β⁻,γ
Silver 110m	253 d	5 d	β⁻,e⁻,γ
Silver 111	7.5 d	—	β⁻,γ
Sodium 22	2.60 years	11 d	β⁺,γ
Sodium 24	15 h	14 h	β⁻,γ
Strontium 85	64 d	64 d	e⁻,γ
Strontium 87m	2.83 h	—	e⁻,γ
Strontium 89	52 d	—	β⁻,γ
Strontium 90	28 years	15 years	β⁻(DR)
Sulfur 35	88 d	44 d	β⁻
Tantalum 182	115 d	—	β⁻,e⁻,γ
Technetium 99	2.12 × 10⁵ years	20 d	β⁻
Technetium 99m	6.0 h	—	e⁻,γ
Tellurium 132	78 h	—	β⁻,e⁻,γ
Terbium 160	72.1 d	—	β⁻,e⁻,γ
Thallium 201	73 h	—	γ (DR)
Thallium 204	3.8 years	—	β⁻,γ
Thorium 230	8 × 10⁴ years	200 years	α,γ
Thorium 232	1.4 × 10¹⁰ years	200 years	α,γ(DR)
Thulium 170	130 d	—	β⁻,e⁻,γ
Tin 113	115 d	—	γ
Tin 119m	250 d	—	e⁻,γ
Titanium 44	48 h	—	e⁻,γ(DR)
Tungsten 185	75 d	—	β⁻
Tungsten 187	23.9 h	—	β⁻,e⁻,γ
Uranium 235	7.1 × 10⁸ years	15 d	α,γ(DR)
Uranium 238	4.51 × 10⁹ years	—	α,e⁻,γ(DR)
Xenon 127	36.4 d	—	e⁻,γ
Xenon 133	5.27 d	—	β⁻,e⁻,γ
Ytterbium 169	32 d	—	e⁻,γ
Yttrium 90	64 h	64 h	β⁻
Yttrium 91	58.8 d	—	β⁻,γ

TABLE 8 (continued)
Radionuclides Listed Alphabetically

Radionuclide	Physical half-life	Effective half-life	Radiation
Zinc 65	245 d	194 d	β^+, e^-, γ
Zinc 69	57 min	—	β^-
Zirconium 95	66 d	56 d	$\beta^-, \gamma(DR)$

Note: DR = daughter radiation, N = neutron.

From *Medical Effects of Ionizing Radiation,* Mettler, F. A. and Moseley, R. D., Eds., Grune & Stratton, New York, 1985. With permission.

Appendix 5

EVALUATION OF NEUTRON EXPOSURE

Evaluation radiation exposure due to neutrons can be done by one of four methods. These are blood analysis for ^{24}Na, a quick sort method, hair analysis for ^{32}P, and finally activation of metal objects such as jewelry. Whole-body neutron doses on the order of 10 rad (0.1 Gy) can be identified by determining the amount of ^{24}Na in blood. Sodium-24 is produced by the neutron interaction with ^{23}Na. With a 30 min count of a 10 ml blood sample, activity as low as 3.9×10^{-5} μCi/cc of ^{24}Na (physical half-life, 15 h) can be identified. The conversion factor is 1.6 times 10 (0.1 Gy) rad of fission spectrum neutrons per microcurie per cc. Of course the time elapsed since exposure needs to be included to correct for the physical decay of ^{24}Na. The formula thus becomes:

$$D = 1.6 \times 10^5 \; C \times e^{0.0462\,t}$$

where D equals dose in rad, C equals the concentration of ^{24}Na in blood in μCi/cc at time t, and t equals time in h between accident and analysis.

The quick sort method can be utilized in cases in which there is no internal or external contamination and only external gamma or neutron exposure. This involves a direct survey of the body with a simple Geiger-type survey instrument held against the abdominal area. Immediately after an accident there will be an error factor in the estimate of dose of as much as 50% caused by activated ^{38}Cl, however this decays quickly and decreases to a 1% error 4 h after the accident. Using the following formula $D = 1.1^{K/M}$ whereas K is the count rate in cpm for a geiger tube instrument (calibrated to indicate a response of 3,200 cpm in a 1 mR/h radiation field from a gamma source), M is the body weight of exposed person in kilograms and D is the first collison neutron dose in rad. Typical sensitivity shows about 65 cpm for one rad (0.01 Gy) in a standard man.[1,2]

Neutron dose to localized areas on critical organs of the body can be estimated by determining the ^{32}P activity in hair and by knowing the neutron spectrum. The reaction ^{32}S (n,p) ^{32}P in body hair produces the activity. Hair samples are often the only ones that can be utilized to indicate the extent of exposure to different parts of the body and the orientation of the patient to the neutron source. Different 1 g hair samples can be obtained from the head, chest, groin, legs, and sometimes even the back area. These should all be carefully labeled. Following chemical separation and evaporation to dryness, the ^{32}P activity can be measured with a low background proportional counter or similar device. Dose in rads = 5.5×10^4A where A equals activity per gram of hair. This formula holds for time = 0 and needs to be corrected for physical decay of the ^{32}P (half-life, 15d) since the time of the accident.[3]

Neutron activation of other materials such as film badge inserts, belt buckles, metal buttons, shoe nails, pocket change, rings, eyeglasses, watchbands, and pens as well assorted tools can all be examined for neutron activation. In order to translate the activation data to personnel exposure one needs to determine the neutron energy range, the activation cross-section for that energy, and the neutron flux.

REFERENCES

1. **Sanders, F. W. and Auxier, J. A.,** Neutron activation of sodium and anthropomorphous phantoms, *Health Phys.,* 8, 371, 1962.
2. **Parker, H. M. and Newton, C. E., Jr.,** The handful criticality accident: Dosimeter techniques, interpretations and problems, in personnel dosimetery for radiation accidence, *IAEA Symp. Proc.* STI/PUB/99, International Atomic Energy Agency, Vienna, 1965, 567.
3. **Peterson, D. F. and Langham, W. H.,** Neutron activation of sulphur and hair, *Health Phys.,* 12, 381, 1966.

GLOSSARY

Absolute risk	See Risk, absolute.
Absorbed dose	When ionizing radiation passes through matter, some of its energy is imparted to the matter. The amount absorbed per unit mass of irradiated material is called the absorbed dose, and it is measured in Gy or rad. See Threshold dose.
Absorbed dose equivalent	See Dose equivalent.
Accelerator	Device imparting high kinetic energy to a charged particle causing it to undergo nuclear or particle reaction.
Actinide series	The series of elements beginning with number 89 and continuing through number 105, which together occupy one position in the periodic table. The series includes uranium, element number 92, and all the manmade transuranic elements. The group is also referred to as the *Actinides*. Compare Lanthanide series.
Activation	The process of making a material radioactive by bombardment with neutrons, protons, or other nuclear particles.
Activity	See Radioactivity, Specific activity.
Acute radiation syndrome	The collective term for the hematopoietic, gastrointestinal, and cardiovascular/central nervous system forms of response to whole-body acute or subacute exposure to radiation. Usually requires absorbed doses in excess of 200 rad (2 Gy). The syndrome is a clinical manifestation of the responses of the individual body systems and their relative sensitivity to radiation. The clinical course is predictable and is divided into prodromal, latent, and manifest periods of illness. If recovery occurs it usually comes 5 to 10 weeks after the radiation exposure.
ALARA	Acronym for NRC operating philosophy for maintaining occupational radiation exposures "as low as is reasonably achievable".
Alpha particle	Nucleus of a helium atom emitted by certain radioisotopes upon disintegration. Contains 2 protons and 2 neutrons.
Annihilation	Reaction between a pair of particles resulting in their disintegration and the production of an equivalent amount of energy in the form of photons.
Annual dose limits	Any of the annual dose equivalent limits for individual members of the public or workers recommended by the International Commission on Radiologic Protection as part of its system of dose limitation.

Annual limit on intake (ALI)	The activity of a radionuclide which, when taken alone, would irradiate a person to the limit set for each year of occupational exposure.
Anticontamination clothing (Anti-C's)	Clothing usually consisting of coveralls, shoe covers, gloves, and hood or cap. These provide protection for the user from getting skin contamination. Sometimes referred to as *protective clothing* although they do not provide protection from gamma or X-rays and only moderate protection from beta particles.
Atom	Smallest unit of an element that can exist and still maintain the properties of the element.
Atomic mass	Mass of a neutral atom usually expressed in atomic mass units.
Atomic mass unit (AMU)	Exactly one twelfth the mass of ^{12}C: 1.661×10^{-24} g.
Atomic number	Number of protons in an atom, the symbol of which is Z.
Atomic weight	Average weight of the neutral atoms of an element.
Attenuation	The reduction in the intensity of radiation as it passes through any material, e.g., through lead shielding or body tissues.
Auger electron	An orbital electron ejected by a characteristic X-ray. The characteristic X-ray is usually emitted following electron capture or internal conversion.
Average life	The mean time during which an atom exists in a particular form. The average life is 1.44 times the physical half-life.
Background	Detected disintegration events not emanating from the sample. Natural background is that radiation which is a natural part of a person's environment, primarily natural radioactivity and cosmic rays.
Battery check	A check to determine that the batteries of a radiation survey meter are charged enough. Generally a battery check position is present on the range knob and if the knob is placed in this position and the batteries are strong enough, the needle will be deflected upwards into the "batt OK" range.
Becquerel (Bq)	The SI unit of radioactivity. One becquerel is one disintegration per second. One becquerel equals approximately 2.7×10^{-11} Ci or 27 picocuries (pCi).
BEIR	Biological Effects of Ionizing Radiation. A series of reports by a Committee of the National Academy of Sciences.
Bent Spear	Term used by the U.S. Department of Defense for a nuclear weapon incident.
Beta particle	An electron of positive or negative charge.
Bioassays	Methods used for determining the amount of internal radioactive contamination.

Boiling water reactor	A reactor system that utilizes a boiling water system to cool the reactor core. The steam generated by the water passing over the core is sent directly to turn the turbines and generate electricity.
Body burden	The amount of radioactive material present in a human or animal.
Bremsstrahlung X-rays	Photonic emissions caused by the slowing down of beta particles in matter.
Broken arrow	Term used by the U.S. Department of Defense for a nuclear weapon accident.
Buffer zone	A zone set up in the hospital radiation emergency area that acts as a buffer between the room in which the patient is being decontaminated and the clean area of the hospital emergency room. The buffer zone is within the controlled area.
By-product material	Radioactive material arising from controlled fission.
Canister (storage)	A container for spent fuel or other high-level radioactive waste material. Usually cylindrical. The material remains in the canister during and after burial in salt or other media. Canister provides physical containment but not shielding. Shielding is provided by the surrounding cask.
Carcinogen	An agent or substance capable of causing induction of a cancer. A complete carcinogen may contain both initiating and promoting capabilities. Other terms involved in the process of carcinogenesis may be:
	Co-carcinogen: An agent which can cause cancer by itself but which, when combined with another carcinogen, produces an effect greater than the sum of either individually (i.e., it is synergistic).
	Initiator: A substance or agent which primes a cell to the development of a tumor. Usually, it will not cause a tumor by itself.
	Promotor: A substance or agent which will not cause a tumor by itself, but will once an initiator has acted on the cell of interest.
Carcinogenesis	The process of induction of cancer in a cell.
Carrier	Quantity of stable isotopes of an element mixed with radioactive isotopes of that element.
Carrier-free	Adjective describing a radionuclide that is free of its stable isotopes.
Cask	A massive shipping container providing shielding for highly radioactive materials. Usually holds one or more canisters.
Cell cycle	The cycle undergone by the nuclear DNA from one cell division to the next. It consists of G1, a period of growth; S, a period of chromosomal DNA replication; G2, period of further growth; and mitosis (M) (G stands for "gap" in DNA replication activity and S stands for "synthesis".)

Central nervous system syndrome

Part of the acute radiation syndrome. Results when there are acute exposures involving the upper portion of the body in excess of 5000 rad (50 Gy). Usually fatal within 48 to 72 h regardless of treatment methods. Manifested by confusion, ataxia, hypotension, and coma.

Centromere

The small constricted region on a chromosome at which identical chromatids are joined and by which the chromosome is attached to a spindle fiber. The position of the centromere determines the length of the arms of the chromosome and, for any particular chromosome, is constant in location.

Chain reaction

A self-sustaining reaction. In a fission nuclear chain reaction a fissionable nucleus absorbs a neutron, then fissions and releases enough more neutrons to enter other fissionable nuclei and keep the reaction going.

Charged particle

An ion or elementary atomic particle that carries a postive or negative electrical charge.

Chromosome aberration

Alteration from normal structure or number.

Chromosomes

Various-sized structural elements in the cell nucleus, composed of DNA and proteins, which carry the genes that convey the genetic information. Chromosomes have a species-specific morphology and number.

Cladding

The outer metallic jacket about nuclear fuel elements. Prevents corrosion of the fuel as well as the release of radioactive fission products into the coolant of the reactor core.

Collective dose equivalent

The collective dose equivalent to a population in units of man-sievert (man-Sv) or man-rem that is the sum of the products of the individual (or per capita dose equivalents) and the number of individuals in each exposed group in a population.

Congenital

Present at birth. Does not imply either genetic or nongenetic causation.

Containment vessel

The heavy metallic receptacle which surrounds and contains the core of a reactor. Also may refer to a receptacle used during transport of radioactive material.

Contamination (radioactive)

A radioactive substance in a material or place where it is undesirable.

Controlled area

An area where entry, activities, and exit are controlled to assure radiation protection and to prevent the spread of radioactive contamination.

Cosmic rays

Radiation of many sorts, but mostly atomic nuclei (protons) with very high energies originating outside the earth's atmosphere. Cosmic radiation is part of the natural background radiation. Some cosmic rays are more energetic than any man-made forms of radiation.

Counts per minute (cpm)	The number of counts or nuclear events detected by a radiation survey device such as a Geiger counter. Since not all events that occur are detected, cpm are always less than actual disintegrations per minute (dpm) emanating from a radioactive material.
Critical organ	(1) Organ of interest; (2) organ most radiobiologically affected by a technique.
Critical mass	The smallest mass of fissionable material that will support a self-sustaining chain reaction under stated conditions.
Criticality	The state of a nuclear reactor when it is sustaining a chain reaction.
Curie	Standard measure of rate or radioactive decay; based on the disintegration of 1 g radium or 3.7×10^{10} disintegrations per second. One curie expressed in SI units is 3.7×10^{10} Becquerels.
Cyclotron	A device consisting of two hollow D-shaped chambers for accelerating charged particles to energies up to 15 MeV or more by periodic accelerations through a potential difference.
Daughter radionuclide	Decay product produced by a radionuclide. The element from which the daughter was produced is called the "parent".
Decay	Radioactive disintegration of a nucleus of an unstable nuclide.
Decay constant (lambda)	The probability per unit of time that a given radionuclide atom will undergo a radioactive transformation.
Decay, radioactive	The spontaneous transformation of one nuclide into a different nuclide or into a different energy state of the same nuclide. The process results in a decrease, with time, of the original radioactive atoms in sample. Radioactive decay involves (1) the emission from the nucleus of alpha particle, beta particles (electrons), or gamma rays; (2) the nuclear capture or ejection of orbital electrons; or (3) fission. Also called radioactive disintegration. See Half-life.
Decay schemes	Diagram showing the decay mode or modes of a radionuclide.
Decommissioning	Preparation of worn-out nuclear facilities for retirement. There is either removal or stabilization of radioactive contamination and items.
Decontamination	The removal or reduction of radioactive contaminants from surface or equipment, for instance, by cleaning and washing.
Delayed neutrons	Neutrons emitted by radioactive fission products in a nuclear reactor over a period of seconds or minutes after a fission takes place. Fewer than 1% of the neutrons are delayed; more than 99%

are prompt neutrons. Delayed neutrons are important considerations in reactor design and control.

Delayed radiation effects	Manifestations of radiation damage that become evident months or years after irradiation. Examples include atrophy, fibrosis, ulceration, cancer, and genetic effects.
De minimus	An expression derived from the Latin "de minimus non jurate lex" (the law is not concerned with trivialities). A *de minimus* level is one that is so low as to be trivial.
Deoxyribonucleic acid (DNA)	The nucleic acid primarily contained within the cell nucleus which carries the genetic information.
Detector	A material or device that is sensitive to radiation and can produce a response signal suitable for measurement or analysis.
Deuterium (symbol: ^{2}H or D)	An isotope of hydrogen whose nucleus contains one neutron and one proton and, therefore, is about twice as heavy as the nucleus of normal hydrogen, which is only a single proton. Deuterium is often referred to as heavy hydrogen; it occurs in nature as 1 atom to every 6500 atoms of normal hydrogen. It is nonradioactive. Compare Tritium.
Diploid	Possessing a paired set of chromosomes, one set from the father and one set from the mother (2n). Characteristics of all somatic cells.
Disintegration	General process of radioactive decay, usually measured per unit time: disintegrations per second.
Dose	A term denoting the amount of energy absorbed. Absorbed dose is the energy imparted to matter by ionizing radiation per unit mass of irradiated material at the point of interest. Usually expressed in rads (conventional unit) or Grays (SI unit). Cumulative dose is the total dose resulting from repeated exposures to radiation.
Dose equivalent (H)	A unit of biologically effective dose, defined as the absorbed dose in rads multiplied by the quality factor (Q). (For all X-rays, the gamma rays, beta particles, and positrons likely to be used in nuclear medicine, the quality factor is 1). The dose equivalent (H) is given by the equation H = DQN, where D is absorbed dose, Q is the quality factor, and N is the product of modifying factors (N is usually 1 also).
Dose equivalent commitment	For any specified decision, practice, or operation, the infinite time integral of the per capita dose equivalent rate for a specified population. In other words, the dose committed over a certain time period resulting from an action.

Dose ranges	Arbitrary designations of dose. Low dose range is roughly 0 to 0.2 Gy (0 to 20 rad) in a single dose or 10 mGy/year (1 rem/year) of uniform whole-body radiation; intermediate dose—roughly 0.2 to 2.5 Gy (20 to 250 rad); high dose—above 2.5 Gy (250 rad).
Dose rate	The radiation dose delivered per unit time and measured, e.g., in rem/h. See Absorbed dose.
Dose rate contour line	A line on a map or a diagram joining all points at which the radiation dose rate is the same at a given time.
Dosimeter	A device that measures radiation dose, such as a film badge.
Dosimeter, pocket	A device used to determine the radiation dose a person has received by utilization of a small air-filled ionization chamber (about the size and shape of a pen). Dose can be read by holding it up to the light and looking through it. Not as sensitive or as accurate as either a film badge or a thermoluminescent dosimeter (TLD).
Dosimeter, thermoluminescent (TLD)	A dosimeter worn by a person to measure radiation dose. Contains a radiation-sensitive crystal that gives off light when heated. Amount of light emitted is proportional to radiation dose. About the size and shape of a film badge.
Dosimetry	The measurement of radiation doses.
Doubling dose (genetic)	That radiation dose estimated to double the spontaneous or natural incidence of any given effect.
Effective half-life	See Half-life, effective.
Electromagnetic radiation	Radiation consisting of associated and interacting electric and magnetic waves that travel at the speed of light, such as light, radio waves, gamma rays, and X-rays. All electromagnetic radiation can be transmitted through a vacuum. Compare Ionizing radiation.
Electron	An elementary particle with a negative electrical charge. Electrons surround the positively charged nucleus of the atom.
Electron capture	Method of radioactive decay in which the nucleus captures an orbital electron, which then interacts with a proton effectively negating the proton and transmuting the nucleus to that of another element.
Electron volt (eV)	A unit of energy equal to the kinetic energy required by an electron when accelerated through a potential difference of 1 volt (1 eV = 1.60×10^{-19} J.
Element	Pure substance consisting of atoms of the same atomic number that cannot be decomposed by ordinary chemical means.

Embryo	The organism in the first stages of development. In humans, this is generally considered to be the period from the end of the second week through the eighth week of gestation.
Encapsulation	A term used to denote an additional fabrication technique often used in preparation of radioactive sources, wherein the basic material is physically placed within sealed high physical integrity capsules to assure that in the event a transport package breaks, there would be little chance of spread of radioactive contamination.
Enriched uranium	Uranium in which the percentage of the fissionable isotope (^{235}U) has been increased above the 0.7% normally found in natural uranium.
Erythema	A medical term for reddening of the skin. Many occur following high doses of radiation received over a short period of time.
Epilation	Loss of hair. May occur transiently or permanently after large exposures to radiation.
Exposure	A term relating to the amount of ionizing radiation that is incident upon living or inanimate material.
Exposure rate	Increment of exposure to expressed per unit time may be expressed in units of R/min or for radioactivity in rad/h.
Fast neutrons	Neutrons with energy greater than approximately 100,000 eV. Compare Delayed neutrons.
FEMA	Federal Emergency Mangement Agency. Federal agency responsible for policy and coordination of civil defense and civil emergency planning, management and assistance.
Fertile material	A material, not itself fissionable by thermal neutrons, which can be converted into a fissile material by irradiation in a nuclear reactor. There are two basic fertile materials, the uranium isotope ^{238}U and the thorium isotope ^{232}Th. When these fertile materials capture neutrons, they are paritally converted into the fissile plutonium isotope ^{239}Pu and the fissile uranium isotope ^{233}U, respectively.
Fetus	Unborn offspring. In humans, refers to the period from 8 weeks after fertilization until birth.
Film badge	Photographic film shielded from light; worn by an individual to measure radiation exposure.
Fissile material	Although used as a synonym for fissionable material, this term has acquired a more restricted meaning; namely, any material fissionable by neutrons of all energies, especially thermal, or slow, neutrons as well as fast neutrons. The uranium isotope ^{235}U and the plutonium isotope ^{239}Pu are examples of fissile material.

Fission	The splitting of a heavy nucleus into two approximately equal parts (which are nuclei of lighter elements), accompanied by the release of a relatively large amount of energy and generally one or more neutrons. Fission can occur spontaneously, but usually it is caused by nuclear absorption of gamma rays, neutrons, or other particles.
Fission products	The nuclei (fission fragments) formed by the fission of heavy elements plus the nuclides formed by the fission fragments' radioactive decay. See Decay, radioactive.
Fuel cycle	The series of steps involved in supplying fuel for nuclear power reactors. It includes mining, refining, fabricating the fuel elements, using them in a nuclear reactor, chemical processing to recover the fissionable materials remaining in the spent fuel (not done in the U.S. as of 1984), re-enriching the fuel material, and refabricating it into new fuel elements.
Fuel element	A rod, a tube, a plat, or other mechanical shape or form into which nuclear fuel is fabricated.
Fusion	The formation of a heavier nucleus from two lighter ones, such as hydrogen isotopes, with the attendant release of energy. It takes energy input to get fusion fuel to fuse, but once fused, it releases much more energy than that put in. Compare Fission.
Fusion fuel	Commonly used fusion fuels for laboratory experiments are isotopes of hydrogen, namely, deuterium and tritium. Hydrogen itself is the fusion fuel of the sun. Other "futuristic" fusion fuels include helium and lithium.
Gamma emission	Nuclear process in which an excited nuclide de-excites by emission of a nuclear photon.
Gamma ray	Radiation emitted from the nucleus having a wavelength range from 10^{-9} to 10^{-12} cm.
Gastrointestinal syndrome	Part of the acute radiation syndrome. Usually occurs following whole-body acute absorbed doses in excess of 500 rad (5 Gy). Manifested in 1 to 4 weeks after exposure by diarrhea, fluid loss, electrolyte imbalance, and sepsis.
Geiger-Mueller counter (tube)	A high-voltage (>1000 V) gas tube used to detect ionizing particles. It is based upon the avalanche effect observed when ions are accelerated by an electric field under appropriate conditions. Can be used to detect gamma and X-rays as well as energetic beta particles. Cannot detect alpha particles. Generally this instrument is used to detect low radiation levels and should not be used in radiation fields >500 mR/h.

Genetic effects of radiation

Radiation effects that can be transferred from parent to offspring. Any radiation-caused changes in the genetic material of germ cells. Compare Somatic effects of radiation.

GeV

One billion electron volts. Also written BeV. See Electron volt.

Giga (G)

A prefix that multiplies a basic unit by one billion (10^9).

GM tube

See Geiger-Mueller tube.

Glove box

A sealed box in which workers, remaining outside and using gloves attached to and passing through openings in the box, can safely handle and work with radioactive materials that emit poorly penetrating radiations (e.g., plutonium).

Gray (Gy)

The SI unit of radiation absorbed dose. One Gray is equal to an energy deposition of 1 J/Kg (100 rad).

Ground state

The state of lowest energy of a system.

Half-life

Radioactive: For a single radioactive decay process, the time required for the activity of a given sample to decrease to half its initial value by that process.

Biological: The time required for the amount of a particular substance in a biological system to be reduced to half of its initial value by biological processes when the rate of removal is approximately exponential.

Effective: The time required for the amount of a particular specimen of a radionuclide in a system to be reduced to half its initial value as a consequence of both radioactive decay and other processes such as biological elimination.

Half-value layer (HVL)

Thickness of absorbing material necessary to reduce the intensity of radiation by one half.

Haploid

Having a single set of unpaired chromosomes (N = 23 in humans) characteristics of the gametes.

Health physics

The science concerned with the recognition, evaluation, and control of health hazards from ionizing radiation.

Hematopoietic syndrome

Part of the acute radiation syndrome. Usually presents following acute whole-body doses >100 rad (1 Gy) and occurs 1 to 4 weeks after exposure. Major manifestations are decreases in circulating platelets, lymphocytes, and granulocytes.

High radiation area

An area where the radiation dose to a person could exceed 100 mrem (1 mSv) in 1 h. There are special requirements for controlling access to such areas.

HVL

See Half-value layer.

ICRP

International Commission on Radiological Protection.

ICRU	International Commission on Radiation Units and Measurements.
Intermediate neutrons	Neutrons having energy greater than thermal neutrons but less than fast neutrons. The range is between 0.5 and 100,000 eV. Also called epithermal neutrons.
Internal contamination	Radioactive contamination within a person's body caused by radioactive material that has been inhaled, ingested, or absorbed through the skin or wounds.
Inverse-square law	The radiation intensity of any source decreases inversely as the square of the distance between the source and the detector (e.g., doubling the distance from a source decreases the intensity by one fourth).
Inversion	A chromosomal abnormality in which a segment of the chromosome recombines in an inverted relationship following breakage.
Ion pair	A closely associated positive ion and negative ion (usually an electron) having charges of the same magnitude and formed from a neutral atom or molecule by radiation.
Ionization	The process whereby a charged portion (usually an electron) of an atom or molecule is given enough kinetic energy to dissociate.
Ionization chamber	A closed vessel used for the detection of radiation energy and containing a gas and two electrodes maintained at a potential difference. Any radiation incident upon this container forms ions that move to the appropriate electrode, producing a current that can be measured.
Ionizing radiation	Radiation that produces ion pairs along its path through a substance.
Irradiation	Exposure to radiation.
Isobar	Nuclides that have the same total number of neutrons and protons but are different elements.
Isomer	One of two or more nuclides having the same number of neutrons and protons in their nuclei, but having different energies. A nuclide in the excited state and a similar nuclide in the ground state are isomers.
Isotones	Nuclides having the same number of neutrons but a different number of protons.
Isotopes	Nuclides having the same number of protons but a different number of neutrons.
Karyotype	A systemized array of chromosomes from a single cell, prepared by photography, that demonstrates the number and morphology of the chromosome complement.
Kerma	Kinetic energy released in material. A unit of quantity that represents the kinetic energy trans-

ferred to charged particles by the uncharged particles per unit mass of medium. Expressed in rads or Grays.

keV
: Thousand electron volts = 10^3 eV.

Joint Nuclear Accident Coordinating Center (JNACC)
: A combined group of the U.S. Departments of Defense and Energy for information and combined assistance in cases of nuclear weapons accidents or incidents.

Lanthanide series
: The series of elements beginning with lanthanum, element number 57, and continuing through lutetium, element number 71, which together occupy one position in the periodic table of the elements. These are the "rare earths" — all having chemical properties similar to lanthanum. They also are called the *lanthanides*.

Latent period
: Usually refers to the time elapsed between radiation exposure and the clinical appearance of an effect (such as appearance of a cancer or cataracts).

LET
: See Linear energy transfer.

Lethal dose
: A dose of ionizing radiation sufficient to cause death. Median lethal dose (MLD or LD_{50}) is the dose required to kill, within a specified period of time (usually 30 d), half the individuals in a large group of organisms similarly exposed. The $LD_{50/30}$ for humans is about 4 to 4.5 Gy (400 to 450 rad).

Light water reactor (LWR)
: May be either a boiling or pressurized water reactor. Uses as coolant ordinary water (H_2O) instead of heavy water (D_2O). LWRs are the most common reactor type in the U.S.

Linear energy transfer (LET)
: Amount of energy lost by ionizing radiation by way of interaction with matter per cm of path length through the absorbing material.

Low specific activity (LSA)
: Radioactive material in which the activity is essentially uniformly distributed and in which the amount of activity is low. Will not present a serious public health hazard if released.

Lugol's solution
: A saturated iodine solution.

Man-rem
: See Person rem.

Mass number (A)
: The sum of neutrons and protons in a nucleus.

Maximum permissible body burden (MPBB)
: The maximum quantity or concentration for activities or radionuclides inside the body, set by requiring that it does not result in doses to critical organs in excess of those specified for external radiation. Note should be made that this level often does not represent a significant medical problem nor should it be used to require intervention or treatment.

Maximum permissible concentration (MPC)
: An obsolescent term for the amount of radioactive material in the air, water, or food that might cause a maximum permissible dose at a standard rate of intake.

Maximum permissible dose (MPD)	The maximum amount of radiation that may be received by an individual within a specified time period with the expectation of no significantly harmful result to himself. For occupational exposures, MPD = 5(N − 18) rem, where N is the age (when the patient is older than 18 years). The pemissible limits of occupational exposures of persons less than 18 years of age are considerably reduced. MPD is a regulatory concept.
Metaphase	The stage of mitosis or meiosis when the centromeres of the contracted chromosomes are arranged on the equatorial plate.
MeV	One million (10^6) electron volts.
Metastable state	An excited nuclear state of a particular isotope that has a finite half-life and decays by gamma emission. Examples: ^{99m}Tc, ^{99}Tc (6 h); ^{38m}Cl, ^{38}Cl (0.74 s).
Micro (μ)	A prefix that divides a basic unit by one million (10^{-6}).
Microcurie (μCi)	That quantity of radioactive material having 3.7×10^4 disintegrations per second. One millionth part of a curie.
Micrometer (μm)	One millionth of a meter; formerly micron.
Milli (m)	A prefix that divides a basic unit by one thousandth (10^{-3}).
Millicurie (mCi)	That quantity of radioactive material having 3.7×10^{-7} disintegrations per second. One thousandth part of a curie.
Mitosis	Somatic cell division by which the mother cell produces two daughter cells, each with the identical chromosome complement as the original cell.
Monitoring	Periodic or continuous determination of the amount of ionizing radiation or radioactive contamination present. Also referred to as *surveying*.
MPC	See Maximum permissible concentration.
MPD	See Maximum permissible dose.
N	See Neutron number. Also used as the abbreviation for the haploid number of chromosomes in the human.
NCRP	National Council on Radiation Protection and Measurements.
Neutron number (N)	Number of neutrons in a nucleus.
Nonstochastic effect	Describes effects whose severity is a function of dose. Some may have an apparent clinical threshold. Examples of nonstochastic effects include skin erythema, cataracts, and bone marrow depression.
Nuclear Regulatory Commission (NRC)	U.S. government agency regulating by-product material.
Nucleons	Any particle commonly contained in the nucleus of an atom.

Nucleus	The small, positively charged core of an atom. It is only about 1/10,000 the diameter of the atom but contains nearly all the atom's mass. All nuclei contain both protons and neutrons, except the nucleus of ordinary hydrogen, which consists of a single proton.
Nuclides	A general term applicable to all atomic forms of the element. The term is often used incorrectly as a synonym for isotope, which properly has a more limited definition. Whereas isotopes are the various forms of a single element (hence, a family of nuclides) and all have the same atomic number and number of protons, nuclides comprise all the isotopic forms of all the elements. Nuclides are distinguished by their atomic number, atomic mass, and energy state.
Packaging (transport)	Transport of radioactive materials occurs at four levels of packaging protection: *Exempt:* Can be sent unlabeled through U.S. mail. Usually less than 10 μCi. *Low Specific Activity:* Must be in strong tight packages or drums. *Type A:* Usually sealed in a container designed to withstand normal accidents. Typical type used for radiopharmaceuticals. *Type B:* Heavy cask type containing dangerous amounts of radioactivity. Packaging designed to withstand exceptionally severe accidents.
Parent radionuclide	Radionuclide that decays to a specific daughter nuclide either directly or as a member of a radioactive series.
Personnel monitor	See Thermoluminescent dosimeter and Film badge.
Person rem	A unit of collective population dose calculated by multiplying the number of persons exposed times their average individual whole-body dose in rems.
Photopeak	The peak (maximum intensity) in a gamma spectrum as measured by a scintillation detector.
Pico (p)	A prefix that divides a basic unit of one trillion (10^{-12}). Same as *micromicro.*
Placarding	Application of an appropriate placard to the transport vehicle (rail or highway) if any package on board bears a radioactive Yellow III label.
Positron	A particle equal in mass to the electron, but with a positive electric charge.
Promotor	See Carcinogen.
Protective clothing	Special clothing worn to prevent radioactive contamination from getting on the skin. Actually a misnomer for anticontamination clothing.

Proton	An elementary particle with a mass 1873 times that of an electron and a positive charge equal to the basic electronic charge.
Quality factor (QF)	Linear energy transfer-dependent factor by which absorbed doses are to be multiplied to account for the varying effectiveness of different radiations. QF for 250 kVp X-rays is equal to 1.
Rad	Radiation absorbed dose. The unit of absorbed dose of ionizating radiation. One rad is equal to 100 erg/g. See also Gray.
Radiation	Energy propagated through space or matter as waves (gamma rays, UV light) or as particles (such as alpha or beta rays). External radiation comes from a source outside the body, whereas internal radiation is from a source inside the body (such as radionuclides deposited in tissues).
Radiation accident	An accident in which there is an unintended exposure to radiation or radioactive contamination.
Radiation area	Any accessible area in which the level of radiation is such that a major portion of an individual's body could receive in any one hour a dose in excess of 5 mrem (50 μSv) or in any five consecutive days a dose in excess of 150 mrem (1.5 mSv).
Radiation emergency area (REA)	A term used by hospitals to refer to the area (usually in or near the emergency room) that has been designated to treat injured and radioactively contaminated patients. This area has access and egress controlled to avoid spread of radioactive contamination.
Radiation Emergency Assistance Center/Training Site	See REAC/TS
Radiation, ionizing	Any radiation that has high enough energy to break apart chemical bonds and cause atoms to form ions (charged particles), e.g., gamma and X-rays.
Radiation, non-ionizing	Radiation from other portions of the electromagnetic spectrum that do not have enough energy to create ions, e.g., microwaves, radar, visible light.
Radiation, penetrating	Radiation that can penetrate deeply into tissues, e.g., gamma, X-rays, beta particles. This term usually only refers to ionizing radiation.
Radiation safety officer (RSO)	A person (often a health physicist or physician) who has the responsibility for overseeing radiation safety in an organization.
Radiation sickness	The prodromal manifestations of acute radiation injury, varying in severity, scope, and etiology, depending upon the conditions of exposure. See Acute radiation syndrome.
Radioactive	See Radioactivity

Radioactive contamination	Deposition of radioactive material in any place where it may harm persons, spoil experiments, or make products or equipment unsuitable or unsafe for some specific use. The presence of unwanted radioactive matter. Also, radioactive material found on the walls of vessels in spent-fuel processing plants or radioactive material that has leaked into a reactor coolant. Often called *contamination*.
Radioactive White I label	A warning label for packages containing radioactive material where the surface dose rate is <0.5 mrem (5 μSv) per hour.
Radioactive Yellow II label	A warning label for packages containing radioactive material when the dose rate at the package surface is <50 mrem (0.5 mSv) per hour and the dose rate at 3 ft from any surface of the package is <1 mrem (10 μSv) per hour.
Radioactive Yellow III label	Same as above except that the dose rate at the surface of the package is between 50 mrem (0.5 mSv) and 200 mrem (2 mSv) per hour or the dose rate at 3 ft from any surface of the package is >10 mrem (0.1 mSv) per hour.
Radioactivity	The property of certain nuclides of emitting radiation by the spontaneous transformation of their nuclei.
Radionuclide	Unstable nucleus that transmutes by way of nuclear decay.
Radionuclidic purity	Amount of total radioactive species in a sample that is the desired radionuclide.
Radiopharmaceutical	Radioactive drug used for therapy or diagnosis.
Radioprotector	Compound which inhibits the radiation response of biological systems.
Radioresistance	A relative resistance of cells, tissues, organs, or organisms to the harmful action of radiation.
Radiosensitivity	A relative susceptibility of cells, tissues, organs, or organisms to the harmful action of radiation.
Radiosensitizer	Substance which enhances the radiation response of biological systems.
Radium (Ra)	A radioactive metallic element with atomic number 88. As found in nature, the most common isotope has an atomic weight of 226. It occurs in minute quantities associated with uranium in pitchblende, carnotite, and other minerals. Uranium decays to radium in a series of alpha and beta emissions. By virtue of being an alpha- and gamma-emitter, radium is used as a source of luminescence and as a radiation source in medicine and radiography.
Radon (Rn)	A radioactive element and the heaviest gas known. Its atomic number is 86 and its atomic weight varies from 200 to 226. It is a daughter of radium in the uranium radioactive series.

Range switch	A switch on a radiation survey meter that changes the scale of the meter, e.g., from 0 to 10 mR/h to 0 to 100 mR/h.
Rare earths	A group of 15 chemically similar metallic elements, numbers 57 through 71 in the periodic table; also known as the lanthanide series.
Rate meter	Device, used in conjunction with a detector, that measures the rate of activity of a radioisotope; usually in units of counts per minute or counts per second.
RBE	See Relative biological effectiveness.
Reactor (nuclear)	A device in which a fission chain reaction can be initiated, maintained, and (preferably) controlled.
REAC/TS	Radiation Emergency Assistance Center/Training Site. A treatment and consultative team for radiation emergencies which also provides training courses and maintains the radiation accident registry. (Oak Ridge, TN, 37831-0117)
Reference man	An "ideal man" utilized for radiation protection purposes. Has defined anatomical and physiological specifications. Defined in ICRP Report Number 23.
Relative biological effectiveness (RBE)	Ratio of the biological response derived from a particular radiation as compared to another radiation exposure.
Relative risk	See Risk, relative.
Rem	See Roentgen equivalent man.
Reprocessing	The process by which spent fuel from a nuclear reactor is separated into waste material, uranium, and plutonium to be reused as a nuclear fuel.
Restricted area	When used in the context of radiation, refers to a controlled access area in which the dose to a person could exceed 2 mrem ($20\mu Sv$) in any 1 h or 100 mrem (1 mSV) in any 1 week.
Ring dosimeter	A thermoluminescent dosimeter worn on the finger in order to be able to measure absorbed dose to the hands.
Risk, absolute	The excess risk attributed to irradiation and usually expressed as the numerical difference between irradiated and nonirradiated populations (e.g., 1 case of cancer per million people irradiated per year per rad). Absolute risk may be given on an annual basis or lifetime (50-year) basis.
Risk, relative	The ratio between the number of cancer cases in the irradiated population to the number of cases expected in the unexposed population. A relative risk of 1.1 indicates a 10% increase in cancer due to radiation, compared to the "normal" incidence. Relative risk is more appropriate to use when considering selected population groups.

Roentgen (R)

Quantity of gamma or X-radiation per cubic centimeter of air that produces one electrostatic unit of charge.

Roentgen equivalent man (rem)

The unit of dose equivalent. The absorbed dose in rads multiplied by the quality factor of the type of radiation. See Sievert.

RSO

See Radiation safety officer.

Scattered radiation

Radiation that, during its passage through a substance, has been deviated in direction and with perhaps an energy loss.

Scintillation counter

An instrument that detects radiation by counting the small flashes of light produced when the radiation interacts with the detector crystal.

Sealed source

A radioactive source sealed in an impervious container, which has sufficient mechanical strength to prevent contact with or dispersion of the radioactive material under conditions of use for which it was designed. Such sources are generally used for radiation therapy and industrial radiography.

Shield (shielding)

A body of material used to reduce the intensity of radiation.

Shielding

Any material used to absorb beta-, X-, and gamma-ray radiation.

SI Units

International system of units. SI refers to Système International d'Unités. Radiation units include J/Kg, Gy, Sv, and Bq.

Sievert (Sv)

The SI unit of dose equivalent. The absorbed dose in Gy multiplied by the quality factor of the type of radiation. One Sievert equals 100 rems.

Somatic effects of radiation

Effects of radiation limited to the exposed individual, as distinguished from genetic effects, which also affect subsequent unexposed generations. Large radiation doses can cause somatic effects that are fatal. Smaller doses may make the individual noticeably ill, may produce temporary changes in blood-cell levels detectable only in the laboratory, or may produce no detectable effects. Also called physiological effects of radiation.

Specific activity

Unit pertaining to the disintegrations per gram of a radioisotope.

Spent fuel

Nuclear reactor fuel that has been irradiated (used) to the extent that it can no longer effectively sustain a chain reaction.

Stochastic effect

An effect whose probability of occurrence in an irradiated population or individual is a function of dose. Commonly regarded as not having a threshold dose. An example is radiation carcinogenesis.

Survey meter	Meter that measures rate of radioactive exposure, usually in units of mR/h.
Thermal neutrons	Neutrons in thermal equilibirum with their surrounding medium. Thermal neutrons are those that have been slowed down by a moderator to an average speed of about 220 m/s at room temperature from the much higher initial seeds they had when expelled by fission. Compare Fast neutrons, Intermediate neutrons.
Thermoluminescent dosimeter (TLD)	Type of crystal used to monitor radiation exposure by emitting light; often used in a body, wrist, or ring badge. Must be processed in order to be read.
Thorium (Th)	A naturally radioactive element with atomic number 90 and, as found in nature, an atomic weight of approximately 232. The fertile thorium isotope ^{232}Th is abundant and can be transmuted to the fissionable uranium isotope ^{233}U by neutron irradiation. See Fertile material.
Threshold dose	The minimum dose of radiation that will repoduce a detectable biological effect.
Transient equilibrium	Equilibrium reached by a parent-daughter radioisotope pair in which the half-life of the parent is longer than the half-life of the daughter.
Transport index	A number placed on a package of Yellow Label materials by the shipper. It is either the highest measured dose rate at three ft from the surface of the package or a number assigned for criticality control purposes.
Transuranic nuclide	A nuclide having an atomic number greater than that of uranium ($>$92). Includes neptunium, plutonium, americium, and curium.
Tritium (^{3}H or T)	A radioactive isotope of hydrogen with two neutrons and one proton in the nucleus. It is man-made and is heavier than deuterium (heavy hydrogen). Tritium is used as a label in chemical and biological experiments. Its nucleus is a triton.
UF conversion	The process of converting the solid uranium oxide (commonly called *yellow cake*) that comes from uranium mining and milling into a uranium fluoride gas.
UNSCEAR	United Nations Scientific Committee on the Effects of Atomic Radiation. A committee of the U.N. General Assembly.
Uranium (U)	A radioactive element with atomic number 92 and, as found in natural ores, an average atomic weight of approximately 238. The two principal natural isotopes are ^{235}U (0.7% of natural uranium), which is fissionable, and ^{238}U (99.3% of natural uranium), which is fertile. Natural uranium also includes a minute amount of ^{234}U. Uranium is the basic raw material of nuclear energy.

Warning labels	See Radioactive White, Radioactive Yellow labels.
Weighting factor (W_T)	The ratio of the stochastic risk arising from a tissue T to the total risk when the whole body is irradiated uniformly. Concept derived for use by the International Commission on Radiologic Protection.
Whole-body counter	A device used to identify and measure radionuclides in the body (body burden) of humans and animals. It uses heavy shielding (to keep out background radiation), ultrasensitive scintillation detectors, and electronic equipment.
Whole-body (total) exposure	An exposure of the body to external radiation, in which the entire body rather than an isolated part is irradiated. Also may occur when a radioactive material is uniformly distributed throughout the tissues of the body.
Wipe test	A test for radioactive contamination by wiping the surface with a filter paper-like material and then measuring the paper with an appropriate radiation detector. Results are often reported in cpm/100 cm² of the area wiped.
Yellow cake	The semirefined product from uranium mining and milling operations that is sent to conversion plants.
Z number	See atomic number.

INDEX

A

Abortion, therapeutic, 223

Absorbed dose, defined and qualified, 80

Accident, see Military radiation accident; Radiation accident

Accident history, importance in identifying appropriate management, 303—304

Accident reconstruction, using TLDs and sectional phantom reconstruction, 304

Acentric aberrations, following ionizing radiation, 111—113

Activated metal, as cause of high-dose exposures, 253

Acute radiation syndrome (ARS)

Chernobyl classification, 70, 72

Chernobyl patients, 288

classification of changes at acute dose levels, 70

clinical course, 70

historical classification, 71

latent period, 83

manifest illness stage, 71

pathogenesis and intricacies, 80, 82—87

prodromal stage, 71

Acyclovir, to treat viral infections, Chernobyl, 289

Adipose tissue, risk estimates for radiogenic tumor induction, 210

Age, as factor in radiation-induced cancer, 208—211

Airborne radioactive contamination, 77

Airplane crashes, potential for nuclear power plant accident, 260

Algeria, accident from radiation device, 23

Alimentary tract, risk estimates for radiogenic tumor induction, 210—211

Alopecia, as parameter for absorbed radiation dose, 43, see also Epilation

Alpha contamination, assessment and measurement, 50—51, 294

Alpha particles

measurement of, 294

penetration and range, 2, 8, 9

Alpha radiation detection equipment, 50, 52, 294

Aluminum-containing antacids, in treatment of internal radionuclides, 162

Ambulance, called to radiation accident, 189

Ambulance personnel, responding to radiation accident, 189

Americium, chelation of by DTPA, 165

Ammonium chloride, used in mobilizing radioactive strontium, 164

Anomalies, risk estimates during pregnancy, 227

Anorexia, symptom of ARS prodromal response, 83

Anticoagulants, in treatment of lesions from burns, 140

Antifibrotic drugs, in treatment of lesions from burns, 140

Antilymphocyte globulin, in treatment of aplastic anemia, 95—96

Anxiety, management of, in radiation accidents, 153—154

Aplastic anemia, medical model for effects of radiation, 94

ARS, see Acute radiation syndrome

Area designation to handle radioactive contamination, factors in choice of, 171

Arteriography, to evaluate vascular status, 216

Assessing risk of radiation injury, possibility of therapeutic abortion, 223

Assessment of absorbed dose, value of TLDs and film badges in cases of lower absorbed doses, 303

Atomic number, 5

Atomic structure, 5

Atrophic skin, after radiation accident, 216

Auxiliary building at Three Mile Island, part in accident, 273

Avulsion injuries, occurrence and treatment, 205—206

Azathioprine, in bone marrow transplant therapy, 101

B

Babcock and Wilcox

manufacturers of pressurized water reactors, 246

representatives at Three Mile Island, 274

Barium sulfate, in treatment of deposition of internal radionuclides, 162

BEIR, see Biological effects of ionizing radiation

Benefit/risk ratio, in assessing safety, 232

Beryllium contamination, in weapons accidents, 53

Beta "burns"

combined with whole-body radiation, Chernobyl, 288

extensive in patients at Chernobyl, 141

to skin as portal for infection, 289, see also Beta emitters; Beta irradiation

Beta contamination, using ionization chamber survey meter to detect, 294

Beta emitters, deaths from, Chernobyl, 288

Beta/gamma radiation, measurement of, 294

Beta irradiation, as cause of significant skin reactions, 141—143

Beta particles, penetration and range, 2, 8—10

Bioassay samples, 327—328

Biological effects of ionizing radiation (BEIR), Committee on, 208, 210, 213

Biological half-life, 6

Biological indicators, in determining overexposure, 110

Birth defects, radiation-induced, Chernobyl, 291

Bladder, risk estimates for radiogenic tumor induction, 210—211

Blocking agents, in treatment of internal radionuclides, 162—163

Blood component therapy

kept minimal after whole-body radiation, 95

required where blood count deficiencies exist, 96

Boiling water reactor, type of light water reactor in U.S., 244, 247

Bone, effects of radiation, 216—217

Medical management of
radiation accidents